4 Week L

nursing
care

an essential guide

Visit the *Nursing Care* Companion Website at
www.pearsoned.co.uk/field to find valuable online resources.

For **students:**

- Multiple choice questions to test your learning
- Essay questions to check your understanding
- An online glossary to explain key terms
- Flashcards to test your understanding of key terms

For **lecturers:**

- Downloadable PowerPoint slides to use in class.

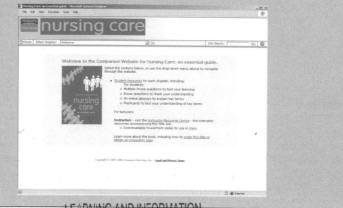

PEARSON EDUCATION

NURSING&HEALTH

FIRST FOR HEALTH

We work with leading authors to develop the
strongest educational materials in nursing,
bringing cutting-edge thinking and best
learning practice to a global market.

Under a range of well-known imprints, including
Prentice Hall, we craft high-quality print and
electronic publications which help readers to understand
and apply their content, whether studying or at work.

To find out more about the complete range of our
publishing, please visit us on the World Wide Web at:
www.pearsoned.co.uk

Linda Field
Warwick Medical School

Barbara Smith
Freelance Consultant and Lecturer

nursing
care

an essential guide

PEARSON
Education

Harlow, England • London • New York • Boston • San Francisco • Toronto
Sydney • Tokyo • Singapore • Hong Kong • Seoul • Taipei • New Delhi
Cape Town • Madrid • Mexico City • Amsterdam • Munich • Paris • Milan

Pearson Education Limited
Edinburgh Gate
Harlow
Essex CM20 2JE
England

and Associated Companies throughout the world

Visit us on the World Wide Web at:
www.pearsoned.co.uk

First published 2008

ISBN: 978-0-13-197652-8

British Library Cataloguing-in-Publication Data
A catalogue record for this book is available from the British Library

Library of Congress Cataloging-in-Publication Data
Field, Linda, 1956–
    Nursing care : an essential guide / Linda Field, Barbara Smith.
        p. ; cm.
    Includes bibliographical references and index.
    ISBN-13: 978-0-13-197652-8 (pbk.)
 1.   Nursing.
    [DNLM: 1. Nursing Care. WY 100 F454n 2008] I. Smith, Barbara, 1954- II. Title.
    RT41.F48 2008
    610.73--dc22

                                                                2008003324

10 9 8 7 6 5 4 3 2 1
11 10 09 08 07

Typeset in 9pt Interstate light by 30
Printed and bound in Great Britain by Henry Ling Limited, at the Dorset Press, Dorchester, DT1 1HD

The publisher's policy is to use paper manufactured from sustainable forests.

I would like to dedicate this book to the memory of my mother Catherine Field (née Buckley), SEN, 1926-2007, who worked as a nurse from 1943 to 2000 and without whose help and inspiration this book would not have been written.
Linda Field

I would like to dedicate this book to the memory of my mother Kathleen Cox. She was a caring and inspirational person. For all those who provided the fantastic community care for my father Kenneth Lindley Cox in March 2008.
Barbara Smith

Contents

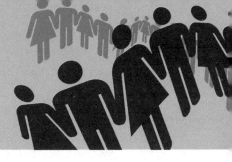

Acknowledgements   xi
Guided tour   xiv
Introduction   xviii

Chapter 1 What is caring?   1

Introduction   1
Learning objectives   2
What do we mean by 'caring'?   2
Quality   9
The assessment process   18
Summary   24
Key points   25
Points for debate   25
Links to other chapters   25
Further reading   25
References   26

Chapter 2 Dignity and privacy   27

Introduction   27
Learning objectives   28
Dignity in care   28
Culturally sensitive healthcare   35
Communication   36
Protecting individuals from abuse   40
Summary   51
Key points   52
Points for debate   52
Links to other chapters   54
Further reading   54
References   54

Chapter 3 Basic observations   56

Introduction   56
Learning objectives   57
The importance of basic observations   57
Pulse   59
Respirations   68
Temperature   77
Summary   87
Key points   88
Points for debate   88
Links to other chapters   89

	Further reading	89
	References	89
Chapter 4	Hygiene	91
	Introduction	91
	Learning objectives	92
	Personal hygiene	92
	Oral hygiene	106
	Infection control	107
	Summary	112
	Key points	113
	Points for debate	113
	Links to other chapters	114
	Further reading	114
	References	114
Chapter 5	Nutrition	116
	Introduction	116
	Learning objectives	117
	The importance of good nutrition	117
	Essential nutrients	118
	Nutritional requirements	122
	Factors affecting nutritional choice	124
	Nutritional assessment	126
	Nutrition in hospital	130
	Feeding patients	133
	Dysphagia awareness	136
	Summary	143
	Key points	144
	Points for debate	144
	Links to other chapters	144
	Further reading	145
	References	145
Chapter 6	Fluid balance and continence care	147
	Introduction	147
	Learning objectives	148
	Fluid balance	148
	Recording fluid balance	155
	Urinary continence	160
	Incontinence	165
	Promoting continence	173
	Catheter care	177
	Problems with elimination of faeces	181
	Summary	188
	Key points	189
	Points for debate	190
	Links to other chapters	190
	Further reading	190
	References	190

Chapter 7 Pain management   193

   Introduction   193
   Learning objectives   194
   What is pain?   194
   How is pain felt?   196
   Government policy developments in pain management   200
   Pain assessment   200
   Pain perception   207
   Pain management   214
   Other methods of pain relief   225
   Summary   229
   Key points   230
   Points for debate   230
   Links to other chapters   231
   Further reading   231
   References   231

Chapter 8 Pressure ulcers   234

   Introduction   234
   Learning objectives   235
   Why study pressure ulcers?   236
   How and why pressure ulcers develop   238
   Avoidance of pressure ulcers   242
   Screening and assessing the possibility of skin damage due to pressure   245
   Pressure ulcer healing   252
   Summary   253
   Key points   254
   Points for debate   254
   Links to other chapters   254
   Further reading   254
   References   254

Chapter 9 Rehabilitation and self-care   256

   Introduction   256
   Learning objectives   257
   What is rehabilitation?   257
   Independence and self-care   261
   Framework for rehabilitation nursing   265
   Factors that impact on individual wellbeing   275
   Summary   279
   Key points   279
   Points for debate   280
   Links to other chapters   280
   Further reading   280
   References   280

Chapter 10 Record-keeping   282

   Introduction   282
   Learning objectives   283
   Overview of record-keeping   283

Purpose of records   285
Legal aspects of record-keeping   287
Nursing documentation   291
Standards for record-keeping   298
Summary   302
Key points   303
Points for debate   303
Links to other chapters   303
Further reading   304
References   304

Index   305

Acknowledgements

I would like to thank my husband Lawrence and my daughter Clare for their constant support and encouragement throughout the writing of this book. Also a big, big thank you to my sister Susan for her patience in reading the chapters and offering enduring support with the re-drafts.

Linda Field

I would like to give a huge thank you to my husband Roger and sons Alex and Lewis for their constant support and encouragement throughout the writing of this book. I would also like to thank Norma Whittal who believed in the Basic Care Course.

Barbara Smith

We would also like to thank the reviewers for their helpful and constructive comments that have helped shape the book:

Caroline Carlisle, Professor of Education in Nursing and Midwifery, University of Manchester

Nicky Davis, Senior Lecturer, UWE

Ann Donnelly, Clinical Skills Tutor at Peninsula Medical School, Universities of Plymouth and Exeter

Andrew Evered, School of Health Science, Swansea University

Nina Godson, Senior Lecturer in Clinical Skills, Coventry University

Ann Lawrie, Lecturer, University of Nottingham

Sian Jones, Head of Division, Acute and Specialised Care, University of Glamorgan

Caroline MacDonald, Senior Lecturer for Clinical Skills Development, The Robert Gordon University, Aberdeen

John Thompson, Principal Lecturer, Northumbria University

Christine Whitehead, School of Nursing and Midwifery, University of Southampton

Publisher's acknowledgements

We are grateful to the following for permission to reproduce copyright material:

Figure 3.1 and Figure 3.4 from pages 7 and 15 respectively, *Foundations of Anatomy and Physiology, 5th Edition*, Churchill Livingstone (Ross, J. and Wilson, K. 1981), copyright Elsevier; Figure 3.2, Figure 3.5 and Figure 6.4 Copyright Clinical Skills Ltd; Figure 3.3 from *Developing Practical Nursing Skills* Hodder Arnold (Baille, L. 2005), copyright 2005 Edward Arnold (Publishers) Ltd, reproduced by permission of the publisher; Figure 4.4, Figure 6.2 and Figure 6.5 from pages 304, 15 and 172 respectively, *Essential Nursing Skills*, Mosby (Nicol, M. et al 2004), copyright Elsevier; Figure 4.5 reproduced with kind permission of the Royal College of Nursing; Figure 4.6 adapted from 'A comprehensive glove choice', copyright

Infection Prevention Society, reproduced by permission; Figure 5.2 copyright Food Standards Agency, reproduced by permission; Figure 6.7 from *British Medical Journal* (1990), 300, 439-40 with permission from the BMJ Publishing Group; Figure 7.1 from 'Descartes Pain Theory', *The Challenge of Pain Revised Edition*, Penguin Books (Melzack, R. and Wall, P.D. 1996), copyright Ronald Melzack and Patrick D. Wall, 1996; Figure 7.4b from 'McGill-Melzack Pain Questionnaire; major properties of scoring methods', *Pain*, 1, 277-99 (Melzack, R. 1975), copyright R. Melzack, reprinted with permission; Figure 8.1 from *Introduction to Human and Social Biology, 2nd Edition*, Murray (Mackean, D. and Jones, B. 1990), copyright D.G. Mackean; Table 8.1 and Figure 8.4 from *Manual of Clinical Nursing Procedures, 5th Edition*, Blackwell (eds Mallert, J. and Doherty, L. 2000).

In some instances we have been unable to trace the owners of copyright material, and we would appreciate any information that would enable us to do so.

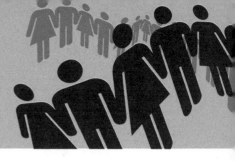

Guided Tour

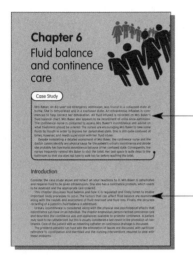

Chapter opening case study: gets you thinking about real nursing practice from the beginning and puts the chapter into context.

Introduction: Provides a brief introduction to the key themes of the chapter.

Learning outcomes: Enables you to focus on what you can gain from reading the chapter.

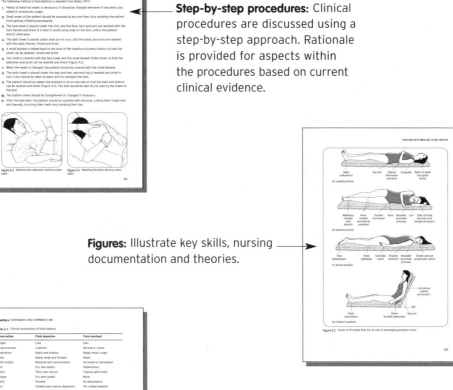

Step-by-step procedures: Clinical procedures are discussed using a step-by-step approach. Rationale is provided for aspects within the procedures based on current clinical evidence.

Figures: Illustrate key skills, nursing documentation and theories.

Glossary: Key words are highlighted in the text and explained in a glossary at the bottom of the page.

Case Studies: Give you a taste of real nursing practice and help you put the theory into context. Encourages you to apply what you have learnt to real-life nursing scenarios.

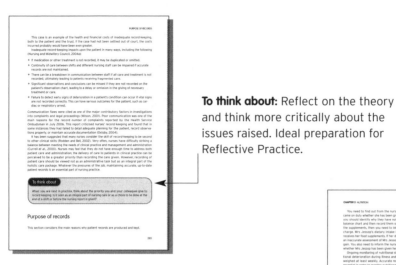

To think about: Reflect on the theory and think more critically about the issues raised. Ideal preparation for Reflective Practice.

Recap: Check your understanding and track your progress with short recap questions at the end of each section.

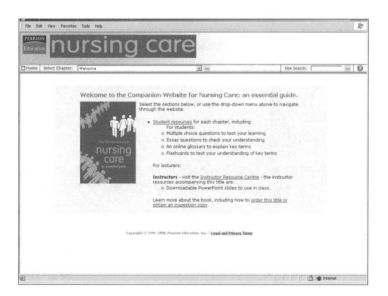

Multiple choice questions: for each chapter there are multiple choice and essay questions on the student companion website at **www.pearsoned.co.uk/field**, giving you a chance to check what you have learnt and get instant feedback.

Summary: Brings together all the key concepts of the chapter to aid your understanding.

Key Points: Summarises the main ideas discussed in the chapter and are ideal for reminder and revision.

Points for debate: Interesting and stimulating questions for you to think about and discuss with other students.

Links to other chapters: Identifies and directs you to related topics in other chapters.

Further reading: Provides a list of other books, journals and websites you may wish to explore to find out more about the areas discussed in the chapter.

References: are included in all chapters and all you to see the evidence base for the material covered within each chapter.

Introduction

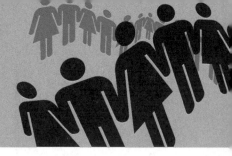

Welcome to *Nursing Care*. This book is to take you on a journey towards the best care that you can give. On that journey you will be able to examine your part in this care-giving process.

This book will teach you how to carry out the most essential nursing skills, explain the theory and rationale behind these skills, and explore how your interactions with patients impact on the care you deliver.

The broad aim of this book is to help you form a view of the reality of nursing. We stress that the contents of the book can be applied to all branches of nursing and to all environments where patients are nursed, whether in hospital, at home or in a care home.

This book has been designed to be a complementary text to other clinical books and is aimed primarily at student nurses, but it may also be of use to other health and social care workers. The content is focused on adult nursing, but it also contains examples and case studies from other branches of nursing. The reason for the emphasis on nursing students is because they are in the unique position of having a 24-hour presence with patients. As a student nurse, you spend 50% of your course in clinical practice. Many of you will be fortunate to be in a variety of diverse placements, from working alongside an acute hospital team to working in a private occupational health setting. The theoretical half of your course exists to back up your practical skills, to ensure that you can make evidence-based care decisions, and to develop your clinical reasoning skills.

Unfortunately, over recent years, there has been increasing disregard of essential and basic care skills and a lack of recognition of the importance of these skills being part of the care/treatment programme. We do not deny the significance and value of more technical care, but in this book we place the emphasis on the *basic* but *essential* nursing skills that are integral to all care and treatment. No other health or social care worker has the same responsibility as a nurse has to ensure that the care given to patients is of the highest quality and meets individual patients' needs.

This book is designed to help you develop a proactive approach to the assessment, planning, implementation and evaluation of the care that you give. It will stimulate your thinking and help you to reflect and develop action learning skills. This will enable you to understand why essential skills are so important and how much of a difference they can make to a patient's wellbeing. The positive effect of this should never be underestimated; it can contribute significantly to a patient's recovery.

Each chapter in this book starts with a case study that sets the scene for the contents of the chapter. These case studies are work-based scenarios that will enable you to link the theory in the book to your work in clinical practice. The case study is followed by a short introduction that explains the content of the chapter. Learning objectives to achieve as you work through the chapters are listed. Throughout the text there are case studies and 'To think about' boxes to encourage you to reflect on what you have read and to apply this to your practice. These features will also help you to explore your interactions with patients. Recap questions let you check that you have understood each section as you work your way through the chapters. Each chapter concludes with a summary and the key points of the text. There are also some issues for debate, so that you can question and engage in critically reflecting on the care you and others give to patients; you may want to discuss these issues with other colleagues or students. Finally, we list the other chapters to which each chapter is linked and offer some suggestions for further reading.

We hope you enjoy reading this book and grasp the importance of the essential and fundamental aspects of nursing care: these are integral to all aspects of nursing.

Chapter 1
What is caring?

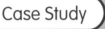

Case Study

Miss Smith was being admitted to hospital for a routine operation. She was anxious and nervous of what was going to happen. On walking into the hospital she was greeted by the receptionist. Immediately Miss Smith felt less anxious. The receptionist introduced herself, wished Miss Smith good morning and asked how she could help. She then directed Miss Smith to the ward. On entering the ward Miss Smith was greeted by a nurse, who showed Miss Smith to a bed and explained the layout of the ward, when meals and drinks were served, where the shop was and about visiting times. Later the nurse formally admitted Miss Smith to the ward and gave her the opportunity to ask any questions. Miss Smith's fears and apprehension disappeared quickly, and she felt confident about the care she was going to receive.

Introduction

Everything in this case study is about showing courtesy to others; it's about making someone feel welcome and showing them that they matter. Miss Smith was frightened and nervous about her hospital admission, even though this admission was for a routine small operation. The receptionist and nurse were understanding; they were efficient but took the time to introduce themselves to Miss Smith, to talk to her and to give her the opportunity to ask questions. Miss Smith felt cared for - but how differently she could have felt had the receptionist and nurse done their duty but not made any extra effort. Miss Smith would then have been left feeling worried and nervous. In this chapter we explore the notion of caring and look at ways in which you can improve the quality of the care you give.

What do we mean by 'caring'?

To think about

Consider a time when you have been ill.

What made you feel cared about?
Why did this make you feel cared for?
What made it a good experience?

Some of the things that made you feel cared for may include being shown kindness, being given drinks or food when you are weak, being made comfortable, warm and safe, and having your needs understood. These behaviours make you feel cared for and that you are *worth* being cared for. Caring behaviours make a difference because they make you feel safe and as comfortable as possible.

It is easy to forget or even not consider the positive effect nurses have on patients. How we treat patients has an impact on the care that they receive. Often it is the smallest details that make the biggest difference. As we saw in the case of Miss Smith, simply greeting the patient, using their name, and knowing why they have been admitted to hospital can allay the patient's

Case Study 1.1

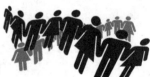

Mrs Vincenzi is an 80-year-old woman who was admitted to a general medical ward a few days ago after a **stroke** (cerebral vascular accident). The stroke has left her semi-paralysed and unable to communicate. She is dependent on the nursing staff for all care.

Mrs Vincenzi is in unfamiliar surroundings. She can hear muffled sounds and occasional bangs and voices, but she is unable to understand where she is and what is going on. She is finding it difficult to focus but is aware that she feels trapped in the bed, unable to move or get up. Mrs Vincenzi is frightened and confused and does not know what is happening to her. She feels very alone and vulnerable and is completely reliant on others. She is thirsty and her lips are sore and dry. She has pain and feels very weak.

fears. Nurses should never undervalue the importance of caring and showing patients that they care. In order to do this, we need to be able to understand the behaviour of caring by exploring and reflecting what caring is. Why are some experiences good and others bad? What are the circumstances that contribute to an experience being good or bad? Consider Case study 1.1.

Now consider the following examples of the care Mrs Vincenzi could receive:

Hello, Mrs Vincenzi. My name is Kathy and this is Fiona. We are nurses and we have come to check that you are comfortable. Is that okay with you? Mrs Vincenzi, is it alright if I change your sheet and help you have a wash? I think you will feel better. Your lips look a little dry; would you like some cream on them? There, how does that feel? Would you like a drink? Have a few sips of water and then I can get you some tea if you would like. Have you any pain? Yes, you have got quite a nasty infection, but you have been started on antibiotics so once these kick in you will soon feel as good as new. You've got quite a temperature; I can get you some paracetamol to help ease the aches and pains and bring your temperature down.

The nurses in this first scenario are caring. They tell Mrs Vincenzi what they are going to do and are efficient and reassuring. They introduce themselves to the patient and ask permission before doing any tasks. They come across as being kind and patient.

Now consider this second scenario:

Come on, Shell. Let's get on and get some of them up. Let's start here. Oh no! She's wet! Let's get her changed. More work: this is a pain. Come on now, roll over and let us get you changed. Fancy wetting the bed! Never mind, eh? Oh no, look what I've just put my hand in! Don't laugh, Lucy. Mind you, if you didn't laugh, you'd cry. Are you going out on your days off? I can't wait to get off this ward. We do an awful lot of shovelling.

Unfortunately, the second scenario is close to an incident that actually happened. The nurses probably did not mean to be unkind and thoughtless – they were simply trying to make light of a difficult situation. However, in doing so they were failing their patient. This is an extreme example of poor care, but unfortunately this does happen in real life. The nurses are being unprofessional and are not considering the patient's feelings in any way. They are just as efficient at cleaning Mrs Vincenzi, but their approach is poor and unkind.

Essential care

> ### To think about
>
> What do you consider to be essential care?
> Why?

A **stroke** results from a bleed into, or a blood clot in, part of the brain.

You will probably have included some of the following:

+ To be listened to and understood, and to understand what others communicate to you
+ To be treated with dignity and respect and to have your privacy respected and maintained
+ To be free from pain
+ To receive adequate, edible food and to have enough to drink
+ To be able to swallow safely
+ To regain independence through restoration and adaptation of physical and psychological functioning
+ To be clean and comfortable
+ To have any infection treated efficiently and not to be put at risk of getting an infection
+ To have your own and your family's and carers' views taken into account
+ If your condition changes, to have this observed and acted upon

All of the above are aspects of care that are important because they deal with basic human needs. The central theme of this book is about the care you give to your patients. It is about ensuring that this care is of the highest quality and is given in a proactive manner so that you are able to anticipate and fulfil your patients' needs.

How can you ensure that you give high-quality care? High-quality care is difficult to define; it is about the difference between good quality and poor quality. Poor quality of care has been a cause for concern for many years. Since 1995, there has been a national commitment to drive up standards of fundamental and essential aspects of care. This has been reflected in government policy following pressure from organisations such as Age Concern and from health and social care practitioners, patients and their families.

To think about

How can good-quality care be defined?
In what ways can the standards of essential care be measured?
How can quality be maintained?

The most effective way of finding out how good care actually is, and the standard to which it is being delivered, is to ask patients and their families how satisfied they are with the care provided. This is about finding out what is important to the patient and what can be improved. Standards of care can be measured in this way and quality can be maintained using this means and through activities such as benchmarking (as we explain in detail later in this chapter).

Patient-centred approach

Patient-centred care puts the person first rather than the illness or the condition. Person-centred care considers the needs, emotions and feelings of the person. A patient-centred approach is about giving the patient the means to have control over their treatment or at the very least to have some say in what is being planned for them. It is about the patient being at the centre of any care or treatment that is provided by healthcare practitioners, from the simplest task to the most complicated technical treatment. In other words, the care revolves around the patient. In such an approach, the patient is an active participant in their care-planning and in the evaluation of that care, so they have a say in whether the treatment is suitable and acceptable to them. Patients are the best people to consult about what services should be available to help them recover. This approach involves the patient and the members of the care team working together. Consider this quote:

> *Empowering patients with information and increasing their contribution to planning services can greatly influence the development of clinical governance. Contributions from patients will affect not just the responsiveness and performance of services but the process through which quality-improvement initiatives are identified and prioritised.* (Halligan and Donaldson, 2001)

This quote shows how patients should be empowered through information so that they can contribute to the planning of services in order to improve quality.

Background to the national drive to improve the quality of care for patients

Since 1997, following intense lobbying from patient pressure groups and because of concerns voiced by practitioners, the UK government has been dedicated to a programme of NHS reform. The aim is for health and social care organisations to be more responsive to the needs of patients. Some of the influential papers that have helped to shape current health-care include the following:

+ In 1999, *Making a Difference: Strengthening the Nursing, Midwifery and Health Visiting Contribution to Health and Healthcare* indicated that services within healthcare should be subject to measurement of quality (Department of Health, 1999).

+ The Department of Health (DH) paper *A First Class Service: Quality in the New NHS* was published in 1998 and set out the government's commitment to improving quality and services for patients (Department of Health, 1998).

+ *The NHS Plan: A Plan for Investment, a Plan for Reform* (Department of Health, 2000a) reinforced the importance of getting the basics right and of improving the patient experience.

+ The National Service Frameworks set out programmes of action and reform to ensure that healthcare meets the needs of patients. Each framework sets out national standards intended to drive up quality and to reduce variations in care and treatment. In particular, the National Service Framework for Older People (NSF Older People) has emphasised the importance of good-quality fundamental and essential care (Department of Health, 2001). Because of this, we look at this particular framework in more detail. The National Service Frameworks provide a structure for healthcare practitioners and managers to follow.

These documents have been a response to growing concerns about the poor standards of care delivered to patients. Although the documents have been produced by the DH, many practitioners and patient groups have been involved and have influenced the development of these. The focus on quality of care tends to be on certain vulnerable groups of people, such as children and young adults, older people, people with learning disabilities and people with mental health issues, because unfortunately it has been reported that care of these people has been significantly poorer than that given to other patients. Mencap (2007) produced a report entitled *Death by Indifference*, which shows how Ollie, a young man with learning disabilities, died through neglect and indifference. This makes compelling reading for any health or social care worker.

To think about

Do you agree that care given to older people has been of a lower standard than the care given to others?
If so, why?

In 1997 the *Observer* newspaper led a campaign calling for 'Dignity on the Ward'. The campaign concerned unacceptably poor-quality essential care being given to older people in hospitals throughout England. The main issue of concern was the lack of basic dignified nursing care, including personalised care, promotion of autonomy, personal hygiene and access to food and drink. Concerns were raised regarding the restrictive and poorly applied care protocols to deal with issues such as swallowing assessment after stroke, when patients were found to be at risk of choking or developing pneumonia because they were not assessed to ascertain whether they could swallow properly. The report also highlighted restrictions on linen supplies causing great discomfort to patients, and a lack of consultation with patients' relatives. Following the campaign, the health secretary Frank Dobson commissioned the Health Advisory Service 2000 (HAS) to investigate these issues and to recommend ways of dealing with them.

The *Observer*'s campaign was significant because of what developed from it; however, on 7 October 2007, a similar report was recorded in the *Mail on Sunday*, ten years after the original campaign.

The HAS investigating team included health advisory staff and representatives from Age Concern, the DH, social services and health professionals from various NHS trusts. The team investigated 16 randomly selected acute hospital wards in general hospitals throughout England. The researchers used different methods to collect information including direct observation of patient care and through questioning and observing patients and staff. The aim of the inquiry was to seek and bring together the views of older patients, their relatives, ward staff and managers about the care given and about the factors that influence the quality of care (Health Advisory Service 2000, 1999). Although this was a fairly small study and the research was **qualitative** rather than quantitative, the resulting report *Not Because They Are Old* had a significant influence on the NSF Older People.

Not Because They Are Old sets out a number of key themes, including lack of satisfaction with care, equipment shortages, poor or inappropriate physical environments, concern about fundamental aspects of essential care, lack of suitable staff training, and dissatisfaction with

Qualitative means not measured numerically.

the patient's journey from admission to discharge. The report sets out a number of recommendations, which are listed in Exhibit 1.1. These recommendations are reflected in all current quality directives.

+ Patients and relatives to be involved in care at every stage
+ Patients, relatives and staff to be able to challenge bad practice
+ Service provision to be geared up for older people
+ Role of ward manager to create a supportive learning environment
+ Better education and training for staff in specific needs of older people
+ Adequate nutrition
+ Multidisciplinary teamwork and secure support systems
+ Improvement in discharge planning and process
+ Adequate numbers of staff
+ Ward environment clean and well maintained
+ Access to specialist and integrated care/treatment
+ Access to rehabilitation and recuperation services in hospital and in the community
+ Consideration of older people's needs when planning and commissioning services
+ A National Service Framework for Older People to focus on the quality of care and service provision

Exhibit 1.1 Recommendations from *Not Because They Are Old*
Source: Health Advisory Service 2000 (1999)

These recommendations are not complex or costly to implement; rather, they are basic rights that should have already been in place. In 1999, Age Concern published a report concerned primarily with age discrimination (Gilchrist, 1999). The report also highlighted incidents of poor-quality care. Over 1500 people were interviewed for the report, and direct quotes from some of the respondents were included. The report found that older people were not always well nourished, clean, comfortable and treated with respect, that many staff were insensitive to the needs of older people, and that staff attitude could be dismissive and disrespectful. Age Concern is a pressure group that campaigns on behalf of older people, and part of its aim is to lobby government to initiate change. This report was influential in the contents of the NSF Older People. We look at this particular National Service Framework in more detail because it highlights the importance of providing good-quality essential care.

National Service Frameworks

The National Service Frameworks set out a strategy for fair, high-quality, integrated health and social care services. They are concerned primarily with improving the quality of care and the promotion of health and independence. The NSF Older People was developed as a response to recognition that older people had been the recipients of poor-quality care and inadequate services (Department of Health, 2001). As with all such initiatives, the success of the implementation of the standards in improving the quality of care is partly dependent on finances; however, health professionals can do much to improve the quality of care despite these financial constraints. The standards are set out in Exhibit 1.2.

Standard 1: rooting out discrimination
Standard 2: person-centred care
Standard 3: intermediate care
Standard 4: general hospital care
Standard 5: stroke
Standard 6: prevention of falls
Standard 7: mental health in older people
Standard 8: promoting an active, healthy life

Exhibit 1.2 Standards from the National Service Framework for Older People
Source: Department of Health (2001)

The Caring Model

The Caring Model™ was developed in 2002 by Sharon Dingman as part of her master's degree. The model helps to give structure to care, enabling health and social care practitioners to focus on and analyse the care they give to patients. Dingman identified five behaviours that practitioners could use to ensure that the care they give to patients is positive (Exhibit 1.3).

+ Introduce yourself to the person and explain your role in their care
+ Call the person by their preferred name
+ Sit at the bedside or with the person at eye level for at least five minutes per shift time to plan and review the person's care or service and review expected/desired outcomes
+ Use touch appropriately (e.g. a handshake, a touch on the arm, holding a hand)
+ Use the mission, vision and value statements (whether personal or organisational) in planning/ reviewing the care or service provided

Exhibit 1.3 Five behaviours of the Caring Model™

These five behaviours can make a significant impact on the care that you give. They are easy to perform but can make a huge difference to the experience of the patient. The model also defines caring, describing it as a set of behaviours that show respect for human dignity and a partnership that is given and received with integrity.

Recap Questions

1. What do we mean by using a person-centred approach?
2. What is the focus of the National Service Framework?
3. What are the five components of the Caring Model? Why do they make a difference?

Quality

Quality in health and social care is about agreeing a set of standards and ensuring the standards are met by way of monitoring and reflection. Quality of care is monitored in health through audit, clinical governance and reflective practice. Healthcare workers are regulated by their professional bodies, such as the Nursing and Midwifery Council (NMC) and the General Medical Council (GMC). Bodies such as the National Institute for Health and Clinical Excellence (**NICE**) and the Commission for Health Audit Improvement (CHAI) evaluate the quality of care. Likewise, by responding to patient commendations and complaints and by fully investigating incidents and near-misses, care quality can be evaluated. Every health and social care practitioner has a duty to provide good standards of care and treatment. Nurses have been seen in the past as providing excellent care in what can appear to be difficult circumstances, such as when time and resources are limited, but reports issued by the media, pressure groups, voluntary groups and the government have shown that this is increasingly no longer the case.

To think about

What does quality mean to you?
How can you ensure your patients receive good-quality care?
How can you maintain quality?

Quality is a difficult word to define. It has been described in various nursing articles over the past couple of decades as:

+ Being excellent – that is, the service is the very best it can be, all those using it are satisfied with it and it cannot be bettered
+ Conforming with requirements, so all standards, protocols and policies are suitable and are complied with
+ Being fit for use or for the purpose it was intended for
+ Being free from defects or imperfections

Why evaluate care and treatment? Evaluation of care is a way of ensuring high-quality care is delivered. Patients, nursing professionals, other professionals, government organisations such as NICE and CHAI, health authorities, and pressure groups such as Age Concern all demand that care/treatment is evaluated (Smith, 1999). Evaluation of care also involves measuring whether care is effective – in other words, whether it is beneficial to the patient and it is fit for the purpose for which it is intended. It is essential that care is provided in an efficient and cost-effective manner. Evaluating services can ensure that care improves, can encourage staff to work harder and can give practitioners a sense of satisfaction and achievement.

NICE is an organisation that gives advice and updates that inform clinical policy and decisions.

A number of tools are available to measure and evaluate care such as through clinical practice benchmarking (Department of Health, 2003). The government has been committed to improving the quality of care and the patient's experience and has issued a number of policy documents and guidance in order to achieve this. These documents have included the White Paper *A First Class Service: Quality in the New NHS* (Department of Health, 1998), which gave details of clinical governance. The aim of clinical governance is to provide structure for NHS organisations to apply to their services in order to ensure that the healthcare they provide is safe and of a high quality and that the patient is put first.

Complaints procedures

Many people have been reluctant to complain about healthcare treatment and many surveys of complaints have therefore, tended to underestimate the extent of patient and relative concerns (Health Advisory Service 2000, 1999). Even today, with a more positive approach to addressing issues, many patients are still reluctant to complain. It is important for organisations to foster a no-blame culture and to be able to learn from mistakes, near-misses, complaints and comments. In order to create this culture, open and honest criticism must be encouraged at all levels of service delivery, from the most menial to the most high-tech. If staff members are supported constructively, they are more likely to seek out and act on patients' comments. The overall level of satisfaction experienced by patients who access health and social care services is often determined by the openness and responsiveness of the organisations in which they work (Redmond, 2004). Consider Case study 1.2.

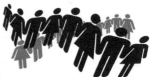

Case Study 1.2

Mrs Jones was recovering from a fractured femur. She was staying in a nursing home. She required assistance to walk and move about (mobilise). She was able to walk independently using a walking frame, but sometimes she did not use the frame appropriately, carrying it around corners rather than using it with all its legs on the floor. While going to the bathroom, Mrs Jones stumbled. The support worker was able to prevent Mrs Jones from falling. The staff nurse in charge decided it was not necessary to record this as an incident.

Do you think this was the right decision?

Even though Mrs Jones did not fall and sustain any injuries, the incident needed to be reported and the incident investigated. Injuries could have occurred both to Mrs Jones and to the support worker, and so action needs to be taken in order to ensure that a similar incident does not happen in the future. Also, it may be that Mrs Jones' mobility needs to be re-assessed and the support worker needs some more education. The incident was reported and an internal investigation took place in the nursing home. On investigation, it was apparent that there were issues that needed to be dealt with. First, on talking to Mrs Jones, it was found that she had difficulty using the frame, that she had discomfort to her feet and legs, and that she was wearing unsuitable footwear. It was also discovered that not all the staff had been on the yearly mandatory moving and handling course. The following actions were initiated jointly by the team and Mrs Jones:

+ Mrs Jones had been becoming more and more anxious about her mobility. She found the walking frame difficult to use and awkward, and she stated that it restricted her rather than helped her.

+ A re-assessment of Mrs Jones' mobility needs was arranged with the physiotherapist, nurse, support worker, occupational therapist, podiatrist and Mrs Jones.

+ Mrs Jones was experiencing pain in her leg, and so her pain relief was re-assessed.

+ On examination, it was found that Mrs Jones' toenails were so long that they were restricting her mobility. This was attended to.

+ Since her admission to hospital, Mrs Jones had not been given suitable footwear. Discussion with Mrs Jones and her relatives remedied this.

+ It was arranged for all staff to attend moving and handling courses. The physiotherapist arranged some in-house training sessions about helping patients to mobilise.

It is clear from this scenario that investigating near-misses and putting into place the necessary actions can improve and inform care and is an integral part of clinical governance.

Governance

Governance of clinical issues, or clinical governance, is about providing a safe and better health service for patients. The aim of clinical governance is to improve the quality of care/treatment that patients receive. This is done in a number of ways, including using reflective practice through a framework such as clinical supervision; investigating complaints, incidents and near-misses; and implementing audits and clinical benchmarking. Clinical governance places the patient at the centre of the service and involves learning from past experiences and preventing mistakes (Hallett, 2002). It is a way of improving care and ensuring that the care provided is safe and suitable for patients.

In 2001, Sir Liam Donaldson, the UK's chief medical officer, and Gabriel Scally, a regional health director, worked on producing some principles of clinical governance. These principles, which we list in Exhibit 1.4, have informed a range of clinical governance models used in healthcare today.

+ To have clear lines of responsibility and accountability for quality of clinical care
+ To give patient satisfaction
+ To have in place information management systems
+ To develop and follow quality-improvement programmes, such as clinical audit, evidence-based practice and clinical guidelines
+ To have in place risk-management policies
+ To educate and train
+ To develop and use ways of identifying and remedying poor practice through professional bodies (e.g. Nursing and Midwifery Council)

Exhibit 1.4 Principles of clinical governance
Adapted from Scally and Donaldson (2001)

Clinical practice benchmarking is a central part of clinical governance. We now look at clinical practice benchmarking in more detail and see how it can be used by practitioners to improve the quality of the care they provide to their patients.

Clinical practice benchmarking

Benchmarking was originally developed as a way of measuring quality of services and goods in industry. In 1998 the DH identified that benchmarking could be used as a way of measuring quality in healthcare (Department of Health, 1998). *The NHS Plan* emphasised the need to get the basics right and to improve the patient's experience (Department of Health, 2000a). In 2001 the *Essence of Care Toolkit* was developed; this toolkit contained eight benchmarks of best practice for essential and fundamental care aspects. In 2003 the toolkit was expanded to contain a ninth benchmark and in 2005 a tenth. Exhibit 1.5 shows current clinical practice benchmarks.

+ Communication
+ Continence and bladder and bowel care
+ Health promotion
+ Personal and oral hygiene
+ Food and nutrition
+ Pressure ulcers
+ Privacy and dignity
+ Record-keeping
+ Safety of patients with mental health needs
+ Principles of self-care

Exhibit 1.5 Clinical practice benchmarks

Clinical practice benchmarks are standards that can be measured. Each contains a benchmark of best practice that healthcare workers can measure against and strive to achieve. All of the clinical practice benchmarks interlink with each other; for example, communication is a common theme throughout every benchmark. The benchmarks are designed so that they complement and relate closely to each other, thus completely covering the important aspects of care giving. The toolkit was developed by DH employees, health practitioners and patients and carers. The aim of the toolkit is to aid practitioners to take a patient-focused and structured approach to providing care and treatment. It enables practitioners to compare and share practice and to work closely with patients and carers in order to develop action plans to improve and maintain good-quality care. Practice can be compared and shared with other health and social care workers. The benchmarks can be used as a way of measuring the work of both individuals and teams. The benchmarks are relevant to all health and social care settings and to all patient and carer groups.

The *Essence of Care Toolkit* can be accessed at the DH website. Each clinical benchmark has an overall patient-focused outcome with a number of factors that are needed in order to achieve the outcome. Each of the factors has a statement of best practice with a continuum of poor to best practice; health practitioners can then measure their practice against this. Each factor has indicators on how best to achieve excellent practice. Exhibit 1.6 shows the stages involved in the benchmarking process. We will now look at an example of using clinical benchmarking in practice.

> *Stage 1*: agree best practice
> *Stage 2*: assess clinical area against best practice
> *Stage 3*: produce and implement action plan aimed at achieving best practice
> *Stage 4*: review achievement towards best practice
> *Stage 5*: disseminate improvements and or review action plan
> *Stage 6*: agree best practice

Exhibit 1.6   Stages of benchmarking

Agreeing best practice

Points for consideration when agreeing best practice include:

+ The patient/carer experience of care – how can this be ascertained?
+ How is current care delivered? Does this need to be changed? If it is satisfactory, how do you know it is satisfactory? Could it be improved?
+ Are you/your team achieving best practice? If not, why not? What evidence is available to demonstrate this?

Assessing the clinical practice/area against best practice

+ Obtain baseline information through observation, listening to patients and using patient surveys. Audit is a way of finding out what is provided or done and ascertaining whether this meets agreed levels or standards. If audits and other systems are already in place, then these can be used as evidence.
+ Construct a portfolio of evidence.
+ Consider the barriers that may be stopping you/your team from achieving best practice.
+ Compare and share best practice with other practitioners and/or teams.

Producing an action plan

The action plan needs to detail:

+ Any changes to practice that need to be made in order to meet the best practice statement of each factor of the benchmark
+ Who is responsible for making any necessary changes
+ The timescale in which to review progress in meeting these changes in practice

It is important to remember that all actions need to be specific, measurable, achievable, realistic and timely (SMART).

Reviewing achievement

+ All activities should be documented, showing details of improvements, problems and unexpected outcomes.
+ Data collected should be analysed: has the patient experience improved? In what way? How has practice changed?
+ Review activities.
+ Share and compare with other practitioners/teams.

Disseminating improvements

+ Discuss changes to practice with others.

+ Initiate change using evidence of benchmarking.

+ Use evidence of benchmarking to challenge bad practice.

+ Use the evidence to help inform service development.

+ Include findings in organisational local business plans.

+ Develop education and training programmes using best practice.

+ Share good practice with other organisations.

Agreeing best practice

+ Continue benchmarking and use benchmarking to maintain good practice.

+ Monitor and disseminate practice continually.

Stages 1, 2 and 3 (see Exhibit 1.6) can be applied to teams and also used by lone practitioners to help them analyse the care they give to patients. Stages 4 and 5 can be used to change practice at a more strategic level. The results of benchmarking can be used to change and influence policies and procedures. Consider Case study 1.3, which shows benchmarking in action.

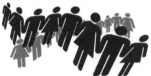

Case Study 1.3

Patients had commented in an exit survey (a questionnaire that asked patients about their experience in hospital) from a ward in a rehabilitation hospital about their dissatisfaction with the meals served. These comments included details of poorly presented meals, dirty tables, patients being unable to access their meals, plates being cleared away before patients had finished eating and meals becoming cold. Clearly action needed to be taken. The ward team decided to use the nutrition benchmark in the *Essence of Care Toolkit* as a way of improving practice. The nutrition patient-focused outcome was:

Patients are enabled to consume food which meets their individual needs (Department of Health, 2003).

How do you think the team was able to do this?

It was decided that representatives would meet together on a monthly basis to assess current practice against the nutrition benchmark, with the aim of formulating an action plan to improve mealtimes for patients.

The team members of the benchmarking group included ward nurses, a dietician, a speech and language therapist, the catering manager, patients and carers. The team met monthly and worked at comparing their current practice against each of the best practice statements for each of the factors that made up the nutrition benchmark. Consequently, a number of changes were made (Exhibit 1.7).

+ Every patient's table was cleaned before meals were served. Nurses agreed to help with the clearing of objects. Catering staff were responsible for wiping down the tables. Patients were encouraged to use the dining room if they were able to do so; assistance was given from nurses to enable them to achieve this.
+ Staff education and training were initiated to help patients with eating and drinking. Topics for the teaching sessions included dysphagia awareness, the importance of fluids and assessment of a patient's nutritional needs.
+ Equipment and aids such as plate warmers and cutlery with special grips were made available for use by patients.
+ A five-point nutrition plan was implemented for every patient, including assessment, positioning, the opportunity to wash hands and go to the toilet, provision of any aids or equipment needed by the patient in order to eat the meal, and ensuring the food meets the patient's nutritional requirements.
+ The use of an agreed assessment and screening tool for patients' nutritional needs was put in place.
+ Changes were made in staffing levels and to ward routines in order to ensure that adequate numbers of nursing staff were available to assist patients at mealtimes.

Exhibit 1.7 Changes made as a result of benchmarking

As a result of the benchmarking group, patient exit surveys showed a vast improvement in the satisfaction rates regarding meals. The group continued to meet regularly in order to monitor and maintain the good practice. The group also disseminated the results of their benchmarking to other groups. This shows a good example of interdisciplinary team working with patients and carers.

As can be seen, clinical practice benchmarking provides a mechanism for structured reflective practice.

Reflective practice

Reflective practice is learning from experience; it is the ability to analyse, assess and change. The goal of reflective practice is to help health professionals to continually improve their practice by identifying what they do well and what areas need improvement (Hallett, 2002). Reflective practice is part of practice development and continuing professional development. Reflecting on practice is to use the knowledge gained from that reflection to develop and improve it (Schon, 1983). Reflective practice is thinking about what you are doing in the context of the care setting and then analysing it through thought, considering why it happened, what influences were there at the time, how and/or why it could have been different and consequently changing one's future practice. Reflective practice can be done in a number of ways, such as keeping a diary, maintaining a profile, using clinical supervision, analysing critical incidents and implementing action learning.

There are many models of reflection that can be used to give structure to reflective thinking. The most important aspect of reflective practice is that the process includes action planning. These actions are then taken forward so that improvements can be made.

> ### To think about
>
> Why might you keep a reflective diary?
> How would you ensure that the diary could help you describe, analyse, evaluate and there-fore inform your practice?

When reflecting it is important to focus on:

+ What you intended to do
+ What actually happened
+ What you felt about this

If you are going to analyse and inform your practice, you also need to critically analyse any incidents:

1. Focus on a particular event.
2. Describe the event in detail.
3. Consider the context of the incident; for example, was the ward short-staffed at the time, or were there a number of admissions or very poorly patients?
4. Note your feelings, your observations and the facts of the event.
5. Think about how you feel about the incident now.
6. Consider what the significant factors were.
7. What have you learnt about this regarding:
   • yourself?
   • your colleagues?
   • the situation/context?
8. What, if anything, are you going to do?
9. What would you do differently next time?

Action learning is about using reflection to analyse events and then taking the necessary action to solve identified problems.

> ### To think about
>
> Use the above or a reflective model such as the Gibbs Reflective Cycle (Gibbs, 1988), shown in Figure 1.1, to reflect on an incident that has occurred in practice. Remember to close the reflective cycle with action learning and problem-solving.

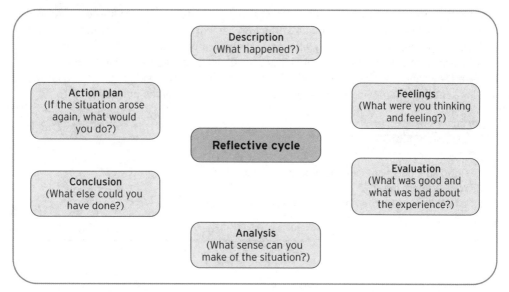

Figure 1.1 Gibbs Reflective Cycle

Clinical supervision

Clinical supervision is a process in which health and social care workers can support each other to reflect on practice and to act as a sounding board to initiate changes in their own practice with the aim of improving quality of care. Clinical supervision is an equal partnership between two or more people who can identify problems, reflect on experiences, learn from experience and implement changes in order to improve quality. Clinical supervision focuses on matters of central importance in the provision of safe and accountable practice (Butterworth and Woods, 1999). Clinical supervision takes place in many healthcare settings and may involve just two people or a whole team.

It is important that student nurses have the opportunity to take part in clinical supervision. Students in clinical placement should be given time to reflect with their mentors on incidences that have occurred in practice. Consider Case study 1.4.

Case Study 1.4

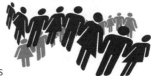

Julie Hilton was a third-year student mental health nurse. She was meeting up with the practice educator to discuss her progress in this clinical placement. During the visit, Julie became very upset when telling the practice educator about an incident that happened when she was in her first year. This clinical incident should have been addressed at the time. Following discussion and by using a reflective model, Julie, supported by the practice educator, was able to analyse and make sense of the incident.

Julie had experienced unnecessary distress that had affected her ability to relate to certain patients. This had had a detrimental effect on her work with a certain ward team and had altered her perception of working with patients with a particular condition. This problem should have been addressed at the time it occurred. Julie needed to be able to reflect on and analyse the incident with her mentor at the time. Clinical supervision is an effective way of making sense and of moving forward particularly for newly qualified nurses.

Recap Questions

1. How is the quality of care monitored nationally and locally?
2. Why evaluate care?
3. Why is it important to report near-misses as well as accidents?
4. What is reflective practice?

The assessment process

What is an assessment?

Assessment is a way of ascertaining the care/treatment and services an individual needs. Assessment explores and identifies these treatments and services through physical, mental and environmental processes that take into account the abilities of the individual. Tools and scales are available to aid assessment. Assessment takes account of the person's spiritual and cultural needs as well as their clinical needs. Most healthcare assessments aim to take into account all aspects of the patient's life rather than their medical needs alone.

Why do we assess?

+ To meet the health and social needs of the patient
+ To facilitate person-centred, holistic care/treatment
+ To collaborate and negotiate with the person to help them identify their problems and/or goals (Creek, 2002)

What is meant by person-centred assessment?

A person-centred assessment is an assessment of a person that takes into account the person's illness, any disability the person has, and other aspects of that person's life, such as their culture, religion, work, school family, friends and personal views and wishes. A person-centred assessment allows practitioners to work together in the best interests of the person.

What makes a good assessment?

+ *Communication*: effective communication is essential for accurate assessments. Effective communication is achieved through:
  - listening and hearing;
  - initiating conversations and giving equal value to each participant;
  - allowing for and accommodating silences;
  - being aware of and responding to non-verbal communication, such as body language;
  - demonstrating empathy.
+ *Understanding what the person wants and needs*: by actively involving the person in all stages of their assessment and treatment.
+ *Being able to respond to the person's expectations*: by providing timely and appropriate assessments.
+ *Collecting accurate and complete information*:
  - gathering information from a variety of sources, including family and friends;
  - using a variety of assessment methods, including observation, tools and scales;
  - documenting all information fully.

Why do we need multi-agency involvement?

Patients' healthcare needs are assessed by more than one health or social care practitioner; for example, nurses, doctors, occupational therapists, physiotherapists and dieticians may work together in the care of one patient. This is known as multidisciplinary working. Multi-agency working is the involvement of more than one agency in the patient's care – for example, a representative from a voluntary organisation such as Age Concern working with a social worker and a nurse.

Multi-agency working is about providing the best care for the patient. Often those care needs include more than just medical aspects. Consider this quote:

> *... some of the causes of [mental] health problems go far beyond the realms of health care and medicine, making it impossible for the nursing profession and the NHS to tackle them independently ...*
> (Alford, 2000)

Each discipline or agency member may approach assessments in a different way, but each has a valuable and unique contribution to the assessment. For example, if a number of practitioners were assessing the mobility needs of a patient, Mrs Wyatt, each practitioner would each assess from a different perspective, as shown in Figure 1.2.

Each of these health professionals contributes to the overall assessment of Mrs Wyatt's mobility. The podiatrist looks specifically at Mrs Wyatt's feet, for example whether her shoes fit properly, whether she has any problems with cuts or sprains, and whether her toenails need attention. The physiotherapist looks specifically at Mrs Wyatt's gait and how she walks. The occupational therapist assesses Mrs Wyatt's home and whether any equipment would be of assistance. The nurse finds out why Mrs Wyatt's mobility is poor, looks at Mrs Wyatt's medication to see whether side effects from this are contributing, and considers Mrs Wyatt's dietary intake. Mrs Wyatt is consulted at every stage of this assessment so that the health and social care practitioners can ensure they take into account her personal preferences, her needs, feelings and emotions.

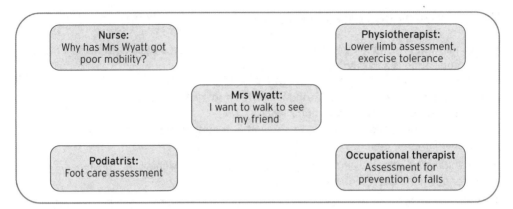

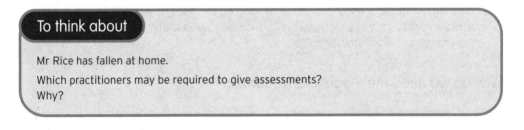

Figure 1.2 Mrs Wyatt's assessment

To think about

Mr Rice has fallen at home.

Which practitioners may be required to give assessments?

Why?

Mr Rice will possibly need assessments from:

+ His general practitioner (GP) regarding Mr Rice's general health
+ District nursing, in order to assess for nursing care input
+ Occupational therapy, for equipment and adaptations
+ Podiatry, for foot care/treatment physiotherapist for mobility
+ Social services, for home care
+ A dietician, for nutrition
+ Housing services

Models of assessment

Assessment is an ongoing process, with treatment/care being constantly evaluated so that outcomes can be achieved and/or renegotiated. The purpose of assessment is to help health professionals to determine the best intervention (Refshauge *et al.*, 2005). Models of assessment give a theoretical structure to treatment and therapy, by providing the means of understanding, assessing, addressing and communicating goals, needs and therapy. An initial assessment commonly uses a process of interview, observation, review and outcome-measuring tools, from which a treatment/therapy plan can be devised.

There are many types of assessment model in use in health and social care settings; however, assessments currently tend to be more patient-focused, so that all health and social care practitioners and other agencies can use the same assessments. The **care programme approach** is used in mental health settings; the **common assessment framework** is used by health, education and social care practitioners working with children; and the **single assessment process** is used in the assessment of people over 65 years of age. These three frameworks are all multi-agency assessment documents. They ensure that there is an integrated assessment of the patient. This means that all the agencies work together so that the patient's care and treatment are integrated. This results in all relevant patient information being shared between the different services that the patient accesses.

To think about

Which agencies may be involved in the assessment process of the following:

A child with asthma?

A young man with a history of drug abuse?

An older person with diabetes?

For the child with asthma the GP, practice nurse, parent and child will be involved initially. Other agencies may include the school nursing service, the child's teacher, a specialist asthma nurse, a physiotherapist, a health visitor and a dietician.

The young man with a history of drug abuse may have input from his GP, family, substance misuse worker, housing officer, hostel worker and social worker.

For the older person with diabetes, there may be input from the GP, practice nurse, district nursing service, consultant, diabetic specialist nurse, podiatrist and dietician.

What is meant by multi-agency assessment?

A **multi-agency assessment** is an assessment of any patient with more than one health, social or educational need. This is an integrated assessment framework so that all those involved with the patient can share relevant information with each other. It is a way of demonstrating integrated care/treatment and of encouraging all agencies to respect and acknowledge the contribution of each professional. The aim is to avoid duplication of information and records and to stop professionals giving conflicting advice. Previously, there have been cases in which failure to share pertinent information resulted in failure to provide the best package of care; in some cases, this has had disastrous consequences, such as the case of Victoria Climbie, a young girl who died following sustained and systematic abuse.

A **care programme approach** is a multi-agency assessment that focuses on the patient and their mental health and social care needs.

A **common assessment framework** is an assessment framework for children in need; the assessment looks at the child's needs in the context of their family life and education.

A **single assessment process** is a multi-agency assessment that looks at the patient's health and social care needs.

The terms **'multi-agency assessment'** and 'common assessment' are interchangeable.

Where does the need for interdisciplinary assessments come from?

The emphasis on all disciplines and agencies using the common assessments and the same patient notes came from the NHS Plan (Department of Health, 2000a) and was incorporated into the National Service Frameworks:

> *The NHS will work together with others to ensure a seamless service for patients. As people age, they have an increasingly complex range of needs which may mean they need a range of services across health and social services. These should be provided in as seamless a way as possible, to avoid confusion for older people and their carers and to minimise duplication of effort.*
> **(Department of Health, 2001)**

Why have interdisciplinary assessments?

+ To ensure that the person is at the centre of the assessment, which is about the person, not the individual agency
+ To address the individual's needs
+ To tailor the care/treatment programme as the patient's needs change
+ To encourage all agencies involved to work together, share information and share values
+ To avoid replication of information
+ To ensure that the person and their carers, friends and family are involved in the process
+ To ensure that care/treatment is a continuous process

To think about

What areas may be part of an assessment? Consider your basic health and social care requirements, such as food, warmth and shelter.

You may have included your health needs, wellbeing, mental health, relationships with others, safety, living environment, work circumstances, clinical background (e.g. any diseases or ongoing conditions) and financial resources. This list is not exhaustive; rather, it shows just how many factors can inform an assessment.

The level or amount of assessment should always be proportionate to the individual's needs. The aim is for all agencies to have access to relevant information about the person so there is no duplication and so that each agency does not hold their own duplicated information, but note that this is different from specialist assessment, which we discuss below. In some circumstances, it will not be appropriate to assess some aspects; however, those aspects may need to be assessed at a later date if the individual's circumstances change.

Consider Case study 1.5, which demonstrates the need for integrated working. Only after integration can issues such as Richard's be prevented from arising.

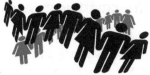

Case Study 1.5

Richard Brown is nine years old. Following surgery to correct a congenital abnormality, he has been left with stress incontinence. Richard has attended an outpatient clinic yearly to monitor his progress. At school, Richard had to go to the toilet immediately and frequently. When he asked the teacher if he could do this, he was told yes he could but that he would receive a detention each time he left the classroom. Richard became distressed and reluctant to attend school. Richard's parents informed the hospital consultant, who supplied the relevant information explaining Richard's condition to the school; the problem was resolved.

Specialist assessments

The common assessment frameworks do not replace the need for specialist assessments. A specialist assessment is an in-depth assessment carried out by an appropriately trained specialist; for example, a person requiring a swallowing assessment will be assessed by a speech and language therapist or other suitably trained support worker. Some people may require more than one specialist assessment. The aim of specialist assessments is to ensure that expert assessment is continued and enhanced.

To think about

Mrs Mills has had a stroke, resulting in a right-sided weakness.

Which agencies/professions will be involved in Mrs Mills' care/treatment?
What will they be assessing?
What specialist assessments will be required in the following situations:
+ At home?
+ On admission to casualty?
+ During Mrs Mills' stay in the stroke unit?
+ On discharge back home?

Mrs Mills will need assessments from many health and social care professionals. Mrs Mills will be assessed by her GP and the paramedics at home. She will be assessed in casualty by a nurse and a casualty doctor. She will be seen by the specialist consultant for the stroke unit. Once admitted to the stroke unit, Mrs Mills will be assessed by a nurse, doctor, physiotherapist, occupational therapist, dietician, and speech and language therapist. She may also be seen by a social worker, housing officer and podiatrist. When discharged home, she will be assessed by her GP and possibly by the district nurse, day unit coordinator and voluntary agency visitor. Thus, potentially there are many people involved in Mrs Mills' care. It is practical that Mrs Mills has one set of notes used by all of these professionals rather than each professional having a slightly different set of notes.

The care/treatment plan

The care/treatment plan is formulated from the assessment. The plan is an integrated document that addresses each identified need and risk. It gives a plan of action to achieve collaborated goals. The implementation of the action plan and the achievement of goals are evaluated at appropriate and timely intervals. New and revised goals and action plans are added as necessary. The purpose of the care/treatment plan is to give overall care/treatment aims for the individual.

Each agency involved will follow its own departmental policy regarding how and when reviews of the care/treatment plan take place. The timing and location of the reviews are influenced by the patient's needs. Good practice dictates an initial review within three months of initial assessment and at least yearly (or before if required) thereafter.

Recap Questions

1. Why do we assess?
2. What makes a good assessment?
3. What is multi-agency assessment?

Summary

In order to ensure that care is of the highest quality, it is essential that health and social care practitioners use strategies such as reflective practice to assess and review the care they give and to take part in clinical practice benchmarking and clinical supervision. The most effective way to measure quality of care is to find out from patients and their families how care-giving can be improved.

This chapter has looked at why the provision of good-quality care is so important. Examples of poor-quality care have centred on some of the more vulnerable members of our society, such as children, people with mental health needs, older people and people with learning disabilities, who, due to age or poor physical and mental health, need more help than certain others. Older people in particular have traditionally accepted what is given to them and consequently have often accepted poor-quality care without question. People with learning disabilities are reaching an increasingly older age, making them even more vulnerable. Children are often not listened to, and people with mental health needs can be ostracised. However, times are changing and older people tend to have better health and are now more active participants in their care. Children have been given a voice through the Children's Act (Department of Health, 1989) and the *National Service Framework for the Assessment of Children in Need and their Families* (Department of Health, 2000b). It is no longer acceptable for these vulnerable people to be given poor-quality care, and it is up to us as health and social care practitioners to make sure that only the highest quality is given. It is the responsibility of health and social care practitioners to ensure that all patients are cared for in the best way possible.

Consideration has been given to the assessment process in this chapter because good assessment is crucial to care. It is important that the patient and family are an active part of this assessment process and that all agencies and practitioners communicate effectively with each other and work towards the achievement of common patient-centred goals. There will always be a place for specialist assessments to complement general assessment frameworks.

> ### Key Points
>
> 1. Nursing is about providing the best possible care to patients.
> 2. All care given should be of the highest quality by ensuring that this care is monitored and evaluated at every stage of the patient's journey.
> 3. Multi-agency and multiprofessional assessments are key to ensuring the highest-quality care is given.

Points for debate

Now that you have come to the end of this chapter here are a few points that you may wish to think about when you are in practice. You may wish to discuss these with your work colleagues or fellow students.

Nurses automatically have compassion; that is why they become nurses.

It is more important to treat the patient's physical symptoms than to waste time getting to know the person.

> ### Links to Other Chapters
>
> Chapter 2   Dignity and privacy
> Chapter 3   Basic observations
> Chapter 4   Hygiene
> Chapter 5   Nutrition
> Chapter 6   Fluid balance and continence care
> Chapter 7   Pain management
> Chapter 8   Pressure ulcers
> Chapter 9   Rehabilitation and self-care
> Chapter 10   Record-keeping

Further reading

Department of Health (1999) *National Service Framework for Mental Health*. London: The Stationery Office.

Department of Health (2000) *National Service Framework for the Assessment of Children in Need and Their Families*. London: The Stationery Office.

Department of Health (2001) *National Service Framework for Older People*. London: The Stationery Office.

Department of Health (2003) *Clinical Practice Benchmarking: A Toolkit for Healthcare Practitioners*. London: The Stationery Office.

References

Butterworth, T and Woods, D (1999) *Clinical Governance and Clinical Supervision Working Together to Ensure Safe and Accountable Practice*. Manchester: University of Manchester.

Clark, C, Bolton, J and Scurfield, M (2000) *Mental Health and the Care of the Older Person*. London: Emap.

Creek, J (2002) *Occupational Therapy and Mental Health: Principles, Skills and Practice*, 3rd edn. Edinburgh: Churchill Livingstone.

Department of Health (1989) *Children Act 1989*. London: The Stationery Office.

Department of Health (1998) *A First Class Service: Quality in the New NHS*. London: The Stationery Office.

Department of Health (1999) *Making a Difference: Strengthening the Nursing, Midwifery and Health Visiting Contribution to Health and Health Care*. London: The Stationery Office.

Department of Health (2000a) *The NHS Plan: A Plan for Investment, A Plan for Reform*. London: The Stationery Office.

Department of Health (2000b) *National Service Framework for the Assessment of Children in Need and Their Families*. London: The Stationery Office.

Department of Health (2001) *National Service Framework for Older People*. London: The Stationery Office.

Department of Health (2003) *Clinical Practice Benchmarking: A Toolkit for Healthcare Practitioners*. London: The Stationery Office.

Gibbs, G (1988) *Learning by Doing: A Guide to Teaching and Learning Methods*. Oxford: Oxford Polytechnic.

Gilchrist, C (1999) *Turning Your Back on Us*. London: Age Concern.

Hallett, L (2002) *Clinical Governance: A Teaching Resource Pack*. London: Emap Healthcare.

Halligan, A and Donaldson, L (2001) Implementing clinical governance: turning vision into reality. *British Medical Journal* **322**, 1413-1417.

Health Advisory Service 2000 (1999) *Not Because They Are Old*. London: Health Advisory Service.

Mencap (2007) *Death by Indifference*. London: Mencap.

Redmond, B (2004) *Reflection in Action Developing Reflective Practice in Health and Social Services*. Aldergate: Ashgate.

Refshauge, K, Ada, L, Ellis, E, eds. (2005) *Science-Based Rehabilitation: Theories into Practice*. London, United Kingdom: Butterworth Heinemann.

Scally, G and Donaldson, L (2001) Clinical governance and the drive for quality improvement in the new NHS in England. *British Medical Journal* **317**, 61-65.

Schon, D (1983) *The Reflective Practitioner: How Professionals Think in Action*. London: Temple Smith.

Smith, M (1999) *Rehabilitation in Adult Nursing Practice*. London: Churchill Livingstone.

Chapter 2
Dignity and privacy

Case Study

Mrs Crevitt was an 86-year-old woman who died on a ward in a small hospital. Before she died, she spoke to her younger sister. Her sister later told the nurses what had been said. Mrs Crevitt spoke of her memories of her childhood: as a young girl with a mother and a father, and brothers and sisters, and of feeling that she was surrounded by love. She remembered herself as a young girl of 16 with dreams for the future. She spoke about how she had married at 20 to the man of her dreams and of how they had raised their children in a secure and happy home. She remembered her sons growing up, marrying and having children of their own. She recalled how she helped with her grand-children and of her love for her husband. Mrs Crevitt recalled her feelings of sadness and loneliness when her husband died and how she dreaded the future to come. She spoke of her anger and frustration of what she had become and how she felt others saw her: an old woman who was not very wise and with a body that was crumbling and falling apart. But Mrs Crevitt wanted to be seen by the nurses as who she really was – someone who had lived a busy and fulfilling life that was full of memories of love, happiness and pain.

Introduction

Consider this case study and reflect on your reactions to it. Mrs Crevitt is crying out for her identity to be recognised and for her feelings to be considered by those who are caring for her. In this chapter we explore why it is necessary for us to give care to our patients that actively promotes dignity. We will explain what is meant by the term 'personhood' – in other words, the things that make a person who they are – their life history, their relationships and their experiences.

We look at the patient–practitioner relationship and explore aspects of communication. We also investigate the topic of abuse, and explore and discuss indicators of abuse and how to manage these.

By the end of this chapter you will be able to:

1. Understand the importance of giving care to patients that actively promotes privacy and dignity
2. Explore issues in communication and the impact of this on care
3. Recognise the health professional's role in safeguarding the interests of their patients
4. Recognise the indicators of abuse
5. Recognise the different types of abuse
6. Understand the need to manage suspected abuse effectively

Dignity in care

In today's healthcare arena there is pressure to ensure that all patients have fast access to effective treatment. This treatment is to be delivered by efficient health and social care practitioners. These practitioners should be able to attend to the patient's physical needs while giving emotional support and treating the patient with kindness and respect. When people are ill or frail, they are often at their most vulnerable and they rely on the integrity of the people caring for them.

How the patient perceives their care can have a huge impact on their recovery. Health and social care professionals face a huge challenge to meet each patient's expectations of how their care and treatment is delivered; these professionals will be working across a vast range of patient perceptions. The Department of Health has worked extensively in the past decades to improve care. Much of this work has been involved with how patients are treated in the day-to-day interactions with staff. Following research, the Caring Model™ was developed by Sharon Dingman (see Chapter 1); this model deals with the components that make up care. The Caring Model gives structure to the processes of caring. The main components of care are maintaining a person's dignity, treating the person with respect and giving the person privacy.

To think about

What do we mean by 'dignity in care'?
What is important to you that may ensure your dignity?

You may have included some of the following in your thoughts:

+ Being put first so that your care is tailor-made for you
+ Being asked about your specific needs and then being listened to
+ Being treated with patience
+ Not being patronised
+ Feeling safe and secure
+ Not being isolated
+ Being given privacy
+ Being encouraged to be independent
+ Having your cultural and religious needs taken into account

As a nurse it is important for you when helping a patient with their most basic and essential care needs, such as feeding, personal hygiene and continence, to maintain the patient's dignity and privacy. There can be problems with achieving this, particularly in poor physical environments and if there is a lack of adequate resources. However, poor care is caused by a failure to recognise each patient's individuality, and this is often due to poor attitudes of staff. The quality of care depends not only on good healthcare but also on respect for the person as an individual (Department of Health, 2001a). The inquiry led by the HAS 2000, *Not Because They are Old* (Health Advisory Service 2000, 1999), concluded that some patients were being treated disrespectfully and that maintaining privacy was perceived as being a major problem. The role of the modern matron is a key aspect to ensuring a positive patient experience. In order to achieve this positive experience, attention must be paid to the promotion of dignity and privacy and to recognising the uniqueness of each person.

It is important that all care follows a whole-person or holistic approach. This is care that addresses the person's physical, psychological, emotional, social, spiritual, religious and cultural needs. It is about putting the person at the centre of everything that a healthcare worker does (this is person-centred care). The needs and emotions of the person are the focal point around which everything else is geared (Tribal Education, 2006a,b).

Personhood

In the past, the care culture has sometimes denied patients their personhood. This applied particularly to the most vulnerable members of society, such as older people, people with mental health problems, people with learning difficulties and young people. Thousands of people have been denied the basic right of dignity and died in poor, inadequately equipped environments staffed by workers who failed to understand the concept of personhood (Kitwood, 1997). An individual's life history contributes to their uniqueness as a person. It is essential that staff working with patients find out about their patients' life histories in order to gain more understanding and to be **empathic** rather than only **sympathetic** to their patients' needs. This enables the nurse to gain an appreciation of the type of person the patient has been and is now. Much can be gained through personal knowledge and through

Empathic means identifying oneself mentally with someone else in order to understand them fully. **Sympathetic** means feeling sorry for the person.

respect of a person's beliefs, but this can be achieved only by encouraging people to express their beliefs, wishes and views, thus giving the patient the opportunity to share their personal uniqueness.

Promoting and maintaining dignity

Health professionals are in a unique position when caring and treating patients. Patients are often in highly vulnerable, helpless and dependent positions and look to nurses for support, understanding and reassurance. Nurses hold the key to upholding patients' dignity and to fostering an atmosphere of respect. The report *Not Because They Are Old* (Health Advisory Service 2000, 1999) found that patients and their relatives were very sensitive to what they perceived as negative attitudes on the part of staff. Consider Case study 2.1, particularly with regard to how the carer responded to the question asked.

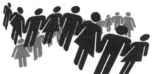

Case Study 2.1

Mrs White attended a day care centre once a week. There were 16 other attendees and two carers (one senior). The local vicar visited the day centre; he held a communion service and chatted to individuals in the group. Most of the attendees were sitting in a circle. One of the carers was in the kitchen area, not far from those seated. Mrs White asked for a plastic apron. The carer in the kitchen replied in a loud voice, 'What do you want with an apron? You don't want an apron.' The carer ignored any reply from Mrs White and busied herself in the kitchen, thereby making herself unapproachable. One of the other attendees remarked to the vicar, 'They always speak to us like this.'

What do you think about this?
How would you ensure this type of incident did not arise in the future?

This staff member displayed a very poor attitude. She was rude and made it clear that she was unapproachable by being far too busy to be interrupted. This gave Mrs White no opportunity to communicate with the carer as an equal. This incident was witnessed by other patients and staff members, and it was evident that the situation needed to be addressed. It was decided that a clinical practice benchmarking group (see Chapter 1) should be set up so that the issues could be tackled in a professional and non-threatening manner. The agreed patient-focused outcome of the clinical practice benchmark for privacy and dignity is 'Patients benefit from care that is focused upon respect for the individual' (Department of Health, 2003). The benchmark of best practice for factor attitudes and behaviours is 'patients feel that they matter all of the time' (Department of Health, 2003). The members of the benchmarking group comprised of patients, relatives, nursing staff (both qualified and unqualified), other health professionals involved in patient care such as the occupational therapist and physiotherapist, and the vicar. The group decided to convene monthly during the existing goal-planning meeting. Discussion ensued and the group was able to deal with this particular issue by exploring the issue further. A suitable staff training programme was developed as a result of the group, and more effective channels of communication were established. Through the benchmarking group, bad practice was highlighted and challenged, and strategies were put in place so that staff and patients could all benefit from good-quality care and where all those giving and receiving care were equal participants.

This was an example of using the benchmarking process to challenge the poor practice of a junior member of staff. It is not always junior staff, however, that are at fault. Consider Case study 2.2.

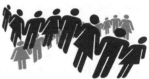

Case Study 2.2

Mr Dudley was an 84-year-old man in a rehabilitation hospital recovering from a short illness. He approached the nursing station where a senior nurse (the deputy ward manager) and the ward clerk were seated.

The nurse was busy with paperwork. Mr Dudley asked to be assisted to the toilet. The nurse replied that she would give assistance in a minute and continued with her writing. A few minutes passed, and so Mr Dudley again approached the nurses' station.

'Yes?' said the nurse, and Mr Dudley repeated his request. Again he was told to wait. Then the nurse shouted across the corridor, 'Oh, don't worry, Mr Dudley. You have got a pad on, so you can always use that.' This incident was overheard by another patient, who reported it to a senior nurse on another ward.

This demonstrates poor nursing practice: the nurse was rude and abrasive, and she made no attempt to assist with Mr Dudley's care or to find someone else to do so. The nurse had no consideration for Mr Dudley; she indicated her paperwork was of far more importance than direct patient care. She treated Mr Dudley without respect. The nurse's attitude and behaviour towards her patient were unacceptable. In fact, she met the worst practice statement of the privacy and dignity benchmark – 'patients experience deliberate negative and offensive attitude and behaviour'. This issue was raised in the benchmarking group and addressed accordingly. The existence of the benchmarking group enabled the group to challenge the poor practice of a senior member of staff in a constructive way.

Sometimes, decisions that put the patient's dignity at risk are made at a strategic level. Consider the following:

To think about

A local primary care trust (PCT) has made a corporate decision that savings are to be made with regard to the continence budget. The decision has been taken to change contractors for incontinence equipment. Predominantly this has affected incontinence pads. Included in this overall decision is that laundry services are to be changed to a different contractor. This decision is having a detrimental effect on patient care at one of the specialist units in the PCT.

What can be done?

Because the patients were suffering as a result of the judgement made at executive level, the frontline staff needed to act on the patients' behalf to challenge and explore the consequences of the decision.

The staff, patients and carers/relatives formed a benchmarking group. It was found that patient care was being compromised by the changes made in supply to laundry provision and with regard to the quality of the continence equipment. Staff were finding frequently that there was an inadequate supply of clean linen. Patients were being treated with no respect or dignity, and priority was being given to cutting expenditure. Action needed to be taken and a compromise to the situation found. The staff were able to challenge the corporate decision by using the continence benchmark together with the documents *Good Practice For Continence Services* (Department of Health, 2000) and *Shifting the Balance of Power* (Department of Health, 2001b). This enabled staff to compile evidence that could then be presented to the executive board in a structured way. As a result of this challenge, a working party was formed that included executives from the PCT, frontline staff, patients and carers. The working party identified that there was a significant lack in staff training and that most of the perceived overspend in the original continence budget was due to inappropriate use of equipment designed to manage continence and to staff having poor assessment skills. Staff training was implemented to cover continence assessment and awareness of managing continence appropriately, such as using the correct pad size. More information was made available for patients and carers. This example illustrates how decisions made at an executive level can be challenged by frontline staff to ensure that patients are treated with dignity and respect.

Compassion and caring

People who work in the care sectors are often seen as compassionate and humane individuals who do not discriminate against others. However, this does not mean that they automatically all treat people fairly. Many people view nurses as dedicated individuals incapable of deliberately harming anyone in their care. But nurses, like other people, may or may not have their own problems. Sometimes these problems can affect how the care worker relates to and treats other people.

To think about

Beverley Allitt, a nurse, was convicted on four counts of murder of children in her care. She was later found to have a rare mental illness, but because she belonged to a 'caring profession' her crimes went undetected for a considerable length of time.

Although Beverley Allitt had been ill for a long time, her illness had not been detected for a variety of reasons. She had qualified as a nurse at a time when newly qualified nurses were not being permanently employed. Consequently, she worked as a temporary nurse and slipped into a permanent job without undergoing an occupational health check and without her references being taken up. Arguably, her illness could have been picked up if procedures had been followed, because investigation showed that all the signs were there from the start. Assumptions were made that Beverley Allitt was fit to practise by virtue of her being a nurse and the expectation was that she was a safe practitioner.

To be compassionate is to understand another's needs. Unfortunately, all too often health professionals fail to do this. Some health professionals even assume that patients are incapable of making their own decisions. Consider Case study 2.3.

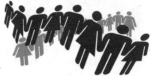

Case Study 2.3

Mrs Mole, an 84-year-old woman, visited her GP's surgery. Mrs Mole's GP was unavailable, and so she saw one of the other doctors in the practice, whom she did not know. Mrs Mole had recently had an operation to relieve the pain of **carpal tunnel syndrome**. The wound healed well, and Mrs Mole appeared to make a good recovery. However, two months later Mrs Mole was experiencing numbness in her hand, which had become swollen and weak. Mrs Mole was due to have the other hand operated on later that month. She was concerned and asked the GP whether she could be referred for a second opinion. She was willing to pay for a private consultation and told the GP this. The GP answered in a condescending, dismissive manner and told Mrs Mole that she could not get a second opinion. The GP gave the impression that Mrs Mole should not have dared to make such a suggestion.

This GP's attitude was very poor. She gave the impression that she was far superior to Mrs Mole and in a position of power. The GP made Mrs Mole feel that she had been wrong to suggest that she could question her treatment or recovery. The GP was wrong: Mrs Mole was perfectly within her rights to request a second opinion.

What are our rights?

We often take our rights for granted and expect them to be met. These rights may include:

+ Caring for oneself as far as this is possible
+ Making choices
+ Making decisions
+ Taking informed risks
+ Having one's cultural, religious, racial, ethnic and sexual identity respected
+ Being supported
+ Having access to information
+ Having one's own space and privacy
+ Being able to complain without fear of victimisation
+ Socialising with whomever you want
+ Being treated with dignity and respect

Carpal tunnel syndrome is compression of inflamed nerves and tendons in the wrist.

> ### To think about
>
> To what extent do people in your care have these rights?
> Do you have more rights than the people you care for?
> Why may it be difficult for some patients to have their rights met?

To be treated with dignity is to be seen as being worthy of respect, and to have privacy is to be seen as being free from intrusion (Department of Health, 2003). Nursing with compassion is about recognising that the patient has a right to make informed decisions and to take risks. It is about not being discriminatory towards patients. Above all, however, it is about understanding the patient and not blaming the patient for being sick.

Privacy

We need to consider how we maintain a patient's privacy wherever the patient is. This includes in acute hospital settings, in the patient's own home and during short outpatient appointments. As a nurse, considering privacy is something you must be aware of at all times. For example, in the patient's home, it is not always acceptable for relatives to be present at every stage of treatment, and the patient's permission for people to be present must always be sought. Exhibit 2.1 shows how nurses can help to maintain a patient's privacy.

> + Patients are protected from unwanted public view
> + Curtains are closed, with no gaps, when personal care is given
> + Staff do not enter a patient's space without first ascertaining permission from the patient
> + Appropriate clothing is available for patients

Exhibit 2.1 Maintaining privacy

The benchmark of best practice is that a patient's care actively promotes their privacy and dignity and protects their modesty (Department of Health, 2003). It is important to remember that for many people mixed-sex wards are embarrassing or culturally unacceptable. Nurses can limit this embarrassment as much as possible by maintaining the patient's privacy at all times.

> ### Recap Questions
>
> 1. What is meant by the term 'personhood'?
> 2. Are all health and social care workers automatically caring and compassionate?
> 3. Why do the attitudes of health and social care workers impact on a patient's care?
> 4. If they do so, in what way?
> 5. Why is privacy an issue for consideration in care?

Culturally sensitive healthcare

Britain is a multicultural country, and this has implications on how healthcare is delivered. It is important that healthcare workers are aware of this multiculture and that they are culturally sensitive when giving care and treatment. Healthcare workers need to familiarise themselves with what is considered acceptable behaviour and then respond accordingly (Timby, 2005). For example, in some cultures it is considered rude to make eye contact or to touch certain areas of the body. It is important that the healthcare worker finds ways of giving transcultural care by learning about cultural beliefs with regard to illness, health and healing. Much of this information is available through NHS healthcare departments, many of which employ staff to deal specifically with cultural and diversity issues. Healthcare staff can also access projects such as the collection of stories recording the experiences of people from the Asian community in Milton Keynes compiled by The Living Archive (www. livingarchive.org.uk) (Quinn, 2001). It is important to remember that even the slightest gesture can be open to misinterpretation, and failing to understand the implications of this can seriously damage the caring/therapeutic relationship (Oxtoby, 2005).

Discrimination

To think about

Have you ever experienced any discrimination?
How did this make you feel?

People suffer from discrimination for all sorts of reasons, including race, ethnicity, gender, age, sexual orientation and disability. Certain groups in society, such as homeless people, unemployed people, lone parents and children, are also at risk of discrimination. Discrimination in treatment occurs when the services received by one patient are different, for example of a lesser quality or shorter duration, from those received by another patient.

In 2001, Age Concern launched its election manifesto *Dignity Security Opportunity* (Lishman, 2001). This was an appeal for older people's rights to be recognised and for strategies and mechanisms to be put in place at a government level in order to meet these rights. The manifesto requested that the government have policies that set older people in the mainstream of society rather than marginalising and discriminating against them. Many of the key issues in *Dignity Security Opportunity* have been included in the NSF Older People (Department of Health, 2001a), such as promoting active health and equal access for all people to services and treatment. How far these issues have been addressed to date is open to interpretation and debate, but some progress has clearly been made.

Recap Questions

1. Why should we as health professionals respect others' personal beliefs?
2. Name six types of discrimination.
3. Which groups of people are more likely to experience discrimination?

Communication

Communication is about imparting information, whether through speaking, writing, transmitting, observing or listening. The ability to communicate effectively is one of the most essential skills a nurse can have. It takes time and effort to develop this skill, but poor communication can have serious consequences that can damage the relationship between the nurse and the patient.

The earlier case studies in this chapter gave examples of poor communication. In Case study 2.1, no attempt was made to explore Mrs White's request and no explanation was given as to why the request was not met. The carer was busy doing other tasks, but this does not excuse her behaviour. In Case study 2.2, Mr Dudley was on the receiving end of inadequate communication. Quality of care depends on the quality of communication used by all those involved in treatment. Poor communication is one of the main reasons for complaints reported to the Health Service Ombudsman (Oxtoby, 2005); this is despite the inclusion of the communication benchmark in the existing *Essence of Care Toolkit* (Department of Health, 2003). The benchmark of best practice for communication is that: 'Patients and carers experience effective communication, sensitive to their individual needs and preferences, that promotes high quality care for the patient' (Department of Health, 2003).

To think about

How can you communicate effectively?
What are some of the skills you may need?

Exhibit 2.2 lists some of the key aspects of good communication (Clarke *et al.*, 2000).

+ Listening and hearing
+ Knowing when and how to start a conversation
+ Taking turns
+ Allowing silences
+ Using non-verbal communication effectively
+ Demonstrating empathy
+ Making eye contact
+ Speaking in a warm tone of voice
+ Using clear speech in everyday language

Exhibit 2.2 Key aspects of communication

These key aspects of communication are all components of active listening.

Physical barriers to communication include:

+ Aphasia
+ Impaired hearing
+ Visual impairment

Aphasia is the loss of ability to speak or understand words. The area of the brain that deals with language may be affected due to certain medical conditions such as stroke and other types of brain injury. When communicating with people with aphasia, certain strategies should be employed, for example using communication aids such as pictures, eliminating all unnecessary noise, giving your message as clearly as possible, allowing the person time to respond, and not making the person feel pressurised or uncomfortable.

There are various degrees of hearing impairment, and different methods of communication are employed depending on the impairment. It is important that the person is not made to feel uncomfortable or pressurised. Simple strategies include eliminating background noise, speaking towards the side of the person where hearing is best, maintaining eye contact, not talking down to or over the person, ensuring that the person can see the face of the person speaking, and finding out whether the person wears a hearing aid and whether it is switched on, working and clean.

For effective communication with people with visual impairment, touch and verbal communication are often important. It is important that health professionals identify themselves and explain what it is they want. It is also important to obtain feedback from the patient and to remember that touch should be used only when appropriate.

Non-verbal communication

As human beings, we are all familiar with non-verbal communication. It is something we are experts in from birth to death, and it is something we practise continually – but we rarely give any thought to the actual mechanics and structure of non-verbal communication until we are faced with a communication problem, either our own or another person's (Perrin and May, 2000). By the age of three years, most children have mastered their own language, in that they can give information and understand the information received. When there is a communication problem, we need to be able to understand how we use different aspects of communication in order to address the issue (Perrin and May, 2000). People communicate by interpreting body and voice, and effective communication involves tone of voice, facial expressions and body language.

Often, challenging behaviour is the result of poor understanding of non-verbal communication. As a society we depend heavily on words, but tied in with this is expressing one thing but meaning another. Therefore, interpretation depends on receiving and understanding the message.

To think about

Mrs Lewis is talking to the occupational therapist. The occupational therapist keeps looking at her watch. Mrs Lewis remarks later to a fellow patient, 'My occupational therapist is very busy with important tasks.'

What message is the occupational therapist really conveying?

There is a mismatch in the message conveyed. Mrs Lewis sees her occupational therapist as being busy and doing important things, but the occupational therapist conveys that Mrs Lewis is of little consequence and of low importance in her busy schedule. The occupational therapist is stating that Mrs Lewis is of low value, and therefore the therapist is controlling and closing down the channels of communication.

Finding out the name that the patient wishes to be known by, and always addressing adults by their title (Dr, Mr, Mrs, Miss) in the first instance and until instructed otherwise by the patient, is important. The use of endearments and nicknames is totally inappropriate, however well meant.

On my last visit, I was informed by a nurse that my grandmother had been a 'naughty girl' because she hadn't eaten her dinner. After the nurse had left, another patient took me aside and informed me that they had placed her food out of reach and simply taken it away later without enquiring whether she needed any assistance, and that this hadn't been the first time.
(Gilchrist, 1999)

Again, such experiences often come down to there being an unequal power balance. The view still persists that patients should be grateful for the care they receive and should behave accordingly, and often health professionals can communicate in paternalistic ways. The document *Shifting the Balance of Power* (Department of Health, 2001b) challenges this preconception and suggests the use of benchmarking and involving patients in their care/treatment plans as a way to address this.

The environment as an aspect of communication

Non-verbal communication is influenced by the person, environment and culture (Perrin and May, 2000). Culture and environment constrain communication, and we have to learn to operate within these constraints. The environment can restrict or enhance communication and it has an effect on a person's consciousness. In the past, older people with mental health problems were often placed in old, run-down wards where little regard was given to a person's individuality. The message given out was: 'You're not worth much. What do you contribute to society? We won't bother to repair your ward or spend any money on it (or you)' (Perrin and May, 2000). Exhibit 2.3 lists the key of for good communication.

Think about Case study 2.1. The care worker disputed Mrs White's need for a plastic apron. Was this really necessary? It is important that people benefit from care that is focused upon the respect of the individual (Department of Health, 2003). Unfortunately, Mrs White was not a recipient of this respect. She was undermined and embarrassed in front of her contemporaries by someone who had power over her. The carer abused her power over Mrs White. The

+ Make eye contact every time you come into contact with the person
+ Try to have a relaxed, friendly expression as you meet the person
+ When you are talking or assisting with care, adopt a calm, unhurried approach
+ Approach the person from the front and at eye level; don't invade the person's personal space without warning
+ Hand objects to the person at eye level and within reaching distance
+ Don't talk over the person to another colleague; always include the person in the conversation
+ Be aware of quiet, less demanding people, who may be starved of human contact; frequent brief contacts can make a difference to a person's wellbeing
+ Validate the person's feelings and experiences whenever you can; try not to get into a disagreement about facts (e.g. if the person says they are hungry, do not dispute this but instead offer a biscuit or a banana)

Exhibit 2.3 Key points of good communication
Adapted from Perrin and May (2000)

carer could easily have spoken to Mrs White in a one-to-one fashion instead of belittling her in front of others. It would appear that the carer was making assumptions about Mrs White's ability to know what she wanted and why. It is important that health professionals interact with patients in a positive rather than a negative way.

Communicating with non-English-speaking patients

Consider Case study 2.4.

Case Study 2.4

Mrs Threadgood was a 70-year-old woman admitted to hospital following a fall. She also had **senile dementia**. She was unable to speak in English and she could now communicate only using German, which was her native tongue. Previously she had been fluent in English. On admission, Mrs Threadgood was very anxious and frightened. The nurses needed to use a hoist to help assist Mrs Threadgood with moving. None of the nurses on the shift had more than a very basic command of the German language.

How would the nurses be able to communicate with Mrs Threadgood?

The nurses used some basic words and phrases to greet Mrs Threadgood. They were able to reassure her with non-verbal communication techniques, such as smiles, touch and the use of body language. The nurses used eye contact so that they could interpret non-verbal cues from Mrs Threadgood. The nurses contacted an interpreter for later episodes of care. In the mean-

Senile means old. **Dementia** is a broad term to describe a range of signs and symptoms of a progressive decline in a person's mental abilities (Tribal Education, 2006a).

time, the nurses acquired some basic German words from friends and relatives. Time was taken to explain the procedure with the use of gestures and pictures, allowing Mrs Threadgood to become familiar with the equipment to be used. The nurses were able to transfer Mrs Threadgood successfully, limiting her anxiety by their relaxed and professional manner.

Most organisations have contact with trained interpreters and people willing to act as emergency translators. It is important when using an interpreter that the health worker looks at the patient rather than the interpreter (Timby, 2005). It is also useful for healthcare workers to develop or obtain translations that describe common procedures, routine care and health promotion (Timby, 2005).

If a patient speaks a small amount of English, the healthcare worker should try to speak slowly but not overly loudly, using simple words and short sentences. This is one situation where the use of direct questions can be of more value than using questions that require long, detailed answers. If the patient appears confused by a certain question, rephrase it rather than simply repeating it. Also, remember to give the person sufficient time for them to respond: be patient (Timby, 2005).

Recap Questions

1. What is good communication?
2. How can you be an effective communicator?
3. What is non-verbal communication?

Protecting individuals from abuse

Protecting patients from abuse is one of the most important aspects of working as a nurse. The NMC states that nurses, midwives and health visitors are responsible for ensuring that they safeguard the interests of their patients at all times. The aim of the NMC is to protect the public, and this includes preventing the abuse of patients (UK Central Council for Nursing, Midwifery and Health Visiting, 1999). Part of the Code of Conduct states that nurses, midwives and health visitors should '... avoid any abuse of your privileged relationship with patients and clients and of the privileged access allowed to their person, property, residence or workplace' (UK Central Council for Nursing, Midwifery and Health Visiting, 1999).

Abuse can happen to any vulnerable individual, whether adult or child. A person is vulnerable whenever their health or usual function is compromised. Vulnerability increases when a person enters unfamiliar surroundings, relationships or situations.

To think about

Have you ever felt vulnerable?
What were the circumstances?

Illness and disability are more likely to lead to a person being vulnerable. Some groups of people are more vulnerable to abuse than others, including people who are physically frail or who have mental health problems, people with learning disabilities, and children of all ages; these groups all require special consideration to protect them from abuse (UK Central Council for Nursing, Midwifery and Health Visiting, 1999).

The term 'vulnerable adult' refers to any person who is aged 18 years or over and who:

+ is unable to take care of themselves;

+ needs care services (e.g. residential, hospital or community) because they have a physical or mental health illness, or sensory or learning disability;

+ is unable to protect themselves against harm or serious exploitation.

Exhibit 2.4 shows some groups of vulnerable people who may be at risk.

+ Children
+ Older people
+ People with visual or hearing impairment
+ People with severe physical illness
+ People with learning disabilities
+ People with mental health problems
+ People with specific illnesses such as human immunodeficiency virus (HIV) or acquired immunodeficiency syndrome (AIDS)
+ People who misuse substances
+ People with specific learning difficulties such as **dyslexia** or **autism**
+ Carers

Exhibit 2.4 Vulnerable people

One of the most vulnerable groups in the UK comprises non-white people with learning disabilities. Often these people do not get the services they need, due mainly to staff not understanding or realising what is required (Department of Health, 2001c).

What is abuse?

To abuse someone is to ill-treat them. As we can see from Exhibit 2.4, abuse can happen to anyone, although certain groups, such as children, are more vulnerable than others. There is no one universal definition of abuse. Warwickshire Vulnerable Adults Committee defines abuse as follows:

> *... the violation of an individual's human and civil rights by another person. It may be physical, psychological or an act of neglect, or occur where a vulnerable person is persuaded to enter into a financial or sexual transaction to which they have not, or*

Dyslexia is a disorder affecting reading, writing and comprehension.

Autism is a disorder that results in a lack of communication and response.

cannot consent. Abuse may be perpetrated as the result of deliberate intent, negligence or ignorance.
(**Warwickshire Vulnerable Adults Committee, 2004**)

Action on Elder Abuse (www.elderabuse.org) defines abuse as follows:

A single or repeated act or lack of appropriate action occurring within any relationship where there is an expectation of trust which causes harm or distress to an older person.
(**Action on Elder Abuse, 2002**)

The aim of Action on Elder Abuse is to prevent abuse in old age by raising awareness, encouraging with education and training, promoting research and collecting and disseminating information.

Prevention of abuse

The most effective way of identifying and preventing abuse is through thorough assessment. The use of an evidence-based assessment framework such as the Single Assessment (Department of Health, 2001) or the Framework for the Assessment of Children in Need and their Families (Department of Health, 2000) will help the nurse to identify who is most at risk of being abused (see also Chapter 1). There are seven main types of abuse (Exhibit 2.5), and it is important to understand that a vulnerable individual may experience more than one type of abuse at the same time.

+ Physical abuse
+ Psychological, including verbal, abuse
+ Financial abuse
+ Sexual abuse
+ Neglect abuse
+ Institutional abuse
+ Discrimination

Exhibit 2.5 Types of abuse

Remember that any act of abuse may also constitute a criminal act.

Physical abuse

Physical abuse is the injury or mistreatment of an individual. The abuse may be intentional or accidental. Physical abuse includes overuse and inappropriate use of medication, such as using medication as a form of restraint, and underuse of medication, such as leaving a patient in pain rather than giving appropriate pain relief. Physical abuse can be inflicted directly, for example with a weapon, fist or foot, or an everyday item such as a rolling pin. Physical abuse also includes handling patients in a rough manner, the poor application of manual handling techniques, and the use of unreasonable physical restraint (UK Central Council for Nursing, Midwifery and Health Visiting, 1999). Injuries may be concealed if the abuser does not want others to know what is happening. Health professionals need to take action if they notice bruising and marks in unusual places.

If a patient has suffered physical abuse, there may be injuries or wounds, even if they are not immediately apparent. The person may be more reluctant than usual to move about, or may not wish to have any physical contact, however gentle. Signs of physical abuse include the following:

+ Cuts, bruises, scratches and burns

+ Injuries that do not match the explanation given for them

+ Injuries and wounds in concealed places

+ Injuries in naturally protected areas, such as the underarm

+ Untreated injuries, for example evidence of old fractures that have healed without medical intervention

+ Repeated injuries

+ Underuse or overuse of medication

Psychological abuse

Psychological abuse is any form of verbal or non-verbal behaviour that demonstrates disrespect for the patient and could be construed as being emotionally or psychologically damaging (UK Central Council for Nursing, Midwifery and Health Visiting, 1999). Action on Elder Abuse (2002) has reported that this is the most commonly reported form of abuse. Psychological abuse may take the form of threatening, bullying, shouting, blaming, mocking, isolating or blackmailing. It includes any remark made to a person that may be conceived as being demeaning, disrespectful, humiliating, intimidating, racist, sexist, homophobic, ageist or blasphemous. It also includes making sarcastic remarks, speaking in a condescending tone of voice and behaving in an overfamiliar manner (UK Central Council for Nursing, Midwifery and Health Visiting, 1999). Consider Case study 2.5.

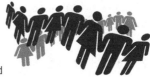

Case Study 2.5

Mrs Johns was a 62-year-old woman with diabetes. She had previously had a below-knee amputation, from which she had made a reasonable recovery. She was re-admitted to hospital for a second below-knee amputation. Mrs Johns was making a fairly good recovery and displayed a positive attitude; she was friendly and chatty with the ward staff. A rehabilitation support worker was overheard saying, in a jovial manner, 'Come on, stumpy.' When challenged by another staff member about the use of this language, the rehabilitation worker replied that she felt Mrs Johns did not mind and it was helping her to accept her condition.

How would you address this situation?
Is this use of language helping Mrs Johns?

Clearly the rehabilitation support worker's behaviour is unacceptable and the situation needs to be addressed. Using any form of nickname is unprofessional and not acceptable. In this particular case, it was clear that the rehabilitation support worker had believed that Mrs Johns did not mind, but it was obvious to any onlooker that Mrs Johns was unhappy and uncomfortable with the label she had been given.

Other forms of psychological abuse include deliberately ignoring a patient and depriving a patient of basic needs and pleasures. In Case study 2.1, Mrs White was denied her request and was subsequently ignored.

To think about

A friend's behaviour changes. She has recently started a new job and has told you that she feels quite afraid of her manager. Over time, she seems to have become far more withdrawn and depressed, and she seems uncommunicative. You suspect there is a serious problem.

What are you going to do?

It may be that your friend is experiencing bullying at work – this is a form of psychological abuse. The signs of psychological abuse are shown in Exhibit 2.6.

+ Withdrawal
+ Depression
+ Agitation
+ Anxiety
+ Anxiousness
+ Isolation

Exhibit 2.6 Signs that may make you suspect psychological abuse

With psychological abuse, there is often an unexpected or unexplained change in the person's behaviour. This may be manifested in various ways, such as the person becoming withdrawn, refusing to eat, not taking an interest in their physical appearance or being reluctant to plan for the future.

Financial abuse

Financial abuse is the second most commonly reported form of abuse against older people (Action on Elder Abuse, 2002). Theft, fraud, forgery and embezzlement can all be forms of financial abuse. Such abuse does not always involve large sums of money; often, it takes the form of small amounts of money, but on a regular basis and over a long period of time. Often, abusers justify their actions because they believe they are entitled to a reward for their 'care' of an individual or they think that the abused person does not need the money. Consider Case study 2.6.

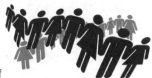

Case Study 2.6

Mrs Jacobs was recently bereaved. Since the bereavement, she had been living with her daughter. She was in receipt of Attendance Allowance, which she had been giving to her daughter. Mrs Jacobs had been living at her daughter's house for the past six months but now felt she would like to return to her own home. Mrs Jacobs' daughter was furious when informed of this intention and became abusive towards her mother. On investigation, it was found that Mrs Jacobs' daughter believed she had a right to receive Mrs Jacobs' Attendance Allowance.

Was she correct in this thinking?

This assumption was wrong. Attendance Allowance is paid to the person who needs care and is not for the carer. The allowance is for the person receiving the care, and it is up to this person to decide how the allowance should be spent. Exhibit 2.7 shows some of the signs of financial abuse.

+ Lack of money for basic necessities, such as food, heating and clothes, despite there being evidence that there is adequate income
+ Unexplained withdrawals or changes in the pattern of withdrawals from the individual's bank account
+ Reluctance on the part of the carer, family, friends or the person in control of the money to pay for food, clothes or furniture
+ A person's inability to explain what is happening to their own income
+ Unexplained or suspicious disappearance of possessions, bank statements or other documents

Exhibit 2.7 Signs that may make you suspect financial abuse

Financial abuse is a contentious subject. We live in a society that actively encourages financial abuse of some of our most vulnerable members of society. Consider the environment in which some people live, particularly those in care settings, and think about whether adequate provision is made for them. Some people are placed in settings that cost them a lot of money but are not necessarily suited to their needs. It can be argued that this is both financial abuse and abuse through neglect.

Sexual abuse

Sexual abuse is any sexual activity that takes place without consent, for example touching a patient inappropriately or engaging in sexual discussions that have no relevance to the patient's care (UK Central Council for Nursing, Midwifery and Health Visiting, 1999). Sexual abuse includes:

+ Sexual assault
+ Rape
+ Sexual harassment
+ Use of inappropriate sexual language

Sexual abuse is an emotive subject, and often people who have been abused find it difficult to talk about their experiences. The person who is told about the abuse may also find the subject difficult to deal with. We discuss how to disclose these issues later in the chapter. Exhibit 2.8 lists some of the signs that may point to sexual abuse.

+ Pain, itching or injury in the genital, anal or abdominal area
+ Torn, stained or bloody underclothing
+ Bite marks and bruises on the breasts, neck or face
+ Venereal disease or recurrent bouts of cystitis
+ Unexplained problems with catheters
+ Difficulty in sitting and walking due to discomfort in the genital area

Exhibit 2.8 Signs that may make you suspect sexual abuse

Neglect

Neglect occurs when there is a lack of care, whereby a person does not fulfil their responsibility of care and allows a vulnerable individual to suffer. Neglect is failing to provide basic necessities such as food, clothing, hygiene and mental stimulation. This can occur in a variety of settings, such as the patient's own home, residential care homes and hospitals. Consider Case study 2.7.

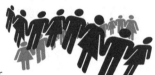

Case Study 2.7

Mrs Barber had recently returned home following admission to hospital for the treatment of an acute infection. She shared her house with her nephew and his wife. She was visited by the health visitor. The health visitor was greeted by the nephew's wife and shown to Mrs Barber's room. The room was in the basement of the house. Mrs Barber was in an armchair in the middle of the room; her bed was by the wall. The bed was unmade and the sheets appeared soiled. There was very little light in the room, but the health visitor could see that the carpet was threadbare; this was surprising, as the rest of the house appeared to be in good condition. The health visitor noticed that Mrs Barber's stockings were around her feet; she asked Mrs Barber whether she would like some help to pull them up, and Mrs Barber agreed. Mrs Barber's legs were cold, red and swollen, her stockings and slippers were soaked with urine. The health visitor washed Mrs Barber's feet; she was unable to find any clean stockings or slippers, so she covered her with a blanket. The health visitor then spoke to Mrs Barber's nephew and his wife; they were reluctant to get any help and they expressed that they felt Mrs Barber was cared for adequately. The health visitor had no alternative but to contact social services, as she believed Mrs Barber was being neglected.

Neglect can be intentional or caused through ignorance. Whatever the cause, it is essential that action is taken to protect the person who is being neglected. Exhibit 2.9 lists some of the signs that may indicate that a person is being neglected.

+ Deterioration in appearance or personal hygiene
+ Unhygienic and unsafe environment
+ Rashes, sores, lesions and ulcers
+ Unexplained weight loss
+ Inadequate food, drink or medical care
+ Lack of social stimulation

Exhibit 2.9 Signs that may make you suspect neglect

Discrimination

Discrimination is a form of abuse caused by a focus on differences. A person may be discriminated against due to their ethnicity, culture, religion, politics, gender, age, sexual orientation or disability (physical or mental), among other things.

Institutional abuse

The types of abuse that can be found in care settings are the same as described in the sections above. However, institutional abuse is more than an individual behaving abusively; rather, it is abuse in an organisational context, such that the delivery of care and the care offered are not adequate for the recipients of that care. Institutional abuse is often a result of poor systems being in place and the misuse of power. Consider Case study 2.8.

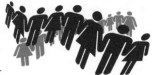

Case Study 2.8

The nurses and care assistants who work overnight in a nursing home ensure that all the patients are clean and dry, any incontinence is dealt with and the residents are ready to eat their breakfast at 8am when the day-shift staff arrive. It is expected that all residents will be ready for breakfast, regardless of how many acutely ill residents there are, and whether they require more or less help. In other words, it is an inflexible task and the end result must always be that the residents are ready when the day-shift staff start work. Therefore, sometimes the night-shift nurses start getting the patients up at 5am in order to make sure that they comply with these instructions.

Case study 2.8 shows that there is a total disregard for the residents' and patients' desires. Do they really want to get up at that time? The patients and residents are being subjected to institutional abuse.

Indicators of abuse

We have considered the different types of abuse. Now we look at the indicators of abuse.

Indicators that may lead you to suspect abuse

+ Difficulty in gaining access to the individual concerned
+ Never being able to speak to the person on their own, because a relative, friend or carer is always there
+ Requests for help to many different agencies or frequent transfers from one agency to another
+ Repeated visits to the GP or accident and emergency department
+ Refusal of support services
+ History of unexplained or repeated falls or injuries

Signs of possible abuse

+ Multiple bruising and/or finger marks
+ Injuries not consistent with their explanations
+ Deterioration of health for no apparent reason
+ Loss of weight
+ Inappropriate or soiled clothing
+ Withdrawal and mood changes
+ Unexplained shortage of money

Location of abuse

+ The person's own home
+ Day centre or day hospital
+ Care home
+ Hospital
+ Sheltered accommodation

Who abuses?

+ Relative (spouse, child, parent)
+ Partner
+ Friend
+ Volunteer
+ Neighbour
+ Another resident or service user
+ Social or health worker

Action on Elder Abuse has reported that family members who are main carers are less likely to be the perpetrators of abuse. Perpetrators are more likely to be family members who are not directly responsible for the victim's care (Action on Elder Abuse, 2002).

To think about

A health worker visits an older woman living in her daughter's home. The woman is in bed and refuses to get up, despite there being no medical reason to do this. The daughter provides all care to her mother. The mother tells the health worker that her daughter is obliged to care for her: the mother feels she has suffered because of her daughter and it is now time to make her daughter suffer.

Who is the abuser?
Who is the abused?

Factors that may lead to abuse

+ Social isolation

+ Poor-quality long-term relationships

+ Pattern of family violence

+ Dependency (of the abuser)

+ Mental illness/substance misuse of the abuser

Preventing abuse

In order to prevent abuse, professional boundaries must be maintained. If any abuse takes place, then it must be acknowledged openly by practitioners and employers. All care workplaces have policies and procedures in place in order to protect both patients and practitioners. Such policies must be adhered to. The implementation of these policies ensures that patients and practitioners are safe. Staff need support both from each other and from their employers; clinical supervision and reflective practice can help as can performance reviews and education and training. Early intervention is crucial if practitioners are thought to be experiencing emotional difficulties or demonstrating impaired emotional functions in their patient relationships (UK Central Council for Nursing, Midwifery and Health Visiting, 1999). Consider Case study 2.9.

Case Study 2.9

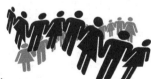

Natalie was a staff nurse employed in a nursing home. She was caring for 12 patients and was assisted by a healthcare assistant. The healthcare assistant noticed that Natalie was getting cross with an elderly patient who was reluctant to eat. The healthcare assistant reported Natalie for bullying. As a result, Natalie was suspended while the incident was investigated.

On investigation, it was found that Natalie was under a lot of pressure and was caring for a lot of highly dependent patients. She was anxious that the patient in the case study would eat properly and was overzealous in her persuasion for him to do so. In this case, it may have been better if the healthcare assistant had offered to take over from Natalie in assisting the patient to eat and then to report the matter to a senior person so that the incident could be investigated.

It is important that any staff member who reports an incident of abuse is supported. Managers who deal with complaints need details of the offender and whether there are any witnesses. The nature of the incident, the date, time and place where the abuse occurred, the circumstances surrounding the events and the action taken, including support given to other staff members, must all be noted (UK Central Council for Nursing, Midwifery and Health Visiting, 1999).

Mechanisms such as criminal record and registration checks help to ensure that the staff employed have no previous records of being abusive.

What to do if you are concerned

+ Always talk to the abused person privately and discreetly.
+ Listen to the abused person, try not to ask leading questions, and be sensitive to the individual.
+ Find out what the person wants to do.
+ Do not challenge the abuser.
+ Follow your employer's policy.
+ Discuss the situation with your line manager or another senior manager as soon as possible.
+ If you are unsure what to do, contact a helpline, such as Victim Support, ChildLine or Action on Elder Abuse.
+ Reassure the abused person.
+ Seek medical treatment for the abused person.
+ Keep accurate records.

Confidentiality

Within an organisation, 'confidentiality' cannot mean absolute secrecy. There may be situations in which someone tells you something that you should pass on, for your, their own or other people's protection. 'Confidentiality' in this situation means that the information disclosed will be treated with discretion within your organisation. It is important that sensitive information is made known only to those with whom it has to be shared so that appropriate decisions can be made and support offered. This is sometimes referred to as the 'need to know'.

Every organisation has a policy detailing information-sharing and with whom information can be shared. However, regardless of policy, suspected abuse must always be disclosed.

Managing disclosure

Don't:

+ Take it lightly or make a joke of it
+ Dismiss or disbelieve what you have been told
+ Change the subject because you feel uncomfortable with it
+ Ignore what has been said
+ Make assumptions
+ Say things such as:
  • 'This can't be true!'
  • 'I don't believe it!'
  • 'That is ridiculous!'

Do:

+ Listen, taking notice of body language
+ Take it seriously - even if it does not make sense to you at first
+ Try not to show you are shocked
+ Explain about confidentiality (e.g. that you are obliged to disclose in order to ensure the safety of the person or other people)
+ Clarify the victim's version, but do not put words into their mouth
+ Report to your line manager
+ Always remember it is not for you to handle this alone

Training in the prevention, recognition and management of abuse is essential for all health-care workers. Abuse of older people is particularly important, as we live in a society with an increasingly older population. Greater dependency and vulnerability often come with age, which in turn can lead to these people being at greater risk of abuse (Smith and Duffy, 2003).

Recap Questions

1. Who might be classed as a vulnerable individual?
2. What are the different types of abuse?
3. What should you do if you suspect abuse is taking place?

Summary

In this chapter we have looked at why it is necessary to give care that actively promotes dignity. How successful we are as carers is dependent on this. By promoting dignity, we can influence the patient-nurse relationship. To treat the patient with respect is to recognise that the patient is an equal partner in care. It shows that we value that person and recognise that the person has rights and beliefs. Personal beliefs and preferences are vitally important to each person and contribute to their individuality. Being aware of these (both your own and the patient's) is an important part of the interaction between a health professional and a patient. The success of each episode of patient care is influenced significantly by how a patient feels they are regarded by staff.

We have considered how the benchmarking process can be used to challenge the bad practice of colleagues in a supportive and non-threatening way. The benchmarking process can also be used to challenge more strategic decisions that affect the patient's dignity.

As nurses, it is important that we understand the meaning of compassion and how this impinges on the care we give. We need to treat our patients as people rather than 'strokes', 'heart attacks' or 'diseases'. We need to care for the whole person, not just the disease.

Western culture depends on and demands high levels of articulate communication, whether spoken or written. If these skills are taken away we are faced with someone who has lost these skills, we often flounder and fail to communicate effectively (Perrin and May, 2005).

We have looked at how it is important to find out the name the patient wishes to be addressed by. We have also seen how, as health professionals, we should not assume that we can call someone by their first name or nickname.

This chapter has considered dignity, privacy and respect in context with cultural aware-ness and communication. Abuse and vulnerability to abuse have been explored. It is important to remember that abuse can take many forms and that it is not always something that you see immediately.

Key Points

1. Treating a patient with dignity and respect are arguably the most important aspects of patient care. This behaviour should underpin every contact that healthcare workers have with patients.

2. Understanding and applying the concept of personhood to every patient ensures that people are treated as individuals.

3. Communication is not only about how you speak to patients. It is about your ability to listen and to interpret visual cues and the environment in which you care for people.

4. It is essential that nurses can protect their patients from all forms of abuse. They can do this only if they recognise the different forms that abuse can take.

Points for debate

Now that you have come to the end of this chapter here are a few points that you may wish to think about when you are in practice. You may wish to discuss these with your work col-leagues or fellow students.

A group of people say they 'look good for their age' (Figure 2.1). What does that mean?

You should always call someone by the first name, whatever their age. It is more friendly and it puts people at ease.

People who come to live in this country should learn to speak English and adopt British customs and values.

Figure 2.1 NHS ageism poster

Links to Other Chapters

Chapter 1   What is caring?
Chapter 5   Nutrition
Chapter 6   Fluid balance and continence care
Chapter 8   Pressure ulcers
Chapter 9   Rehabilitation and self-care

Further reading

Department of Health (2001) *Learning Difficulties and Ethnicity*. London: The Stationery Office.

Gilchrist, C (1999) *Turning Your Back on Us*. London: Age Concern.

Mencap (2007) *Death by Indifference*. London: Mencap.

References

Action on Elder Abuse (2002) *Time for Action on Elder Abuse*. London: Action on Elder Abuse.

Clark, C, Bolton, J and Scurfield, M (2000) *Mental Health and the Care of the Older Person*. London: Emap.

Department of Health (2000) *Good Practice in Continence Services*. London: The Stationery Office.

Department of Health (2001a) *National Service Framework for Older People*. London: The Stationery Office.

Department of Health (2001b) *Shifting the Balance of Power*. London: The Stationery Office.

Department of Health (2001c) *Learning Difficulties and Ethnicity*. London: The Stationery Office.

Department of Health (2003) *Essence of Care: Patient-Focused Benchmarks for Clinical Governance*. London: The Stationery Office.

Gilchrist, C (1999) *Turning Your Back on Us*. London: Age Concern.

Health Advisory Service 2000 (1999) *Not Because They Are Old*. London: Health Advisory Service 2000.

Kitwood, T (1997) *Dementia Reconsidered: The Person Comes First*. Buckingham: Open University Press.

Lishman, G (2001) *Dignity Security Opportunity*. London: Age Concern.

Oxtoby, K (2005) Reaching a clear understanding. *Nursing Times* **101**, 20.

Perrin, T and May, H (2000) *Wellbeing in Dementia: An Occupational Approach for Therapists and Carers*. London: Churchill Livingstone.

Quinn, S (2001) *Meri Kahani My Story: Asian Voices*. Milton Keynes: Living Archive Press.

Smith, R and Duffy, A (2003) *Responding to Elder Abuse*. London: Community and District Nursing Association.

Timby, B (2005) *Fundamental Nursing Skills and Concepts*. Philadelphia, PA: Lippincott Williams & Wilkins.

Tribal Education (2006a) *Certificate in Dementia Awareness*. York: Network Publishing.

Tribal Education (2006b) *Palliative Care*. York: Network Publishing.

UK Central Council for Nursing, Midwifery and Health Visiting (1999) *Practitioner-Client Relationships and the Prevention of Abuse*. London: UK Central Council for Nursing, Midwifery and Health Visiting.

Warwickshire Vulnerable Adults Committee (2004) *No Secrets: Briefing Session Papers*. Coventry: Warwickshire County Council.

Chapter 3
Basic observations

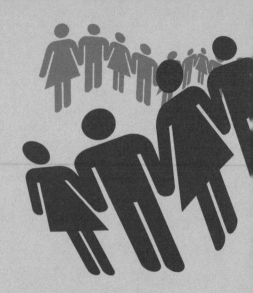

Case Study

Nurse James comes on duty and decides to go round and check all the patients in her care. She discovers Mrs Pywell slumped in her chair. This was surprising as she had just been informed from the nursing report that Mrs Pywell was 'doing well'.

Initial assessment of the situation revealed that Mrs Pywell's colour was pale and ashen and unlike her usual colour. Her breathing was shallow and slightly laboured. She was conscious but looked dehydrated. Nurse James spoke to Mrs Pywell and asked her whether she was alright. Mrs Pywell responded in a feeble voice, indicating she felt 'awful'. She was put back into bed immediately and moved to a single room. Her vital signs were subsequently recorded. Her radial pulse was 116 per minute (significantly faster than normal) and felt weak and thready. Her respirations were 32 per minute and she was having difficulty with breathing, using her abdominal and accessory chest muscles to help her. Her axilla temperature was raised to 39.5 °C.

The doctor was informed immediately of these observations. Meanwhile, Nurse James tried to make Mrs Pywell more comfortable by placing a fan close by to help lower her temperature. Her vital signs were monitored half-hourly until the doctor arrived. Mrs Pywell was given fluids to help correct her dehydrated state. Once the doctor arrived and examined Mrs Pywell, a chest X-ray was subsequently ordered, which revealed that she had a purulent chest infection that had developed into pneumonia. If Mrs Pywell's vital signs had been recorded more frequently (they had not been recorded for several days), her condition would have been detected sooner and she probably would not have developed pneumonia.

Introduction

Consider the above scenario and reflect on your reactions to it. It demonstrates how important it is to regularly monitor a patient's vital signs as this can tell us a great deal about the patient's condition. As indicated in the case study, Mrs Pywell's vital signs should have been recorded more frequently – they had not been monitored for several days. Her chest infection would then have been detected and treated much sooner, and Mrs Pywell would not have developed pneumonia, which can have serious consequences, such as **septicaemia**, severe respiratory distress and even respiratory arrest (the patient stops breathing). This chapter considers the importance of monitoring and recording basic observations of pulse, respirations and temperature. The reasons why basic observations are made and the abnormalities that can be detected are discussed. The procedure for carrying out these observations is outlined.

LEARNING OBJECTIVES

By the end of this chapter you will be able to:

1. Recognise the importance of accurately recording patients' vital signs: pulse, respirations and temperature

2. Indicate the reasons why the pulse, respirations and temperature are recorded, and identify the normal ranges for each vital sign

3. Explain the associated anatomy and physiology related to the pulse, respirations and temperature

4. Describe the factors that can affect the pulse, respirations and temperature, and identify the different sites used to assess the pulse and temperature

5. Discuss the characteristics/aspects that should be included when assessing the pulse, respirations and temperature

6. Outline the procedure for recording the pulse, respirations and temperature

The importance of basic observations

Performing a comprehensive physiological assessment entails the taking and recording of patients' observations and is usually one of the first procedures nursing students and healthcare assistants learn. Although the taking and recording of 'routine' or basic observations of temperature, pulse and respiration (TPR) can sometimes be viewed as a mundane aspect of nursing care, it is vital that these tasks are carried out in order to detect changes that can indicate a deterioration in a patient's condition. Basic observations are sometimes referred to as 'nursing observations', as essentially they are undertaken by trained nurses, student nurses or healthcare assistants deemed competent to perform them. Basic observations must be documented accurately in order to give a clear picture of a patient's progress. The most common reasons for recording basic observations are outlined in Exhibit 3.1.

Septicaemia is a severe systemic infection of the blood that can spread and infect different parts of the body.

> + To obtain baseline physiological information on admission or before medical intervention
> + For early identification of deterioration in a patient's condition
> + To assist in the diagnosis
> + To assess the effects of treatment

Exhibit 3.1 Common reasons for recording basic observations

The nursing management of patients is becoming increasingly complex, and ward staff are more and more likely to care for acutely ill patients (Docherty, 2002). The formation of **critical care outreach teams** has resulted in more acutely ill patients being cared for in the ward environment. As a consequence, many NHS trusts are now focusing more on the importance of basic observations and have introduced tools for monitoring patients. These help to identify patients whose condition may be likely to deteriorate based on the information obtained from their observations. Educational packages are produced by some trusts to train staff in assessing and managing acutely ill patients (Trim, 2004).

To think about

When you are next in practice, identify those patients whose basic observations are being recorded frequently. Look at the recordings and ask one of your trained colleagues to help you interpret the readings.

Did you identify any patients who you thought needed to have their basic observations checked more frequently?

If so, why did they need to be monitored more frequently?

Research has identified deficiencies in the ability of both nurses and doctors to carry out and interpret basic observations. The main causes, as outlined by Trim (2004), include:

+ Changes in the pre-registration curriculum
+ The growth of high dependency and critical care units (Department of Health, 2000; Docherty, 2002)
+ Perception that making observations is a mundane task (Kenward *et al.*, 2001)
+ Unpredictable and busy workloads (O'Neill and Le Grove, 2003)
+ Inadequate documentation (Alcock *et al.*, 2002)
+ Insufficient knowledge of associated physiology (Casey, 2001; Stoneham *et al.*, 1994)
+ Misinterpretation and mismanagement of patients (McQuillan *et al.*, 1998)

A **critical care outreach team** is a team of healthcare professionals who liaise between a critical care unit and an associated ward.

When you are carrying out basic observations on a patient what information do you need to enable you to analyse/interpret your findings? You may wish to discuss this with a trained work colleague.

In order to be able to undertake and analyse any basic observation, nurses need knowledge of the following:

+ The associated anatomy and physiology
+ The meaning of the measurements
+ How all the measurements are interrelated

In some cases, cardiorespiratory arrest or admission to a critical care unit can be prevented if a patient's vital signs are recorded accurately (Alcock *et al.*, 2002). For example, McQuillan *et al.* (1998) found that half of the admissions to intensive care units could have been prevented by closer and more accurate monitoring of vital signs (TPR) in the preceding hours and days. Up to 84% of patients show warning signs in the hours before respiratory or cardiac arrest (Schein *et al.*, 1990; Smith and Wood, 1998). Sadly, according to some research, survival to discharge following a cardiac arrest on a general ward is only 5% (Smith and Wood, 1998). Therefore, one of the important aims of routine or basic observations should be to reduce the incidence of avoidable cardiac and respiratory arrest (Kenward *et al.*, 2001).

To summarise, basic observations are essential in providing information on which many clinical decisions are based. They help to ensure patients' continued recovery and assist in identifying when any nursing or medical intervention is required. Consequently, they need to be recorded accurately, and any changes from the norm need to be recognised and reported to the necessary health professional as soon as possible so that action can be taken.

In the following sections we consider each of the vital signs, focusing on the associated anatomy and physiology, factors that can affect the signs, what we assess when monitoring the vital signs, and finally how to carry out the procedure.

Pulse

The pulse is one of the most important of all the basic observations. It is taken to assist with the assessment of a patient's cardiovascular function - in other words, how well the heart and circulation are functioning. If taken and recorded correctly the pulse can give a wealth of information about a patient's condition. The pulse is recorded for three main reasons:

+ To obtain information on the heart rate, pattern of beats and strength of pulse
+ To determine the individual's pulse on admission - that is, to establish a baseline with which further readings can be compared
+ To monitor changes in the pulse

Anatomy and physiology

The pulse is created by a series of pressure waves within the arteries, caused by contraction of the left ventricle. These pressure waves result in expansion of the walls of the arteries, which forms the pulse. Thus, each pulse wave corresponds to each contraction of the left ventricle (called the heart beat). The pulse can be felt at the point where an artery crosses a bone near the surface of the body. Generally the pulse wave represents the volume output, which is the amount of blood that enters the arteries with each ventricular contraction. The pulse is strongest in arteries close to the heart and becomes progressively weaker as it passes through the arterial system, disappearing in the capillaries. Compliance of the arter-ies relates to their ability to contract and expand. Sometimes arteries lose their elasticity, as can happen in old age, resulting in greater pressure being required to pump the blood around the arteries. Cardiac output is the volume of blood pumped into the arteries by the heart and equates to the stroke volume (SV) multiplied by the heart rate (HR) per minute. For example:

$$\text{Cardiac output} = 65 \text{ mL (SV)} \times 70 \text{ beats (HR)} = 4.55 \text{ L/min}$$

When an adult is resting the heart pumps about 5 L of blood per minute. The pulse reflects the heart beat and therefore equates to the rate of the ventricular contraction of the heart. However, in some types of cardiovascular disease, the heart beat and the pulse may differ. In this instance, the heart may produce very weak or small pulse waves that cannot be detected in a peripheral pulse far away from the heart. Examples of where a peripheral pulse can be detected are the foot, wrist and neck. The apical pulse is a central pulse located at the apex of the heart (Figure 3.1).

Factors affecting the pulse

The pulse rate is expressed in beats per minute (bpm). According to Kozier *et al.* (2004), the pulse rate can be influenced by a number of factors:

+ *Age*: the pulse rate decreases gradually with age (Table 3.1).
+ *Gender*: the average male pulse rate is slightly lower than the average female pulse after puberty.
+ *Exercise*: the pulse increases with activity. It is worth noting that the rate of increase in a professional athlete is often less than that in the average person due to the athlete's greater cardiac size, strength and efficiency. Therefore, an athlete's pulse does not increase as much during activity and is usually slower at rest (i.e. naturally bradycardic) compared with the average person.

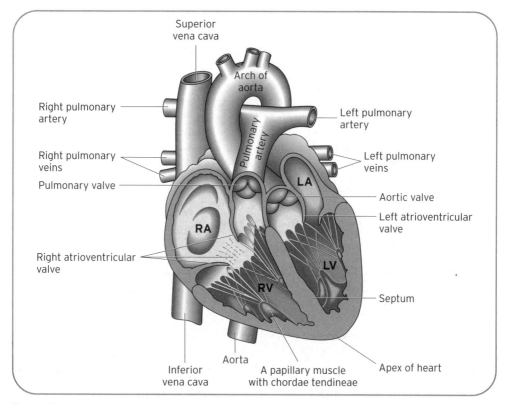

Figure 3.1 Internal structure of the heart
Source: Ross and Wilson (1981)

+ *Fever*: the pulse rate increases (i) in response to the lowered blood pressure that results from **peripheral vasodilation** associated with elevated body temperature and (ii) because of the increased metabolic rate.

+ *Medication*: some medications decrease and others increase the pulse rate. For example, cardiotonics (e.g. digitalis preparations) decrease the heart rate, whereas epinephrine (adrenaline) increases it.

+ *Hypovolaemia (reduced blood volume)*: loss of blood from the vascular system normally increases pulse rate. In adults, the loss of circulatory volume results in an adjustment of the heart rate to increase blood pressure as the body compensates for the lost blood volume. Adults can usually lose up to 10% of their normal circulating volume without adverse effects.

+ *Stress*: in response to everyday intensive stress, sympathetic nervous stimulation increases the overall activity of the heart. Stress increases both the rate and the force of the heart beat. Fear, anxiety and the perception of pain stimulate the sympathetic system.

Peripheral vasodilation is an increase of the lumen of blood vessels supplying the peripheries of the body.

+ *Position changes*: when a person is sitting or standing, blood usually pools in the lower blood vessels of the venous system due to the effects of gravity. This pooling results in a transient decrease in the venous blood return to the heart and a subsequent reduction in blood pressure and increase in heart rate.

+ *Pathology*: certain diseases such as some heart conditions and conditions that impair oxygenation can alter the pulse rate, particularly when the person is at rest.

Table 3.1 Normal heart rate in different age groups

Age group	Beats per minute
<3 months	100-180
3-24 months	80-150
2-10 years	70-110
10-16 years	55-90
Adult	60-100

Recording the pulse

The pulse can be felt with the fingers as a wave-like sensation over arteries close to the surface. The most common site to feel/palpate the pulse is at the wrist, in line with the thumb; this is called the radial pulse. Other pulses that are recorded are (Figure 3.2):

+ *Ulnar*: at the wrist, in line with the small finger (this is rarely used)
+ *Carotid*: to the front of the neck
+ *Brachial*: in the join of the elbow (usually used for recording blood pressure)
+ *Femoral*: in the groin
+ *Popliteal*: behind the knee
+ *Apical*: a stethoscope is used to listen to the heart rate
+ *Dorsalis pedis*: on the top part of the foot, between the big toe and leg
+ *Posterior tibial*: just to the lower side of the inner aspect of the ankle

To think about

Try to find as many of these pulse sites as you can, either on yourself or on a colleague, and try to work out when and in what conditions they would be used to detect and record the pulse.

You have probably discovered that some of the pulse sites are easier to detect than others mainly due to their accessibility. The radial pulse tends to be used the most in adults, mainly because it is easy to locate and is non-invasive. The radial pulse can also be used in older children (age 10-16 years), whereas, the brachial pulse tends to be used in younger children (age 2-10 years). For very young children (under age 2 years), the apical pulse (see Figure 3.1 for

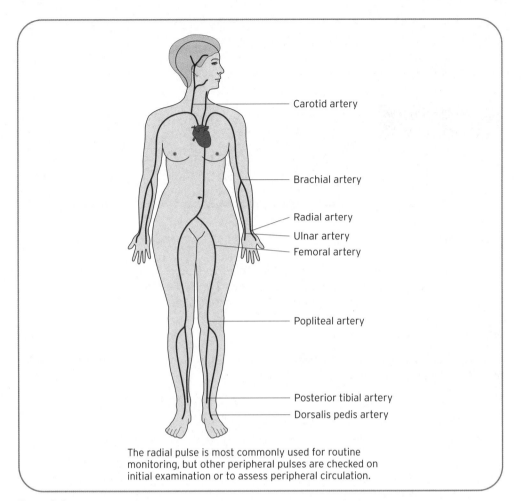

The radial pulse is most commonly used for routine monitoring, but other peripheral pulses are checked on initial examination or to assess peripheral circulation.

Figure 3.2 Pulse sites
Source: © Clinical Skills Ltd

the location of the apex of the heart) is often recorded by listening through a stethoscope, as children of this age are often reluctant to keep still for a whole minute and the radial and brachial pulses can be more difficult to detect. The normal heart rates in relation to age are shown in Table 3.1.

The carotid and femoral pulses are used in emergency situations where a person has collapsed and may be having a cardiac or respiratory arrest. In this case, the peripheral pulses are difficult to detect. The pulse in the lower legs (popliteal, dorsalis pedis and posterior tibial) tends to be used to assess circulation in conditions where the blood flow to the limbs, particularly the lower limbs, is impaired.

Due to increases in nursing workload and improvements in technology, most patients nowadays have their pulse assessed using a machine such as a pulse oximeter. However, such devices are unable to detect pulse irregularities or strength as they tend to provide only an average value. Furthermore, the reading could be inaccurate and provide no information about heart rhythm (Trim, 2004). Therefore, to ensure a comprehensive assessment the pulse should be taken manually for 30 or 60 seconds, depending on the rate and any rhythm irregularity. For example, if the pulse is slow and irregular it should be taken for 60 seconds; otherwise it should be counted for 30 seconds and then the reading doubled. If the pulse rate is irregular, Docherty (2002) recommends that an apical and a radial pulse check be conducted in order to identify any deficit; both readings should then be recorded.

To think about

When assessing the pulse what are you actually measuring? What information do you need to carry out an accurate assessment of the pulse? You may like to discuss this with your work colleagues.

Assessment

We now consider how to assess the pulse. The full procedure of how to take and record the pulse is outlined later, but first you need to understand what you are looking for. This includes the rate, rhythm and amplitude (strength) of the pulse.

Rate

This is measured as the number of beats per minute. The rate varies with age (see Table 3.1) and the patient's condition:

+ The normal/resting pulse rate in a healthy person is about 65-80 bpm.
+ Tachycardia means a rapid resting pulse - over 100 bpm.
+ Bradycardia means a slow resting pulse - under 60 bpm (Tortora and Grabowski, 2002).

The causes of each of these abnormalities are outlined in Exhibit 3.2. You may find that you do not have sufficient knowledge of some of the conditions indicated in Exhibit 3.2 and need to study further in these areas or discuss them with your clinical colleagues or mentors.

Tachycardia
+ Hypovolaemia: due to blood loss or peripheral vasodilation, and characterised by a fall in blood pressure and compensatory increase in pulse to maintain cardiac output
+ Stress or anxiety
+ Pyrexia (for definition, see section on temperature later in this chapter)
+ Pain
+ Sympathetic stimulation (O'Neill and Le Grove, 2003)
+ Respiratory distress because oxygen demand is increased
+ Arrhythmias, such as atrial fibrillation. Rapid tachycardias of more than 140 bpm may compromise ventricular filling, with a subsequent drop in blood pressure (Docherty, 2002)

Bradycardia

+ Vasovagal stimulation following suctioning via a tracheostomy. If sustained, hypotension may follow the drop in heart rate and the patient may lose consciousness.
+ Ischaemic heart disease: reduced blood flow to the vessels supplying the heart
+ Cardiac medication, for example beta-blockers
+ Hypovolaemia
+ Hypoxia

Exhibit 3.2 Causes of tachycardia and bradycardia
Adapted from Trim (2004)

Rhythm

Rhythm is the sequence of beats, including the intervals between the beats. In good health, the heart rhythm is regular (Pritchard and Mallett, 2001). Disturbance to the heart's normal **conduction system** can cause irregular heart rhythms, for example **atrial fibrillation**. A pulse with an irregular rhythm is called a dysrhythmia or arrhythmia.

Amplitude

The pulse amplitude is the strength/volume of the pulse and reflects the elasticity of the arterial wall (Pritchard and Mallett, 2001). Normally the pulse volume is the same for each beat, but it can range from absent, weak and thready to bounding. If the pulse feels weak and thready, this may indicate hypovolaemia (reduction in blood volume). A strong and bounding pulse can indicate infection (Trim, 2004). With experience, detecting the amplitude/strength of the pulse becomes easier.

Procedure

A watch or clock with a second hand is needed to carry out the following procedure of assessing the pulse:

1. Explain the procedure to the patient – even if he or she is unconscious.
2. The patient should be resting, either lying down or sitting.
3. Adhere to local infection control policies and ensure appropriate handwashing before touching the patient.
4. Ensure the patient is comfortable and relaxed, as anxiety and distress can alter the pulse rate. Allow the patient time to rest after physical activity, emotional upset or smoking.
5. Note whether the patient is taking any medication that might alter the pulse rate.

The **conduction system** is made up of a network of specialised cells and pathways that control the electrical activity and contraction of the heart.

Atrial fibrillation is loss of the conduction ability of the heart's atria, with consequent impairment of the heart rhythm.

6. Generally the radial pulse is recorded, as it is easily accessible (Figure 3.3). Place your first and second fingers along the artery. Apply light pressure until you feel the pulse. Do not use your thumb, as this has a pulse that could be mistaken for the patient's pulse.

7. Looking at a watch or clock with a second hand, count the number of beats for either 30 seconds if the pulse is regular (and then double the number) or 60 seconds if the pulse is irregular (Nicol *et al.*, 2004).

8. While counting, assess the pulse rhythm and volume/strength of the pulse.

9. Ensure the patient is comfortable after the procedure.

10. Document the rate and any rhythm and amplitude/strength abnormalities. Any irregular pulse must be recorded.

11. Report any changes from the previous reading to the nurse in charge.

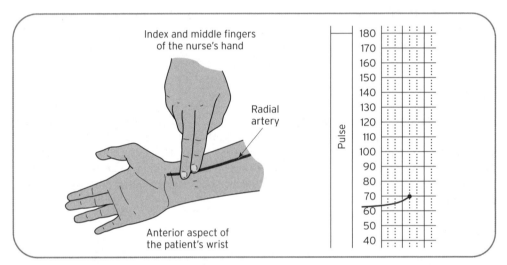

Figure 3.3 Correct position for taking the radial pulse
Source: Baillie (2005)

Frequency of recordings

When and how often the pulse is recorded depends on the patient's condition and illness. For example, a patient who is critically ill or in a coronary care/intensive care unit has their pulse and heart rate recorded continuously via a cardiac monitor. The pulse is taken on admission to hospital in order to establish a baseline with which further recordings can be compared. The pulse may also be monitored on a daily basis or every four hours if the patient has an infection.

It is important to remember that the pulse is not assessed in isolation. When recording the pulse, other aspects of the patient should be noted, such as the colour of the lips, nail beds and mucous membranes. Look for signs of cyanosis (lack of oxygen) indicated by a bluish colour to the skin and nail beds, and observe the patient's skin for pallor, flushing, sweating or coldness. Such signs may be indicative of cardiovascular or respiratory disease. Assessment of the pulse is part of an integrated assessment that includes respiration, temperature and, if required, blood pressure.

Now you have read about why, where and how the pulse is taken, consider Case studies 3.1 and 3.2.

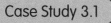

Case Study 3.1

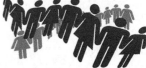

Mrs Ford is a 50-year-old woman admitted to your ward for major abdominal surgery. She is to have a bowel resection with the possibility of a **stoma**. You are asked to assess her vital signs as part of the admission process. She appears to be very anxious. You count her pulse and it is 115 bpm.

What would you do next?

There are several things you can do, but it is necessary to prioritise. First, do you think Mrs Ford's pulse rate is acceptable? We know that a normal resting pulse for an adult is between 70 and 80 bpm, so this woman's pulse is raised. We need to identify why it is raised. Look back to the factors that can affect the pulse. The information on Mrs Ford states that she appears anxious, and this could be causing her pulse rate to increase. As far as we know, she has not been exercising, which would also raise the pulse rate. Patients are often very anxious when they first arrive on a ward, especially if they are going to have surgery, as Mrs Ford is. For this reason, it is a good idea to allow the patient to settle in before going through the admission process and recording their vital signs.

Second, it is worth checking that Mrs Ford does not have a medical condition that could account for her raised pulse. Tachycardia can occur in some heart conditions (see Exhibit 3.2). This information may be obtained directly from the patient or from the patient's medical records. However, consider whether it is necessary to inform the patient that their pulse rate is raised, as this could increase their anxiety further.

Once you have tried to establish why Mrs Ford's pulse rate is raised, inform the nurse in charge and then return later and record the pulse again, giving the patient time to calm down and become familiar with her new surroundings. If you find that the pulse is still raised, then inform the nurse in charge promptly.

Case Study 3.2

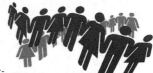

Mr Urovitch is a 35-year-old man who works as a physical trainer at the local gym. He has been admitted to the accident and emergency unit following a knee injury sustained during a gym session. You are asked to obtain personal details from the patient and to assess and record his vital signs. His temperature and respirations are fine but his pulse is only 48 bpm. He appears to be well, apart from his painful knee.

What would you do next?

A **stoma** is a refashioning of a portion of the bowel to form an external opening on to the skin's abdominal surface.

Mr Urovitch's pulse rate appears to be below the average rate for an adult. His other vital signs are within normal range, so why do you think he has a bradycardia/slow pulse? If we consider some of the factors that can affect the pulse, you may recall that athletic people tend to have a lower pulse following exercise and also at rest. These people are described as being naturally bradycardic. You need to ask Mr Urovitch what his pulse rate normally is and then record this information on his basic observation flow chart and his admission form for future reference. You also need to inform the nurse in charge of the patient's naturally low pulse rate.

This section has considered the pulse and factors that can affect it. We have highlighted how and where to take the pulse, what you are looking for when carrying out this procedure and what the measurement means.

Recap Questions

1. What are the main reasons for recording the pulse?
2. What factors can affect the pulse rate?
3. When taking the pulse, what three factors are assessed and what do they measure?

Respirations

Taking note of a patient's respiratory rate provides essential information about the patient's cardiopulmonary state. By recording the respiratory rate, you can determine whether the patient is taking in enough oxygen to ensure the lungs and circulatory system can function correctly. Respirations are recorded for the following reasons:

+ To establish a baseline on admission
+ To monitor a patient with breathing problems
+ To assist in the diagnosis of disease
+ To evaluate a patient's response to medication that affects the respiratory system

Revision

Before reading the next section, you need to revise the anatomy and physiology of the respiratory system, with particular reference to internal and external respiration.

Anatomy and physiology

Respiration is the act of breathing. It involves two processes: external respiration and internal respiration. External respiration involves the interchange of oxygen and carbon dioxide between the **alveoli** in the lungs and blood in the pulmonary circulation. Internal respiration takes place throughout the body and involves the interchange of these same gases between the circulating blood and the cells of the body tissues. Figure 3.4 shows the human respiratory system.

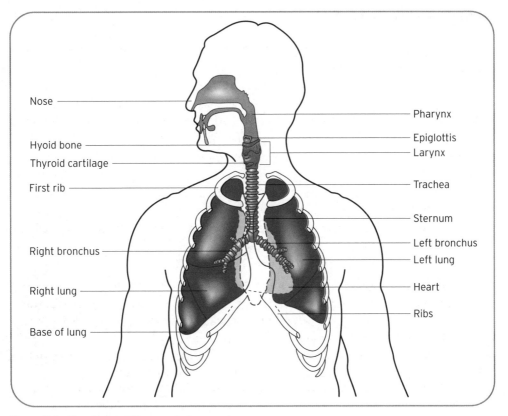

Figure 3.4 Structures of the respiratory system
Source: Ross and Wilson (1981)

The function of the respiratory system is to supply adequate oxygen to the tissues and remove carbon dioxide. This is achieved with the inspiration and expiration of air. Ventilation is the term used to describe the movement of air in and out of the lungs. One respiration is made up of one inspiration (breathing air in) and one expiration (breathing air out). Thus, when we count the respiratory rate, this equates to one inspiration and one expiration.

To think about

Your breathing rate can alter frequently throughout the day. Try monitoring your own respiratory rate and make a note of the factors that affected your breathing.

Alveoli are microscopic air sacs in the lungs.

Factors affecting respiration

Several factors influence the respiratory rate, many of which are similar to those that affect the pulse rate (Kozier *et al.*, 2004):

+ *Exercise*: the respiratory rate increases during exercise (the increase in metabolism means more oxygen is required). Long-term fitness training has an effect on the respiratory rate, such that it takes longer for the rate to increase in a fit person compared with an unfit person.

+ *Stress/anxiety*: the sympathetic nervous system stimulates the respiratory system by increasing the respiratory rate to prepare the body for action – the so-called 'fight or flight' syndrome.

+ *Environmental temperature*: a rise in external temperature increases the respiratory rate, while a drop in external temperature reduces the respiratory rate.

+ *Lowered oxygen concentration*: this occurs at high altitudes. The respiratory rate increase in an attempt to get more oxygen into the body.

+ *Medication*: certain medications, such as morphine, can lower the respiratory rate.

+ *Sleep*: the respiratory rate falls to its lowest normal level in deep sleep.

+ *Increased intracranial pressure*: any condition that causes an increase in **intracranial pressure**, such as a head injury, can lead to a fall in the respiratory rate, due to pressure on the respiratory control centre in the brain.

+ *Age*: the normal respiratory rate alters with age. The rate is highest in young babies and decreases over the age of 12 years (Table 3.2). Babies and children up to 6 years of age rely predominantly on **diaphragmatic** movement to breathe. This leads to greater abdominal movements during normal breathing in children compared with adults. The nurse needs to be aware of this when assessing respirations on babies and young children.

Table 3.2 Normal range for respiratory rates in children

Age (years)	Respiratory rate (breaths per minute)
<1 year	25-35
1-5 years	20-30
5-12 years	20-25
>12 years	15-25

Adapted from Hull and Johnson (1999)

Intracranial pressure is the pressure within the skull bone.

The **diaphragm** forms a large dome-shaped partition that separates the thoracic cavity from the abdominal cavity. It consists partly of muscle and partly of membrane. It is a very important muscle of respiration, contracting during inspiration to enlarge the thoracic cavity and relaxing during expiration.

Recording respirations

Respirations are counted by observing the rise and fall of the chest wall. One rise and one fall equate to one respiration. Chest movements should be bilateral, equal and symmetrical (Ahern and Philpot, 2002). This means both sides of the chest should rise and fall and take in equal amounts of air per breath. There is usually a short pause between inspiration and expiration (Bennett, 2003).

To think about

Try counting your friend's or a colleague's respirations for one minute. Did you find it difficult? If so, in what way was it difficult? When you are next in practice, have a look at the patients' observation charts. Is the respiratory rate always recorded; if not, why not?

Discuss your findings with your friends or work colleagues.

Recording respirations seems like a simple procedure to carry out, but unfortunately respiratory activity is often a neglected basic observation: some authors claim that respiratory rates are rarely recorded (Kenward et al., 2001). One study found that 55% of patients had not had their respiratory rate recorded for at least 8 hours; in the same timeframe, 36% had not had their oxygen saturation recorded (Trim, 2004). As a consequence of such findings, Kenward et al. (2001) devised an education programme to address some of the issues. They had found before the implementation of their programme that nurses were consistently not recording the respiratory rate, even on patients who were clearly unwell and who deteriorated to cardiac or respiratory arrest. Concerns about such patients' shortness of breath had been documented by doctors and nurses, and yet the patients' respiratory rates had not been monitored or recorded on the patients' charts.

Why was the respiratory rate recorded so infrequently? Kenward and colleagues (2001) claimed this was due to an 'over-reliance on monitoring technology', in particular pulse oximetry used to measure ventilation function. We discuss oximetry later in this chapter. The monitors used on wards are not configured to record respiratory rate; thus, it is important to remember that monitors and pulse oximetry provides only limited information about a patient's condition and the respiratory rate still needs to be counted and recorded.

Assessment

To undertake a full assessment of respirations, the rate, depth and pattern of breathing should be monitored. The process of how to count and record a patient's respiratory rate is discussed later. First, it is important to understand what you are looking for when carrying out this procedure.

Rate

The respiration rate is measured in breaths per minute. As with the pulse, the respiratory rate varies with age (see Table 3.2). The normal range for a healthy adult is between 12 and 20 breaths per minute (Blows, 2001). The rate should be regular, with an equal pause between each breath. Normal respiration (eupnoea) is quiet, rhythmic and effortless. The pattern of breathing should also be noted. Any irregularities, such as those outlined below, should be noted and reported to the nurse in charge. When observing respiratory rate, the colour of the patient's lips should be noted. The lips may be cyanosed (blue) or discoloured if the patient has respiratory problems. Cyanosis can also be observed in the nail beds, the tip of the nose and the ear lobes (Woodrow, 2000). The following abnormalities may be detected:

+ *Tachypnoea*: quick and shallow breaths above 20 per minute
+ *Bradypnoea*: abnormal slow rate, with fewer than 12 breaths per minute
+ *Apnoea*: absence of breathing for several seconds, leading to respiratory arrest
+ *Dyspnoea*: difficulty in breathing – the patient may gasp for air and use accessory muscles of respiration, such as the neck and abdominal muscles. The patient may mouth-breathe as there is less resistance to airflow through the mouth than the nose, but this can lead to drying of the oral mucosa; therefore, good oral hygiene is essential
+ *Orthopnoea*: the person is unable to breathe unless they are upright
+ *Cheyne-Stokes respiration*: breathing is very slow, shallow and laboured, with periods of apnoea (lasting 15–20 seconds) – often seen in dying patients
+ *Hyperventilation*: the patient breathes rapidly due to a physical or psychological cause such as pain or panic. During hyperventilation, the carbon dioxide levels reduce in the blood, causing tingling and numbness in the hands. There may also be dizziness and fainting as a result of the low carbon dioxide levels, leading to cerebral **vasoconstriction.** This can often lead to further distress. In adults, more than 20 breaths per minute is considered to be moderate hyperventilation. More than 30 breaths per minute is considered severe hyperventilation (Mallett and Dougherty, 2000).
+ *Hypoventilation*: a decrease in respirations, leading to reduced oxygen content in the body (hypoxia) and particularly in the blood (hypoxaemia).

It is worth noting that a sleeping adult's respiration can fall to fewer than 10 breaths per minute. Therefore, other vital signs also need to be recorded in order to accurately assess the patient's condition.

It is quite common for infants to have an irregular breathing pattern, with alternating short (a few seconds) periods of rapid breathing and apnoea.

The causes and symptoms of some of the above abnormalities are given in more detail in Exhibit 3.3.

Depth

This refers to the depth/volume of the breath and is known as the tidal volume (TV). The TV is usually about 500 mL per breath (Blows, 2001). The TV increases during strenuous exercise to as much as 1500 mL per breath and also varies according to gender and weight. For example, a woman weighing 50 kg may have a TV of 500 mL, and a man weighing 75 kg may have a TV of 700 mL. Prolonged, rapid, deep ventilation is called hyperventilation. This can occur in a person having an anxiety attack. When the breathing becomes slow and shallow, this is called hypoventilation and results in inadequate gaseous exchange. It is important to note whether both sides of the chest are expanding equally on inspiration. If the person has sustained a chest injury, then the lung on the affected side could have deflated. Similarly, if the lung has collapsed as a consequence of infection, this leads to absence of lung expansion on the affected side. Furthermore, lung collapse can lead to **pneumothorax**, an emergency situation that requires urgent medical intervention.

Bradypnoea

Causes

+ Respiratory depression
+ Fatigue
+ Hypothermia
+ Central nervous system depression
+ Opiates

Symptoms

+ Rate below 12 breaths per minute
+ Inadequate oxygen saturation/hypoxia
+ Cyanosis
+ Drowsiness

Tachypnoea

Causes

+ Anxiety, stress
+ Hypercapnia (raised CO_2 levels)

Symptoms

+ Rate above 20 breaths per minute
+ Inadequate oxygen saturations

Cheyne-Stokes respiration

Causes

+ Left ventricular failure
+ Cerebral injury
+ Imminent death

Symptoms

+ Irregular rate and depth of reading
+ Periods of apnoea (no breathing)

Exhibit 3.3 Causes and symptoms of altered breathing
Source: Bennett (2003); Stevenson (2004)

Rhythm

This refers to the regularity of the inspirations and the expirations. Normally the respirations are evenly spaced. The rhythm may be regular or irregular. An infant's respiratory rate may be less regular than an adult's (Kozier *et al.*, 2004). Abnormalities in respiratory rhythm are usually associated with lung disease. For example, rapid, shallow breathing can indicate restrictive lung disease in which airflow is impeded and which may lead to respiratory failure.

Respiratory quality or character

This denotes any aspects of breathing that are different from normal, effortless breathing, including the effort a patient must exert to breathe and the sound of the breathing. Breathing should require no noticeable effort, but some patients are able to breathe only with decided effort. This is known as laboured breathing.

The sound of breathing is also significant. Normal breathing is silent. Abnormal sounds such as a wheeze (a high-pitched sound that occurs when air is forced through narrowed respiratory air passages) can be heard by the nurse when counting respirations. A person with asthma may present with a wheeze heard on expiration. This is caused by air being forced

Vasoconstriction is a narrowing of the blood vessels, with a consequent reduction in blood flow.

Pneumothorax is air in the pleural cavity.

through narrow airways due to asthma-induced **bronchoconstriction**. When the larynx (voice box) is obstructed, a harsh, high-pitched sound known as a stridor can be detected. Crackles – high-pitched rustles – can be heard at the end of expiration and may indicate **pulmonary oedema**. If crackles are heard during both inspiration and expiration, then the person may have **pneumonia**. Generally, all of the abnormalities outlined above are associated with problems related to the respiratory system.

> ### To think about
>
> When you are in practice, have you seen patients having their oxygen saturation levels recorded? Why were they being recorded?
>
> You may wish to discuss your findings with a work colleague.

Oxygen saturation

The amount of **haemoglobin** in arterial blood that is saturated with oxygen can be measured indirectly through pulse oximetry. This procedure is simple and non-invasive. A probe is placed on the finger, ear lobe, toe or nasal septum. The probe is two-sided and transmits red and infrared light through the tissue. The light that is not absorbed by the tissue is detected by sensors and is indicative of the percentage of oxyhaemoglobin present in capillaries. Normal values are 95–98%. A value of 90% or less can be indicative of respiratory failure leading to inadequate amounts of oxygen reaching the body cells. However, if the patient has **chronic obstructive pulmonary disease**, their usual oxygen saturations may be 85–90%; this should be considered when recording oxygen saturation.

Oxygen saturation is usually recorded when a patient has a respiratory condition that results in less oxygen being inspired and there is less oxygen circulating in the blood.

The nurse should not rely on oxygen saturation alone when assessing a patient's respirations, as it gives information only on how much oxygen is carried by haemoglobin, and not how much haemoglobin there is or how well the oxygen is being delivered (Casey, 2001). To obtain a more accurate assessment of a patient's oxygen levels, the doctor will request blood gas analysis to be carried out. This blood test measures the amount of oxygen and carbon dioxide in the blood, allowing the doctor to determine the levels of these gases and what treatment to prescribe.

> **Bronchoconstriction** is narrowing of the bronchioles/air passages and a subsequent reduction in airflow.
>
> **Pulmonary oedema** is fluid in the lungs.
>
> **Pneumonia** is inflammation of the alveoli in the lungs.
>
> **Haemoglobin** is the oxygen-carrying component of red blood cells.
>
> **Chronic obstructive pulmonary disease** is a chronic respiratory disease in which the air passages narrow as a result of chronic inflammation. It causes debilitating breathlessness and affects daily activities.

Procedure

This section outlines the steps involved when recording a person's respiratory rate. A watch or clock with a second hand is needed to carry out this procedure:

1. Explain the procedure to the patient - even if he or she is unconscious.

2. Adhere to local infection control policies and ensure appropriate handwashing before touching the patient.

3. Ensure the patient is comfortable and as relaxed as possible, because stress and anxiety can increase the respiratory rate.

4. It is a good idea to monitor and record respirations immediately after taking the pulse. This can give a more accurate recording, as the patient is unaware that you are observing their breathing. If the patient is aware that you are assessing their respirations they may become conscious of their breathing and the rate may change.

5. Observe the rise and fall of the chest (inspiration and expiration). This counts as one breath. In infants and young children, abdominal movements should also be observed. This can be achieved by placing the hand gently against the lower part of the chest to feel any movement. A stethoscope can be placed on the infant's chest to record the respiratory rate if you are unable to monitor the rate because the infant is wriggling a lot.

6. Count the respirations for a full minute to give an accurate recording. If the respirations are regular, even and unlaboured, it is acceptable to count the respirations for half a minute and then multiply by two in order to calculate the rate for one minute. However, if the respirations are abnormal, they should be counted for a full minute. In infants under 1 year of age, whose breathing is often irregular, the respirations must be counted for a full minute in order to ensure that an accurate picture is obtained.

7. Note the pattern of breathing and the depth of the breaths.

8. Document the findings on the patient's observation chart.

9. Report any changes from the previous recording to the nurse in charge. If you are unsure during any stage of the assessment, seek guidance from a qualified nurse who is more experienced in carrying out this procedure.

10. Ensure the patient is comfortable after the procedure.

When carrying out this procedure, the following points should be considered:

+ Is the patient breathing through the mouth?

+ Are the patient's lips pursing on expiration?

+ Are the abdominal muscles being used?

+ Are the nostrils flared? In children and babies, this is indicative of acute respiratory distress (Field, 2000)

Frequency of recordings

The frequency at which the respiratory rate should be recorded depends on the patient's condition. Recordings should always be taken on admission in order for the hospital to establish a baseline with which further recordings can be compared. Respirations are usually recorded when the pulse is taken, so the frequency is likely to be daily, four-hourly or continuously if the patient is critically ill.

Now you have read about assessing a patient's respirations, consider Case studies 3.3 and 3.4.

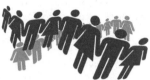

Case Study 3.3

Mr Thomas is a 76-year-old man admitted to your ward with a chest infection. He has chronic obstructive airways disease. He is a heavy smoker and lives alone in a ground-floor flat. His daughter visits him regularly in hospital and is trying to get him to stop smoking with help from the nursing staff. You are doing routine observations on Mr Thomas and find his oxygen saturation to be 88%. His respiratory rate is 36 breaths per minute and he is struggling for breath, although he tells you he is feeling okay. He is apyrexial, although his pulse is 125 bpm. On recording the respirations on his chart, you note that Mr Thomas's respiratory rate has not been recorded since his admission yesterday.

What would you do next?

There are several things you need to do, including reporting your findings immediately to the nurse in charge, even though you note that Mr Thomas's oxygen saturation was 88% at the last recording taken on the previous day. He has very low oxygen levels, which need to be dealt with urgently. It is essential to count his respiratory rate for one minute and record clearly on the chart and also notify the nurse in charge of the result. As Mr Thomas has a chest infection, it is imperative that his respirations are recorded at least every four hours, particularly in view of him having chronic obstructive airways disease. As this patient's oxygen saturation is only 88%, there is inadequate oxygen supplying the body cells. However, patients with chronic obstructive pulmonary disease can have usual oxygen saturations of 85–90%, and this needs to be considered in Mr Thomas's case. The nurse in charge should notify the doctor straight away, who may decide to administer oxygen to Mr Thomas in order to raise his oxygen levels, but this needs to be monitored carefully because of his pulmonary condition. Blood gas analysis may also be ordered to provide an accurate assessment of both Mr Thomas's oxygen and carbon dioxide levels.

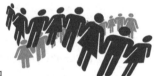

Case Study 3.4

Nicholas is a 7-year-old boy admitted to the ward following an acute asthmatic attack at school. He was in the middle of sitting his SATs test when the attack occurred. On arrival on the ward, he is still very breathless and looks pale and anxious. He is given oxygen therapy by the trained nurse. You are asked to record Nicholas's vital signs every 15 minutes and to keep an eye on his oxygen saturation levels. He is accompanied by his father, who is also very distressed. You record Nicholas's vital signs: his respiratory rate is 38 breaths per minute, his pulse is 140 bpm and his temperature is 30 °C.

What would you do next?

You should report your findings to the nurse in charge and then continue to monitor Nicholas's vital signs, paying particular attention to his respiratory rate. You would also need to assess his skin colour and nail beds for signs of cyanosis, which would indicate that his oxygen levels are falling. He will be seen by the doctor as soon as possible, who will prescribe medication to improve Nicholas's breathing, probably along with oxygen therapy. Oxygen saturation levels may need to be monitored as a consequence. Nicholas's father needs to be reassured and informed of his son's condition and subsequent treatment. This is the responsibility of the trained nurse, but you can give support by offering tea and kind words.

This section has considered the vital sign of respirations. The associated anatomy and physiology have been outlined briefly. Factors that can affect respiration have been considered, along with the aspects of respiration that need to be monitored when assessing and recording a patient's respiratory rate. Breathing abnormalities have been highlighted, and the procedure for observing and recording respirations has been described.

Recap Questions

1. What are the main reasons why respirations are recorded?
2. What factors can affect the respiratory rate?
3. To carry out a full assessment of respirations, what aspects of breathing need to be noted?
4. What abnormalities in breathing can be detected?

Temperature

Recording body temperature can provide vital information about a patient's physiological state. A rise or fall in temperature indicates changes in bodily function – for example, a rise in temperature can indicate infection. The temperature is recorded for a number of reasons:

+ To establish a baseline
+ For intraoperative (during an operation) and postoperative (after an operation) monitoring
+ To monitor response to infection
+ To monitor patients with hypothermia or hyperthermia (we discuss these terms later in the chapter)
+ To monitor critically ill patients
+ To monitor patients receiving blood transfusions

Revision

Before reading the next section, you need to revise the temperature regulatory system, with particular reference to the difference between core and surface temperature and how the body gains and loses heat in order to maintain a constant body temperature.

Anatomy and physiology

Body temperature reflects the balance between heat gain and heat loss from the body and is measured in units called degrees. There are two kinds of body temperature: core temperature and surface temperature. The core temperature is the temperature of the deep tissues of the body, such as in the abdominal, cranial and pelvic cavities. The core temperature remains relatively constant in a healthy person, within the range of 36–37.6 °C. The surface temperature refers to the temperature of the skin, subcutaneous tissue and fat. The surface temperature fluctuates in response to the environment; consequently, there can be a great variation in recordings between core temperature and surface body temperature (Figure 3.5).

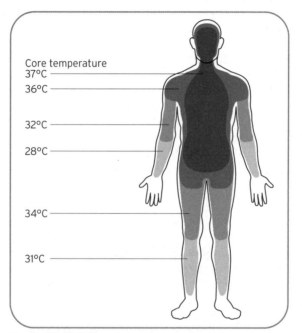

Figure 3.5 Variations in body temperature from the core to the surface
Source: © Clinical Skills Ltd

The body temperature needs to remain constant in order to produce an environment that enables normal cellular activity to occur. To ensure a constant temperature is maintained, the body maintains a balance between heat loss and heat production. The body produces heat as a by-product of metabolism, which can be affected by a number of factors.

To think about

What factors do you think might affect how the body produces heat? Consider what would happen to you if you were sitting in a cold room with no clothes to keep you warm.

Heat production

The body's production of heat can be affected by the following:

+ *The basal metabolic rate (BMR)*: this is the rate at which energy is used to maintain essential activities such as breathing. The metabolic rate tends to decrease with age.

+ *Muscle activity*: any sort of muscle activity, including shivering, increases the metabolic rate and thus produces more body heat.

+ *Thyroxine*: increased levels of **thyroxine** increase the cellular metabolism throughout the body, therefore producing more body heat.

+ *Adrenaline*: when released in the body, this hormone causes an immediate increase in cellular metabolism in many body tissues, in particular in the liver and muscle cells.

To think about

How is heat lost from the body?
What happens to you on a very hot day or following strenuous exercise?

Heat loss

Heat can be lost from the body through the following four main processes:

+ *Radiation*: this is the transfer of heat, mostly in the form of infrared rays, from a warm body to relatively colder objects without any contact. For example, radiation accounts for 60% of the heat lost by a nude person standing in a room at normal room temperature.

+ *Conduction*: this is the transfer of heat from the hotter to the cooler of two objects in contact with each other. For example a dog lying on a floor with a temperature lower than that of the dog's body will lose heat to the floor by conduction. Similarly, a person sitting in a cold room will lose heat to the floor and chair. Conduction normally accounts for minimal heat loss, as it is dependent on the temperature difference and the amount and duration of the contact.

+ *Convection*: this is the movement of air resulting from local pockets of warm air being replaced by cooler air, and vice versa. These air movements speed up loss of heat by radiation and evaporation.

+ *Evaporation*: when liquid changes to a vapour, the process is accompanied by cooling. Evaporation of water from the surface of the body depends on various factors, such as temperature, humidity and air currents. Evaporation can account for a substantial loss of heat. For example, a person in a room of temperature 21 °C can lose 25% of heat by evaporation.

Thyroxine is a hormone produced by the thyroid gland to regulate the BMR.

The processes involved in heat production and heat loss are summarised in Table 3.3.

Table 3.3 Factors contributing to heat production and heat loss

Heat production	Heat loss
Basal (body) metabolism	Radiation
Muscular activity (shivering)	Conduction/convection
Thyroxine and adrenaline (stimulating effects on metabolic rate)	Evaporation (vaporisation)

Adapted from Kozier et al. (2004)

Body temperature is regulated by the hypothalamus in the brain. Specialised heat detectors/sensors are able to pick up changes in body temperature. When these sensors detect heat, they send out signals intended to reduce the body temperature by decreasing heat production and increasing heat loss. These signals initiate sweating and **peripheral vasodilation**, and the person perspires more and becomes flushed. Conversely, when the detectors sense cold, the sensors send out signals to increase heat production and decrease heat loss, thus initiating **peripheral vasoconstriction** and shivering in an attempt to conserve heat. This whole process is called thermoregulation.

Factors affecting body temperature

As with other basic observations several factors can affect body temperature, including:

+ *Age*: the thermoregulatory mechanisms of newborns and infants are not fully developed. Therefore, such patients are greatly influenced by the environmental temperature and must be protected from extreme changes. Children's body temperatures are more variable than those of adults, and young children tend to have a slightly higher body temperature due to their increased metabolic processes producing more heat. This tends to last until puberty. Older people tend to have a slightly lower body temperature, as the metabolic rate falls after the age of 50 years. People over 75 years of age are at risk of developing hypothermia for a variety of reasons, including inadequate diet, loss of subcutaneous fat, lack of activity and reduced thermoregulatory efficiency.

+ *Diurnal variations (circadian rhythms)*: body temperature normally varies by as much as 1.0 °C throughout the day between the early morning and the late afternoon. The point of highest body temperature is usually reached between 8pm and midnight, and the lowest point is reached during sleep between 4am and 6am.

+ *Exercise*: hard work and strenuous exercise can raise the temperature to as high as 38.3–40 °C.

Peripheral vasodilation is an increase in diameter of the lumen of blood vessels supplying the peripheries of the body.

Peripheral vasoconstriction is a decrease in diameter of the lumen of blood vessels supplying the peripheries of the body.

+ *Metabolic rate*: metabolic processes in the body produce heat. A person with a high metabolic rate, which could be associated with an overactive thyroid gland, may have a higher than normal body temperature. Conversely, underactivity of the thyroid gland leads to a low metabolic rate, which may cause a low body temperature.

+ *Hormones*: women usually experience more hormone fluctuations than men. In women, progesterone secretion at the time of ovulation raises the body temperature by about 0.3-0.6 °C.

+ *Stress*: stimulation of the sympathetic nervous system can increase production of adrenaline and noradrenaline, which in turn increases metabolic activity and heat production. Nurses should be aware of this and appreciate that a highly stressed or anxious patient could have a raised temperature for that reason.

+ *Environment*: extremes in temperature can affect a person's temperature regulatory system.

+ *Drugs*: sedatives and narcotic drugs such as morphine may reduce the perception of cold and the appropriate bodily responses to cold. Alcohol also has a similar effect by impairing shivering and causing vasodilation, which leads to a fall in body temperature.

+ *Eating*: the body temperature can be raised slightly following eating, as the process of digesting and metabolising food produces heat.

When interpreting the results of temperature recordings, the nurse needs to consider the effects of all of the above factors.

Recording body temperature

The temperature can be measured orally (in the mouth), in the axilla (armpit), in the tympanic membrane (eardrum) and rectally (in the rectum). The procedure for recording the temperature is discussed later in this section.

Traditionally, mercury-in-glass thermometers were used to record body temperature. However, there is the potential for these to break and, for health and safety reasons, the following alternatives are now used:

+ Disposable single-use thermometers
+ Tympanic thermometers
+ Electronic thermometers

The choice depends on the patient's condition and what is available in your place of work.

Assessment

The normal body temperature is 36-37.5 °C, varying according to the site where the temperature is measured. For example, the core temperature can be more than 0.4 °C above oral temperature and 0.2 °C below rectal temperature (Jamieson *et al.*, 2002). It is important to remember that body temperature alters in response to environmental temperature and fluctuates at different times of the day, as we described earlier.

When recording the temperature, the following abnormalities may be detected:

+ *Hypothermia*: this is defined as a core temperature below 35 °C. It can occur when the body loses too much heat or cannot maintain its thermal balance. Hypothermia causes the metabolic rate to decrease. Children and elderly people are more at risk of hypothermia because of their immature and altered thermoregulatory mechanisms, respectively. Other risk factors for hypothermia include a cold environment, burns, overdose of medicines that lead to immobility (particularly in elderly people) and surgery. It is imperative that the patient's core temperature is monitored closely in order to detect changes that will allow the nurse to implement and evaluate strategies to prevent further heat loss and re-warm the patient. If left untreated, hypothermia can lead to death quite rapidly especially in elderly patients (Jevon, 2001a).

+ *Pyrexia*: this is a significant rise in core body temperature. There are three grades of pyrexia, as outlined in Table 3.4. When a person is pyrexial, vasoconstriction and shivering can occur. There is increased oxygen demand, and carbon dioxide excretion is also raised (Trim, 2005).

Table 3.4 Grades of pyrexia

Pyrexia grade	Causes
Low-grade pyrexia: normal to 38 °C	Inflammatory response due to mild infection, allergy, disturbance of body tissue through trauma, surgery or thrombosis
Moderate- to high-grade pyrexia: 38–40 °C	Wound, respiratory tract or urinary tract infection
Hyperpyrexia: above 40 °C	Bacteraemia, damage to the hypothalamus or high environmental temperatures

Source: Dougherty and Lister (2004)

Sites used for temperature recording

The temperature can be recorded at various sites. We consider these in the following sections.

Oral temperature

This is the most frequently used site, except in young children, breathless patients, patients who are confused, unconscious or uncooperative, and patients with oral pain, trauma or a history of convulsion. The temperature is detected via **thermoreceptors** in the posterior sub-lingual pocket of the mouth (i.e. under the tongue at the back of the mouth), which respond to changes in core temperature. Certain factors can affect the oral temperature, including a respiratory rate above 18 breaths per minute, eating and drinking immediately before a reading is taken, smoking within 15 minutes of a reading, and the patient moving the thermometer in their mouth.

Thermoreceptors are specialised cells that are sensitive to temperature change in the body.

Axilla temperature

This site is rarely used, as temperature readings taken from a patient's armpit are considered unreliable (Trim, 2005). There needs to be good contact between the two skin surfaces to get an accurate reading, and this is generally difficult to achieve, especially in thin people.

Tympanic temperature

This is a convenient site for temperature recording and tends to be the most commonly used nowadays. Temperature is detected using a special thermometer that senses body heat through infrared energy given off by the tympanic membrane (eardrum). The thermometer works by using infrared light to detect thermal radiation. A probe is gently inserted into the outer ear, adjacent to (but not touching) the tympanic membrane (Nicol *et al.*, 2004). The infrared light detects heat radiated from the tympanic membrane and provides a digital reading. This usually takes only a few seconds; an audible signal indicates that the reading is complete. Factors that can impair readings include the size of the ear canal, the presence of wax, the patient's position (for example, if the patient has been lying on the ear that is used) (Jevon, 2001b) and the operator's technique (Carroll, 2000). It is important that the thermometer probe is placed correctly so that it can detect heat from the tympanic membrane. If placed incorrectly, it can detect heat from the ear canal, which can be 2 °C lower, and thus give an inaccurate reading. Education and training are needed before the device is used, in order to ensure that the correct technique is followed.

Rectal temperature

The rectal site is used rarely nowadays, due to its invasive nature and the possible risk of bowel perforation. However, rectal readings are considered to be more accurate than oral and axillary readings (Trim, 2005).

Procedure

The equipment required includes a thermometer, a watch or a clock with a second hand, a thermometer cover if using an electronic thermometer, and gloves and wipes if recording rectal temperature. Disposable thermometers can be used and are becoming increasingly available.

The procedure varies slightly depending on which recording device is being used.

Oral recordings using an electronic thermometer

This consists of a probe placed in the patient's mouth (Figure 3.6a). The probe is usually connected to a power supply and display unit. When the probe is ready to give a reading it produces an auditory signal. The following explains how to take the temperature using an electronic thermometer:

1. Wash your hands and explain the procedure to the patient. Oral thermometers should not be used if the patient is unconscious or uncooperative, as mentioned earlier.
2. Apply a plastic sheath if required, making sure you follow the manufacturer's guidelines.
3. Ask the patient to open their mouth. Place the probe under the tongue, next to the frenulum. This is adjacent to a large artery (sublingual artery), so the temperature will be close to the core temperature.

(a)   (b)

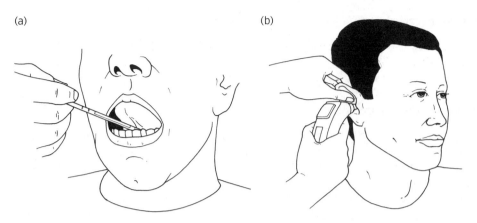

Figure 3.6 Recording a patient's temperature using (a) an oral electronic thermometer and (b) a tympanic membrane thermometer

4. Ask the patient to gently close their mouth.
5. Remove the thermometer on hearing the audible tone (usually one minute).
6. Record the temperature on the patient's observation chart. Report any differences from previous readings, and any temperature not within the normal limits, to the nurse in charge.
7. Dispose of the plastic sheath and wash your hands.

Ear canal recordings using electronic (tympanic membrane) thermometer

You will need an infrared thermometer (Figure 3.6b) for this procedure:

1. Wash your hands and explain the procedure to the patient, even if they are unconscious.
2. Refer to the manufacturer's guidelines for correct use of the thermometer.
3. Ensure there is good access to the patient's ear.
4. Apply the disposable cover.
5. Gently place the probe into the ear, ensuring that it fits well.
6. Record the temperature on the patient's observation chart and compare with previous readings and normal values.
7. Dispose of the cover and wash your hands.

Axilla recordings

This procedure is used only occasionally these days:

1. Wash your hands and explain the procedure to the patient, even if they are unconscious.
2. Ensure the patient's privacy.
3. Loosen any clothing for easy access to the axilla.
4. Prepare the thermometer and ensure the axilla is clean and dry.
5. Place the probe in the axilla and position the thermometer.
6. If the patient is able, ask them to hold their arm across the chest to help keep the probe in position.
7. Remove the probe after the required time, according to the manufacturer's guidelines.

8. Clean or dispose of the used thermometer according to local policy.

9. Record the temperature on the patient's observation chart.

10. Wash your hands.

Rectal recordings

This procedure is used only occasionally these days:

1. Wash your hands and explain the procedure to the patient, even if they are unconscious or confused.

2. Ensure the patient's privacy and dignity.

3. Refer to the manufacturer's guidelines for correct use of the thermometer.

4. Ask the patient to lie on his or her side, with the knees bent.

5. Apply gloves and then gently insert the thermometer probe 2–4 cm into the patient's anus (Jamieson *et al.*, 2002).

6. Remove the probe after the required time, according to the manufacturer's guidelines.

7. Wipe around patient's anus if required and ensure the patient is comfortable.

8. Dispose of the gloves.

9. Wash your hands.

10. Clean or dispose of the used thermometer according to local policy.

11. Record the temperature on the patient's observation chart.

Frequency of recordings

The frequency at which temperature should be recorded depends on the patient's condition and the reason for recording the temperature. The temperature should not be considered in isolation; rather, the nurse should include other general observations such as whether the patient looks flushed or pale, whether the skin feel hot, cold, dry or clammy, whether the patient is sweating or shivering, and whether the patient is confused.

It is important to use the same type of thermometer and the same body site each time you take a particular patient's temperature in order to ensure consistency.

Now you have read about why, where and how the body temperature is taken, consider Case studies 3.5 and 3.6.

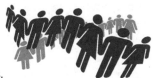

Case Study 3.5

Miss Smith is a 20-year-old Afro-Caribbean student with diabetes mellitus. She has been admitted for stabilisation of her diabetes. She tells you that her appetite has been poor, that she has not been eating properly and that she has given herself **less insulin than usual**. She states that she feels very hot and nauseous and is sweating profusely. Her **blood glucose** is 22 mmol/L, which is very high. You are recording her vital signs. When you take her temperature using an oral electronic thermometer, the result is 38.1 °C. Her pulse is 120 bpm and her respirations are 24 breaths per minute.

What would you do next?

Miss Smith is showing a reading that indicates she has a moderate- to high-grade pyrexia (see Table 3.4). This generally means that the patient has some kind of infection. It is worth talking to Miss Smith and asking how she feels. She may tell you about other signs and symptoms that will help you to identify where the infection is. For example, if she is coughing a lot or producing sputum, this could indicate a chest infection. If Miss Smith is passing urine frequently and mentions pain or irritation when passing urine, she could have a urinary tract infection. Also check that she has not had a hot drink in the past 15 minutes (although this is unlikely to cause such a high reading). It would be a good idea to check the patient's previous temperature reading and whether it was raised or whether it is increasing, which could indicate that her infection is worsening and needs prompt treatment. Although it is not the nurse's responsibility to diagnose infection, the nurse must inform the doctor of Miss Smith's raised temperature, along with other symptoms that will assist the doctor in the correct diagnosis. Because the patient has diabetes, any infection will greatly interfere with her condition and may have lead to her being admitted to hospital to help stabilise her blood glucose levels and insulin requirements. Therefore, it is imperative that Miss Smith's pyrexia is reported to the nurse in charge immediately so that appropriate action can be taken. Miss Smith's raised temperature must be recorded and checked on a frequent basis, probably every two to four hours, in order to monitor any changes.

Case Study 3.6

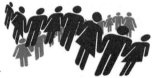

Mrs Mary Broadbent is an 87-year-old woman admitted to the ward in a hypothermic state. She was found at her home by a neighbour, who had not seen her for a few days and had become concerned. Mrs Broadbent had fallen and had been lying on the floor for some time. Mrs Broadbent was unable to get up as she had injured her leg quite badly. On admission, her temperature is 34.5 °C. Her pulse is 50 bpm and her respirations are 12 breaths per minute. You try to talk to Mrs Broadbent, but she is quite confused.

What would you do next?

You should report Mrs Broadbent's low body temperature to the nurse in charge. The doctor should be informed of the low reading. Mrs Broadbent's body temperature is very low and needs to be raised by applying warming-up measures, including covering her with a **space blanket**. However, the warming-up process must be done slowly in order to increase the body temperature gradually to normal. Mrs Broadbent's temperature needs to be monitored frequently to ensure that the warming-up measures are taking effect. Once Mrs

Even if a person with diabetes eats **less than usual**, they should not reduce their **insulin** intake, as this can have dire effects on their condition.

The normal **blood glucose** level is 4-7 mmol/L.

A **space blanket** is a blanket made of foil-like material that helps to insulate the body and raise the temperature.

Broadbent's confusion improves, she could be offered a warm (not very hot) drink and possibly some warm cooked food. Mrs Broadbent's vital signs and fluid balance need to be monitored and recorded frequently to assess her overall physical state, and any changes must be reported to the nurse in charge and the doctor.

Recap Questions

1. Why is the body temperature recorded?
2. What factors can affect body temperature?
3. What abnormalities can be detected when recording body temperature?
4. What sites are used to detect body temperature, and what are the main differences in the procedure for each site?

Summary

It is very important that patients' vital signs are taken and recorded properly. These signs can give a wealth of essential information about a patient. The nurse needs to know not only how to carry out the procedure but also how to interpret the measurements and what to do if they are abnormal. Major clinical decisions are made based on this interpretation. Accurate recordings of basic observations are essential to ensuring good-quality patient care. Therefore, attaining appropriate observations using the correct technique is paramount to the accuracy and reliability of the patient assessment. Furthermore, it enables practitioners to piece together a picture of the patient's condition and compare a series of observations in order to monitor the patient's condition over time.

This chapter has considered each vital sign separately but has then discussed the same factors in relation to each measurement. Reasons why the clinical measurements are made have been highlighted. Emphasis has been placed on the associated anatomy and physiology of each vital sign, as the authors feel that this is imperative to understanding each clinical measurement and any abnormalities that may be detected.

Several factors influence the clinical measurements discussed in this chapter. The nurse needs to be aware of these when analysing results.

The anatomical sites where the vital signs can be detected have been addressed, and an outline of aspects to consider when carrying out the clinical assessment has been given. For example, when assessing a patient's pulse, the rate, rhythm and amplitude/strength are noted.

The procedure has been presented in a concise instructive way so that the reader can appreciate the step-by-step method required to carry out monitoring and recording of each vital sign accurately. Pictorial representation will help the nurse to remember the different procedures.

Finally, the case studies in this chapter help to put the recording of vital signs into a clinical context and enable the reader to understand and apply the information they have learned in each section. Historically, nurses were taught the importance of being observant throughout their whole shift. With the advent of technology, perhaps some of the skills of observation have been subsumed by the use of technical gadgets to record vital signs. To illustrate this point, the author draws the reader's attention to the following quote, extracted from an article focusing on the history of nursing. Here, the ward sister is speaking to a junior nurse:

'You have not yet learnt the difference between seeing and observing', she said. 'It is one of the most important lessons you will ever learn during your training and one which may be vital in your patient's treatment and recovery. Watch his expression, how he breathes, feel his pulse and what it is telling you. How does he lie in bed – is he taking an interest in what is going on around him? And when you speak to him, is he taking in what you say? Your patient can tell you so much about himself without having to say a word ...
(Baker, 2002)

This quote emphasises the importance of good observational skills and how a lot can be gleaned about a patient's condition through vigilant observation. It is not enough just to be able to carry out the procedure of recording basic observations it is far more important to understand what the outcome of the recording is telling you about the patient's condition and what to do about it.

Key Points

1. Taking and recording basic observations should be seen not as a mundane aspect of nursing care but rather as an essential and informative task that tells us a lot about the patient's condition.

2. The nurse needs to be aware of the reasons why the pulse, respirations and temperature are taken and be aware of the normal ranges for each vital sign so that he or she knows when to report changes to the nurse in charge.

3. The nurse needs knowledge of the factors that can affect the pulse, respirations and temperature and must take these into consideration when interpreting readings.

4. An awareness of the sites used to record vital signs and being able to decide when to use them is essential.

5. The nurse needs to be able to discuss the characteristics/aspects that should be included when assessing the pulse, respirations and temperature.

6. The nurse should be able to outline the procedure for recording all of the basic observations.

Points for debate

Now that you have come to the end of this chapter here are a few points that you may wish to think about when you are in practice. You may wish to discuss these with your work colleagues or fellow students.

Taking and recording basic observations can be seen as a mundane and useless aspect of nursing care. Do you agree?

The taking and recording of basic observations tends to be carried out by untrained nursing staff, i.e. healthcare assistants, who often are not aware of the meanings of abnormal readings and indeed what to do about them.

It has been said by some trained nurses that basic observations do not need to be done on a daily basis, as information about the patient can be detected merely by looking at them. Do you agree?

Links to Other Chapters

Chapter 1   What is caring?
Chapter 2   Dignity and privacy
Chapter 10   Record-keeping

Further reading

Blows, WT (2001) *The Biological Basis of Nursing: Clinical Observations*. London: Routledge.

Skinner, S (1996) *Understanding Clinical Investigations*. London: Baillière Tindall.

References

Ahern, J and Philpot, P (2002) Assessing acutely ill patients on general wards. *Nursing Standard* **16**, 57-64.

Alcock, K, Clancy, M and Crouch, R (2002) Physiological observations of patients admitted to A&E. *Nursing Standard* **16**, 33-37.

Baker, M (2002) Every breath you take. *Nursing Times* **98**, 28.

Bennett, C (2003) Nursing the breathless patient. *Nursing Standard* **17**, 45-51.

Blows, WT (2001) *The Biological Basis of Nursing: Clinical Observations*. London: Routledge.

Carroll, M (2000) An evaluation of temperature measurement. *Nursing Standard* **14**, 39-43.

Casey, G (2001) Oxygen transport and the use of pulse oximetry. *Nursing Standard* **15**, 46-53.

Department of Health (2000) *Comprehensive Critical Care: A Review of Adult Critical Care Services*. London: The Stationery Office.

Docherty, B (2002) Cardiorespiratory physical assessment for the acutely ill: 1. *British Journal of Nursing* **11**, 750-758.

Dougherty, D and Lister, S (2004) *The Royal Marsden Hospital Manual of Clinical Nursing Procedures*. Oxford: Blackwell.

Field, D (2000) Respiratory care. In: Sheppard, M and Wright, M (eds) *Principles and Practice of High Dependency Nursing*. Edinburgh: Baillière Tindall.

Hull, D and Johnston, DI (1999) *Essential Paediatrics*, 4th edn. Edinburgh: Churchill Livingstone.

Jamieson, EM, McCall, J and Whyte, L (2002) *Clinical Nursing Practice*, 4th edn. Edinburgh: Churchill Livingstone.

Jevon, P (2001a) Hypothermia assessment: 1. *Nursing Times* **97**, 45-46.

Jevon, P (2001b) Using a tympanic thermometer. *Nursing Times* **97**, 43-44.

Kenward, G, Hodgetts, T and Castle, N (2001) Time to put the R back in TPR. *Nursing Times* **97**, 32-33.

Kozier, B, Ebb, A, Berman, A and Snyder, S (2004) *Fundamentals of Nursing: Concepts, Process and Practice*, 7th edn. Upper Saddle River, NJ: Prentice Hall.

Mallett, J and Dougherty, L (eds) (2000) *The Royal Marsden Hospital Manual of Clinical Nursing Procedures*, 5th edn. Oxford: Blackwell Science.

McQuillan, P, Pilkington, S, Allan, A and Taylor, B (1998) Confidential inquiry into quality of care before admission to intensive care. *British Medical Journal* **316**, 1853-1858.

Mooney, G (2004) Respirations. In: Shuttleworth, A (ed) *Monitoring and Assessment*. London: Emap Healthcare.

Nicol, M, Bavin, C, Bedford-Turner, S, Cronin, P and Rawlings-Anderson, K (2004) *Essential Nursing Skills*. London: Mosby.

O'Neill, D and Le Grove, A (2003) Monitoring critically ill patients in accident and emergency. *Nursing Times* **99**, 32-35.

Pritchard, A and Mallett, J (2001) *The Royal Marsden Hospital Manual of Clinical Nursing Procedures*. Oxford: Blackwell Science.

Schein, R, Hazday, N and Pena, M (1990) Clinical antecedents to in-hospital cardiopulmonary arrests. *Chest* **98**, 1388-1392.

Smith, A and Wood, J (1998) Can some in-hospital cardiac arrests be prevented? A prospective survey. *Resuscitation* **37**, 133-137.

Stevenson, T (2004) Achieving best practice in routine observation of hospital patients. *Nursing Times* **100**, 34-35.

Stoneham, M, Seville, G and Wilson, I (1994) Knowledge about pulse oximetry among medical and nursing staff. *Lancet* **344**, 1339-1342.

Tortora, G and Grabowski, S (2002) *Principles of Anatomy and Physiology*, 10th edn. New York: HarperCollins.

Trim, J (2004) Performing a comprehensive physiological assessment. *Nursing Times* **100**, 38-42.

Trim, J (2005) Monitoring temperature. *Nursing Times* **101**, 30-31.

Woodrow, P (2000) *Intensive Care Nursing*. London: Routledge.

Chapter 4
Hygiene

Case Study

Mrs Reed had been diagnosed with breast cancer. Despite treatment, she was very poorly. She was weak and needed assistance to maintain her personal hygiene. She was being cared for in her own home by her husband and the district nursing team. Sometimes she felt so unwell that she did not have the strength even to wash her face. Despite feeling like this, Mrs Reed wanted to keep some control over the level and type of personal assistance she was given. Fortunately, most of the regular nursing team seemed to know instinctively how much care to give. Occasionally, nurses and care workers who were not permanent members of the team would care for Mrs Reed in a way that she found upsetting: they gave expert physical care but paid little attention to her emotional and psychological needs. Because of the distress this was causing Mrs Reed and her husband, they were considering refusing any further outside help.

Introduction

Mrs Reed needed assistance with her personal hygiene, but she needed to be in control of this. She wanted to be able to make choices regarding how much or little assistance should be provided. Her condition was such that her level of need varied from day to day. She also wanted the staff to understand that she had personal preferences and her own particular likes and dislikes. She was relying on the nurses to realise that it she did not just want them to deal with her physical care; she also wanted them to address her feelings and emotional needs. She wanted the healthcare workers to be able to identify her strengths and weaknesses so that at times she could participate in her own care.

In this chapter we look at how we can support patients with their personal care needs. The level of assistance given varies from individual to individual and at different times in a person's life. Personal care is not only a matter of keeping clean; in this chapter we explore some of the issues that have an influence on this.

By the end of this chapter you will be able to:

1. Explore issues relating to personal hygiene in the context of practice
2. Identify the roles of the nurse and other health professionals and explore the value of intra-agency work
3. Identify aids and equipment used
4. Explore physical, emotional, spiritual and cultural aspects of giving personal care
5. Discuss the involvement of patients and carers in planning and evaluating personal care
6. Develop awareness of the prevention and control of infection in healthcare settings

Personal hygiene

Helping to maintain a person's personal hygiene is one of the most important jobs a nurse does. To enable a person to regain independence of their washing and dressing is to give the person control over a fundamental and essential part of their everyday life. When assisting a patient with these tasks, the nurse is in a unique position to observe and communicate with the patient and be aware of any changes in the patient's condition. Helping with personal hygiene gives opportunities for the nurse to assess the patient. The nurse works together with the patient, and in some instances alongside carers and other health and social care practitioners, such as occupational therapist, care workers, dental nurses, podiatrists and physiotherapists. These practitioners work together to produce a full assessment that is implemented and evaluated in line with the patient's needs.

To think about

What do we mean by 'personal hygiene'?
Why is it important to maintain personal hygiene?
To whom is personal hygiene important?

What is personal hygiene?

Hygiene is essential for all people. *Baillière's Nursing Dictionary* describes the science of hygiene as 'a condition or practice, such as cleanliness, that is conducive to the preservation of health' (Weller, 1971). Hygiene is a basic right for all people rather than a luxury for people in developed countries. When a person is unable to maintain their own hygiene needs, intervention is required; this is a basic nursing duty. During the time taken to attend to or assist with a patient's hygiene, the nurse has a unique opportunity to observe, assess and monitor the patient's condition. All nursing models, such as those of Roper *et al.* (2000) and Orem (1991), make reference to meeting the patient's hygiene needs; this is an activity of everyday life. The Roper model is constructed around activities known as activities of daily living. The emphasis of the Orem model is about self-care. This model gives a structure to assist the patient to achieve the activities associated with everyday life independently. Using models such as these enables the nurse to organise the patient's care and treatment. The nurse assesses the patient's hygiene needs, taking into consideration any deficits that the patient may have that affect their ability to care for themselves. The assessment and monitoring of the patient enable the nurse to carry out appropriate interventions and evaluate the effectiveness of any care and treatment given. Continual assessment ensures that appropriate hygiene care can be given. It is important that this is negotiated with the patient in order to ensure that their needs are being met fully. The definition of personal hygiene in the *Essence of Care Toolkit* (Department of Health, 2003a) states that this is the 'physical act of cleansing the body to ensure that the skin, hair and nails are maintained in optimum condition'. The patient-focused outcome of the benchmark for personal and oral hygiene is: 'Patients' personal and oral hygiene needs are met according to their individual and clinical needs' (Department of Health, 2003a). The following quote, from a patient's relative to Age Concern, shows why the *Essence of Care Toolkit* included personal hygiene:

> *She was left to lie in her excrement and urine, and the staff informed us she was doubly incontinent. We informed them that she would be if no one came to see if she needed to go to the toilet and she couldn't see anyone, being flat on her back on a large busy ward. She was confused and frail, but before she went into hospital she was not incontinent ... She deteriorated so rapidly that you could be forgiven for thinking she had had a bad stroke ... The ward was a disgrace. Dirty sheets, obstacles such as walking frames and trolleys strewn all over ...*
> (Gilchrist, 1999)

Clearly, this situation is totally unacceptable and immediate action should be taken. It is every nurse's duty to ensure patients are cared for appropriately. Being clean, dry and warm are fundamental human rights. The patient's immediate needs should always be dealt with in the first instance. Second, any obstacles should be removed, and areas should be made safe for patients and for staff to work in. Inadequate bed linen is due to poor ward management – all too often, lack of resources is used as an excuse for poor nursing care, but this is unacceptable and a clear action plan needs to be implemented in order to avoid a similar situation happening.

Historically, if a person was unable to meet their own hygiene needs on a temporary or permanent basis due to illness or disability, nurses intervened. Sometimes, this intervention was detrimental, leading to patients becoming unable to look after themselves. In particular, hospital routine resulted in many patients having no control over their own personal hygiene. However, latterly poor assessment together with a disastrous interpretation of nursing duties by a considerable number of nurses have resulted in the hygiene needs of patients not being met at all, which in turn has led to many patients suffering in unacceptable and even inhumane conditions due to neglect.

There have been numerous newspaper and television reports of poor care. Consider this statement taken from the *Daily Telegraph*:

> *Nurses were laughing and chatting at the nurse's station while my mother was dying lying in squalor.*
> (Sergeant, 2003)

This patient had been neglected and her daughter found her mother in awful conditions. The daughter could see members of staff on duty, and yet her mother's personal hygiene had not been attended to. This is distressing for both the relative and the patient.

Many media reports relate particularly to the failure of nurses in meeting patients' hygiene needs. In 1997, the *Observer* newspaper drew attention to the care of older people in hospital; the focus was on basic or essential care, of which personal hygiene was one of the main areas of concern. Unfortunately, despite various taskforces being set up, the work of the Health Advisory Service 2000 (HAS), and official reports and documents that have led to a government determination to improve clinical standards, as set out in the National Service Framework for Older People (Department of Health, 2001), it would appear that little has changed. The Channel 4 (2005) programme *Dispatches* showed evidence of poor nursing care with particular regard to meeting patients' personal hygiene needs. In this programme, an undercover investigator worked as a nurse and exposed extremely poor practice by other nurses, particularly with respect to many aspects of basic care and hygiene issues.

Consider Case study 4.1.

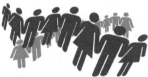

Case Study 4.1

Mrs Smith had come to visit her brother. He had been admitted to a general medical ward with a severe infection. On visiting her brother, Mrs Smith found him wearing dirty clothes and sitting in a chair. He appeared unwashed and unshaven. Mrs Smith was very upset. She told the nurse in charge that her brother had always been a man who took pride in his appearance. He was normally well-dressed, always wore a tie and shaved every day.

What can be done?
How could this situation be avoided?

Inadequate assessment, together with poor communication and a lack of awareness of the patient and his life history, contributed to this problem. Unnecessary distress was caused to Mr Smith's sister. She felt that her brother was being cared for badly, that the nurses were slapdash in their approach to patients, and that the nurses did not value their work or their patients. This in turn caused her to question all of Mr Smith's treatment. If the nurses did not care, then did the doctors or other health professionals? Was her brother receiving the best treatment available, or did he not matter?

Assessment of hygiene using a person-centred approach

Appropriate assessment (see also Chapter 1) of the patient could have helped to prevent the distressing situations discussed above. The best practice benchmark statement for the hygiene clinical practice benchmark in the *Essence of Care Toolkit* (Department of Health, 2003a) states: 'All patients are assessed to identify the advice and or care required to maintain and promote their individual personal hygiene.' It is important to find out about the patient, either from the patient or from their relatives. The patient and/or their relatives need to inform the assessment process and should be involved in all stages of care. Staff need to engage with relatives regularly, and not only when they need them to solve a problem or help out in a crisis.

Sometimes care workers need to be aware of the boundaries of care; for instance, the patient may want a relative rather than a nurse to carry out a certain task. These boundaries may require careful negotiation and can be a sensitive issue that needs to be handled with care (Health Advisory Service 2000, 1999). Assessment of a patient's personal hygiene should always be the responsibility of a suitably trained, and ideally a registered, person – in most cases, this is a nurse. Unqualified staff, students and carers can assist with the assessment process if they have received the appropriate education and training and if they have been assessed as competent to undertake such assessments, but **accountability** remains with the registered practitioner (Department of Health, 2003a).

The assessment undertaken should incorporate the identification of the patient's individual needs and any risk factors, such as infection control. Assessment needs to be undertaken at appropriate times, such as when the nurse first comes into contact with the patient and if the patient's condition changes. Assessment may need to be a continuous process: as the patient's condition changes, so should the assessment. The assessment, the care and treatment to be given, and the evaluation of that care and treatment should be documented clearly in the patient's records so that consistency with other carers and treatment providers is maintained. The assessment needs to encompass all members of the interdisciplinary team, such as podiatrists, occupational therapists and voluntary agencies, as well as the patient and any informal carers. The provision of education and training in assessment is essential for all staff contributing to the maintenance of the patient's hygiene.

Teamworking

Many different health and social care practitioners may be involved in helping a patient maintain their personal hygiene.

> ### To think about
>
> Who might be involved in helping a patient with their personal hygiene?

Nurses have an important role in assessing, assisting and monitoring the patient's hygiene. The qualified nurse is responsible for supervising the assistance given by the healthcare assistant. The occupational therapist may assess and help the patient to develop ways to become self-caring through teaching and through the introduction of different equipment. The physiotherapist may be involved in helping the patient with posture and mobility. The podiatrist may help the patient with any foot problems. Continence and oral health specialists may be involved in certain aspects of the patient's care. In addition, social care workers, volunteers, and formal and informal carers may have roles to play. All of these people need to work together to develop and carry out the patient's care/treatment plan.

Accountability means being answerable for something or to someone.

Care-planning

The best practice statement for Factor 2a of the benchmark is that 'planned care is negoti-ated with patients and or carers and is based on assessment of their individual needs' (Department of Health, 2003a). To meet this, care must be evidence-based and all staff involved with the implementation of this care/treatment must have education and training to enable them to contribute to the assessment and evaluation process. All members of the team must recognise the value of each member's contribution. The care given needs to be reviewed continually in order to be kept up to date. Effective care-planning ensures that care is negotiated between the team, the patient, the informal carers and the relatives; in this way, the care may be shared in order to meet the patient's needs. The patient's age and culture influence the care/treatment plan.

The patient's ability and mobility will most likely need continual assessment. The role of the nurse or health care assistant is in helping the patient to select the washing items, to pre-pare the washing area, to ascertain what the patient can or is willing to do, and to assist with the washing technique. Assessing the procedure throughout ensures the safety of the patient and minimises any risk.

Consider Case study 4.2.

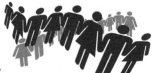

Case Study 4.2

Mr Bennett sometimes failed to meet his own hygiene needs. He was often found to be dirty, unshaven and smelling strongly of body odour. Mr Bennett's wife and daughter insisted that the visiting nurse would make him clean and tidy, but it was evident that Mr Bennett found this distressing and he refused to have his clothes changed. On being told by the nurses that they could not force Mr Bennett to accept care, his relations said they would inform the press that their care was poor. The team manager was concerned about the effect this would have on the Trust's reputation.

How could the nurses have handled the situation more constructively?

The ward team needed to work together with Mr Bennett and his wife to develop a plan of action that would ensure Mr Bennett achieved an acceptable level of hygiene while at the same time taking into account why Mr Bennett found it distressing to have assistance with washing and dressing. The case study shows that the skills required for washing and dressing are complex. Mr Bennett did not want to be dressed by other people; he preferred to remain unwashed rather than to have help. The ward team needed to take all of this into account when planning and implementing Mr Bennett's care in order that they could do so sympa-thetically. Mr Bennett's initial care showed that this had not been done.

Assisting with personal hygiene

In order for a patient's individual hygiene needs to be met, it may be necessary for the patient to have assistance from other people. Assistance can come from nurses, support workers, therapists, care workers and informal carers. The statement for best practice is:

'Patients have access to the level of assistance that they require to meet individual personal hygiene needs' (Department of Health, 2003a). This level can alter, and so continuous assessment that includes the patient and their relatives is important. The people assisting with hygiene require appropriate training, access to information, aids and adaptations, and (if not qualified as health professionals) support and verification from a registered practitioner. Effective communication is required between the patient and all those involved with assisting with personal hygiene in order to maintain the person's dignity, meet their cultural and religious needs, and take into account age-related matters and any other special needs (Department of Health, 2003a).

The skills needed for washing and dressing are physical, cognitive, sensory and expressive. Consider the amount of stamina the patient has: perhaps the patient needs only minimal help or wants help later rather than at first. The patient's coordination (or lack of) may also be an issue. Consider the patient's range of movement; for example, can they do up a zip or use buttons? Can the patient stand at a sink without overbalancing? If the patient needs a chair, can they reach the taps? Do they have the strength and grip to turn the taps on and off?

Consider the patient's decision-making. Can they determine how hot the water should be and what to wear? Will the patient remember to test the water before getting into the bath? Can the patient concentrate and organise themselves? Do they have the knowledge to perform the task? What are the patient's preferences? Think about Mr Bennett in Case study 4.2: he preferred not to have help, but the consequences of this were that he was unkempt.

The sensory skills of sight, touch, smell and hearing are all used for personal hygiene. Loss of any of these skills alters the task. For example, not being able to see dirt or to feel the temperature of water can cause significant problems. Patience is needed if a patient is relearning a skill such as tying shoelaces. The attitudes of staff can affect the task: if the patient feels belittled or dirty, this may have an effect on their self-esteem and motivation.

It is common for nurses to find themselves in some fairly challenging situations with regard to personal hygiene. Consider Case study 4.3.

Case Study 4.3

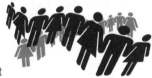

Mrs Chinn had multiple sclerosis. As a result, she needed assistance with bowel care. The district nurse visited regularly to assist by giving Mrs Chinn an enema. On one occasion, as the nurse was carrying out the procedure, some shelves in the room started to collapse. Mr Chinn ran into the room on hearing the noise. Mrs Chinn was very upset that her husband had seen her having an enema.

This was a very sensitive situation. There is no right or wrong solution here; the care worker simply has to be aware that this type of situation can occur.

The environment

The best practice statement for Factor 3 is: 'Patients have access to an environment that is safe and acceptable to the individual' (Department of Health, 2003a).

> ### To think about
>
> When you are washing and dressing, what do you consider to be an acceptable environment?

It may be that you would like privacy and warmth. You probably like a place with adequate facilities such as hot and cold running water. The environment also needs to be safe. The challenge for the practitioner is in ensuring that the environment helps to maintain the patient's dignity and privacy and meets any special cultural, religious and age-related needs. A safe environment is one that addresses a patient's physical and psychological aspects, minimises infection, and has available any equipment on hand that may be required, such as moving and handling equipment and bath seats (Department of Health, 2003a). It is important to take account of any risk factors; these need careful consideration and negotiation in the care-planning process. This in turn enables the patient to make informed choices with regard to taking risks at a level that is acceptable to them. It is important that the nurse is aware that the patient's circumstances may change at any time and must be prepared to renegotiate the treatment plan.

Nurses often have to work in some very badly equipped places, particularly people's homes. Consider Case study 4.4.

> ### Case Study 4.4
>
>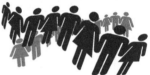
>
> The paediatric district nurse was asked to visit William Otty, a 3-week-old baby living with his 17-year-old mother in a run-down flat. On visiting, the nurse found the flat to be in a very poor condition. The flat was damp and dirty. Although it was heated adequately, the water heater had broken. Ms Otty was very independent, but it was obvious that she needed help with William, who had a skin infection. The bathroom in the flat was dirty but in working order. The paediatric nurse and health visitor worked together to assist Ms Otty with William's care. They were able to arrange for the water heater to be fixed and they notified the landlord of the dampness in the flat. The nurse and health visitor visited William and his mother regularly, supporting her and teaching her about the importance of keeping both the flat and William clean.

William's mother needed more support than what would normally be given because of the environment in which she and her baby lived.

Provision of toiletries

Over recent years, the provision of toiletries in hospitals has become less common. The main reason for this was to save money, but it was also seen as a way to minimise infection. The benchmark best practice statement of Factor 4 states: 'Patients are expected to supply their own toiletries but single use toiletries are provided until they can supply their own' (Department of Health, 2003a). It is important that patients and their relatives are aware which toiletries are required, that they keep these toiletries for their personal use and that they do not share them with other patients.

Information and education to support patients

Factor 6a concerns information and education to support patients in meeting personal hygiene needs, particularly if these are changing or have to be met in unfamiliar surroundings. The benchmark of best practice is: 'Patients and or cares are provided with information and education to meet their individual personal hygiene needs' (Department of Health, 2003a). This information needs to be up-to-date, evidence-based and available in formats that make it accessible to understand. The information must also be culturally appropriate. Some patients, for example following radiotherapy, may require specific information. The practitioners giving the information need to ascertain that the information is understood by the patient and all the other agencies involved with meeting the patient's personal hygiene requirements.

Evaluation and re-assessment

Appropriate and effective evaluation and re-assessment can be achieved only by a good patient–carer (informal or formal) partnership. Clear verbal and written communication and inclusion of all the agencies involved are key. The best practice statement stresses: 'Patients' care is continuously evaluated, reassessed and the care plan renegotiated' (Department of Health, 2003a). This can be achieved through the use of evidence-based care, keeping documentation up-to-date, using appropriate tools to assist in re-assessment and evaluation, ensuring that re-assessment and evaluation take place in a timely manner, and maintaining and monitoring the skills and competencies acquired by the patient and the team throughout the care programme.

Aids and adaptations

A number of different adaptations can be made to a person's home to aid personal hygiene, such as installing a stair lift to enable the person to access upstairs rooms. A plethora of equipment is also available, such as high toilet seats, bath seats and adapted taps. It is essential that any adaptations and aids are safe and that infection control issues are met.

To think about

What adaptations may be used?
How can these adaptations be accessed?
What equipment may be used?
Where can you obtain this equipment?
How can the environment be made safe?

The healthcare worker needs to be aware of these adaptations and aids and how the patient or their family can obtain them. Some NHS and social services equipment supply equipment such as bath boards, shower seats (Figure 4.1), bath steps, grab rails and tap levers. Some equipment can also be bought from specialist shops and large pharmacies. Details of specialist shops and equipment stores are usually available at local libraries, GP practices and hospitals. The book *A Practical Guide for Disabled People or Carers* (Department of Health, 2003b) is updated yearly and gives information on services and equipment available for disabled people. This book also gives current accurate information about disabled people's rights and lists some useful organisations.

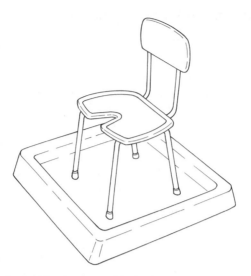

Figure 4.1 Shower seat in the home

It is the nurse's responsibility to ensure that any equipment used by the patient is safe. It is advisable for users to seek advice from a qualified practitioner. All equipment and adaptations should also comply with British and/or European Standards.

Sometimes expensive adaptations and equipment are not needed. Consider Case study 4.5.

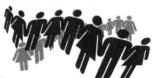

Case Study 4.5

Mrs Ralph had been admitted to an acute hospital with an infection. The infection was severe, and Mrs Ralph's recovery was slow. She was discharged from the acute hospital after 10 days and admitted to a rehabilitation hospital. A rehabilitation programme was put in place. Mrs Ralph was given physiotherapy to help with her mobility and encouraged by the nurses to wash and dress herself. After 3 days she was able to wash herself using a bowl of water that the nurses took to her bedside. Her mobility improved gradually, but she needed assistance from one other person as well as her walking frame. A bank (relief) nurse came to the rehabilitation ward and was helping to care for Mrs Ralph. The bank nurse asked Mrs Ralph if she would like to go to the bathroom for her wash. Mrs Ralph agreed and confided in the nurse that this had been the first time since her admission to the two hospitals that she had seen herself in the mirror.

Mrs Ralph needed very few aids or adaptations in order to meet her rehabilitation plan, although she did need help to get to the bathroom. It was quicker for the nurses to hand her a washing bowl. However, to prepare Mrs Ralph for her home life, they needed to help her regain her independence. This case study shows that Mrs Ralph's rehabilitation programme was incomplete and that her needs had not been considered when her care/treatment plan was put together. She was more of a passive recipient. It took a nurse outside the team to realise that Mrs Ralph's needs were not being met. In this case, the professionals had made inappropriate decisions.

Therapeutic approach to washing and dressing

The aim of any therapeutic approach to washing and dressing is to assist the patient to gain maximum independence and to provide appropriate equipment and adaptations if necessary. The nurse's role is to encourage the patient and/or carer to have a positive attitude, so they can work together to achieve goals, to identify any problems that may hinder the achievement of these goals, and how to solve these problems. There is an opportunity for health and social workers to give the patient information and also to educate and counsel the patient if required to do so during the time spent with washing and dressing. Washing and dressing is an activity of everyday life. The skills to perform this task are acquired throughout childhood and improve with practice. How we perform this task is influenced by our environment: think back to William in Case study 4.4 – his mother was finding it difficult to keep him clean because of the environment in which she lived. Our ability to keep ourselves clean is also dependent on our mental and physical state. We take these activities for granted when we are able-bodied, but washing and dressing can be difficult if we become ill, disabled or frail. When assisting with washing and dressing, the nurse needs to consider the following:

+ *The patient:*
  - What is the patient's ability?
  - Has the patient any deficits that would affect their ability to meet their personal hygiene needs?
  - What are the patient's needs?
  - What are the patient's diagnosis and **prognosis**?
  - What is the patient's mobility/strength?

+ *The environment:*
  - Does the environment inhibit or assist the process?
  - How private is the environment?
  - Is it conducive to maintaining the patient's personal hygiene?
  - Is it warm and free from draughts?
  - Is there adequate space?
  - What equipment, such as a bath seat or high toilet seat, does the patient need?

+ *Timing:*
  - When should this take place?
  - Have you allowed adequate time to perform the tasks?

+ *Clothing:*
  - Has the patient chosen what they want to wear? This simple act gives the patient some degree of control.
  - Have you considered what clothes the patient already owns? For example, it may not be financially viable to buy a new wardrobe of clothes, but you can adapt what is available.
  - Have you given thought to the patient's lifestyle? For example, a businessperson may not take notice of advice to wear jogging pants because they are easy to take on and off.

The **prognosis** is the expected progression of the patient's illness.

All of these issues need to be considered when devising a care/treatment plan for the patient. The safety of the patient and practitioner is paramount throughout, as is deciding with the patient the level of risk that they may wish to take. These factors, together with the evaluation and re-assessment, determine how much help is given.

Lewin and Reed (1998) formalised the process of washing and dressing by dividing it into the following components:

✦ *Performance area:* this is the actual tasks of grooming, oral hygiene, foot care, bathing, showering, toilet hygiene, dressing, mobility, communication, safety and risk.

✦ *Performance components:* sensory awareness and sensory processing, taking into account the person's senses of touch, smell, sight, hearing and taste.

✦ *Performance context:* this includes the person's age, their development or maturity, where they are in their lifecycle, their disability or illness state, and consideration of the physical, social and cultural aspects of the individual's environment.

Bed-bathing

Bed-bathing is a common nursing procedure, particularly when caring for unconscious patients, very ill patients and patients near to death. It is important that bed-bathing is carried out with expertise and sensitivity. The basic principles of this procedure are as follows:

Equipment

✦ Soap
✦ Two flannels – one for the face, one for the body
✦ Two towels – one for the face, one for the body
✦ Toothbrush and toothpaste
✦ Tooth beaker and receiver
✦ Hairbrush and comb
✦ Towel, sheet or small blanket to cover the patient
✦ Washing bowel of hand-hot water (a good way to test the temperature of the water is to dip in your elbow to see whether it feels comfortable to the skin; always ask the patient whether the water is at the correct temperature for them)
✦ Clean bed linen
✦ Clean clothes
✦ Soiled linen bag
✦ Yellow bag for clinical waste

Preparation of the patient

The nurse should gain full cooperation from the patient. The procedure should be explained and conducted in privacy. Throughout the procedure, you should talk to the patient, asking them to participate and informing them of what you are intending to do. Any nearby windows should be shut to prevent draughts. The patient should have the opportunity to go to the toilet before bathing commences. The patient should be covered with a bath blanket or sheet. The bed clothes should be placed on a chair. If possible, any extra pillows should be removed, leaving the patient in a semi-recumbent position. If the patient has breathing difficulties, they should be left in an upright position. The patient should then be helped to undress.

Method

The following method of bed-bathing is adapted from Bates (1971).

1. Plenty of hand-hot water is necessary. It should be changed whenever it becomes cool, soiled or excessively soapy.
2. Small areas of the patient should be exposed at any one time, thus avoiding the patient from getting chilled unnecessarily.
3. The face towel is placed under the chin, and the face, neck and ears are washed with the face flannel and dried. It is best to avoid using soap on the face, unless the patient directs otherwise.
4. The bath towel is placed under each arm in turn, and the hands and arms are washed with the body flannel, rinsed and dried.
5. A small blanket is folded back to the level of the umbilicus (tummy button) so that the chest can be washed, rinsed and dried.
6. The chest is covered with the face towel and the small blanket folded down so that the abdomen and groin can be washed and dried (Figure 4.2).
7. When the water is changed, the patient should be covered with the small blanket.
8. The body towel is placed under the legs and feet, and each leg is washed and dried in turn. Care should be taken to wash and dry between the toes.
9. The patient should be asked and assisted to lie on one side so that the back and bottom can be washed and dried (Figure 4.3). The bed should be kept dry by placing the towel on the bed.
10. The bottom sheet should be straightened or changed if necessary.
11. After the bed-bath, the patient should be assisted with dressing, cutting their fingernails and toenails, brushing their teeth and combing their hair.

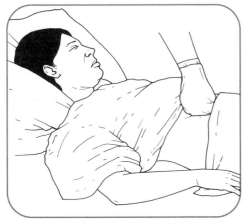

Figure 4.2 Washing the abdomen during a bed-bath

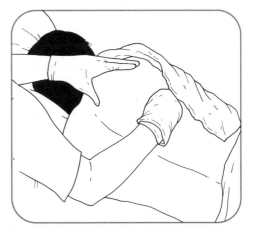

Figure 4.3 Washing the back during a bed-bath

12. The small blanket is replaced with the top bedclothes, and the pillows are made comfortable.

13. Personal belongings such as magazines and drinks and the call bell should be replaced within the patient's reach.

14. The equipment used should be cleaned and returned for further use.

As with most nursing procedures, the principles can be modified to suit each individual patient. It is interesting to note that this is taken from a clinical skills book first published in 1971. This demonstrates that the principles of bed-bathing have not changed over the past three decades or so.

Bed-bathing as a therapeutic activity

The process of bed-bathing can be very beneficial and calming for patients. Very ill people often find the procedure comforting. A study in the *Journal of the American Geriatrics Society* found that bed-bathing people with dementia reduced the number of aggressive incidents compared with continuing normal bathing or showering arrangements. Aggressive incidents were reduced by more than half (Sloane *et al.*, 2004). Bed-bathing was also found to reduce the patients' self-rated discomfort levels by 25% (Strachan-Bennett, 2004).

Compression stockings

The use of compression stockings, or surgical stockings, reduces the incidence of deep vein thrombosis, which can be caused by immobility or restricted mobility. Compression stockings are also prescribed as part of the treatment of **venous ulcers,** leg **oedema** and low blood pressure. Middle-aged and older people undergoing surgery or those on prolonged bed-rest are usually prescribed compression stockings. The stockings are used as part of a patient's treatment and are intended for use for a specified amount of time. Relatively fit patients may wear the stockings for only a few hours, but other patients may be advised to wear them for a number of days or weeks. Graduated compression hosiery is also available on prescription for mobile patients (Dilks *et al.*, 2005).

Compression stockings are available in a variety of sizes and lengths. Careful assessment is necessary to ensure that the patient receives the correct size and level of pressure to suit their medical needs. The nurse needs to identify the correct size of stocking for the length and circumference of the patient's leg, and whether below-knee or thigh-length stockings are required. It is important that the stockings are not too tight or too loose, although you may need to explain to the patient what is meant by 'too tight'. Figure 4.4 demonstrates the method of putting on compression stockings.

A variety of aids are available for use with compression hosiery, to help users put the stockings over their feet and pull them up over the legs. These aids aim can enable individuals with physical limitations and/or restricted movement to be more independent (Dilks *et al.*, 2005).

Consider Case study 4.6.

A **venous ulcer** is a breakdown of the skin caused by poor circulation or wounds. Venous ulcers are often difficult to heal and chronic.

Oedema is swelling of legs due to poor lymphatic circulation.

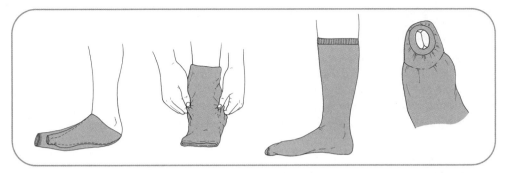

Figure 4.4 Putting on anti-embolic stockings
Source: Nicol (2004)

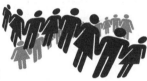

Case Study 4.6

Mr Brown was a recently bereaved man who had been admitted to hospital for a hernia repair. Following the operation, his wound became infected and his discharge was delayed for 6 weeks while the infection was treated. He was discharged home and district nursing visits were arranged. At the first of the district nurse visits, Mr Brown's wound was re-dressed. The nurse asked Mr Brown to remove his compression stockings. Mr Brown replied that he had been told that the stockings were not to be removed and that he had not had the stockings changed since his operation. The district nurse explained that the stockings could be removed for up to 30 minutes each day for skin care and personal hygiene. Removal of Mr Brown's stocking revealed a deep pressure ulcer on his heel. This ulcer took months to heal and severely restricted Mr Brown's mobility and lifestyle. Before his hernia operation, Mr Brown had been fit, active and independent and had enjoyed going dancing regularly.

How could this situation have been avoided?

The nurses in the acute hospital were not aware of how to care for a patient wearing compression stockings. They needed education and training on how to do this. Stocking manufacturers give clear instructions on the use of their products. Some produce training materials such as videos to address this issue, and some send out representatives to train staff in the use of compression stockings. Most employers, including primary care trusts, have local procedures for the care of wearing compression stockings. Exhibit 4.1 gives some guidelines on caring for a patient wearing compression stockings.

+ Ideally, each patient should have at least two pairs
+ Accurate measurement is necessary to ascertain the required size
+ Stockings should be fitted to the leg, with no creases or wrinkles
+ The hole in the foot of the stocking should be placed under the ball of the foot
+ Stockings should be checked daily with regard to fit
+ The stockings should be removed every day for up to 30 minutes
+ The patient's washed and dried legs should be checked for lesions and discoloration
+ Stockings should be washed at least every three days (more frequently if soiled) at 60 °C or lower

Exhibit 4.1 Compression stocking care

Recap Questions

1. Why is personal hygiene important?
2. What is a therapeutic approach to washing and dressing?
3. Where can you obtain equipment and adaptations?
4. What care is necessary for a patient wearing compression stockings?

Oral hygiene

In order to maintain a healthy mouth, the teeth and gums need to be cleaned twice daily. It is important that patients are assisted to meet their oral hygiene needs. A variety of grips for toothbrushes and sculptured handled toothbrushes are available from specialist equipment shops and large pharmacies to help people with restricted hand movement, for example due to arthritis. Exhibit 4.2 offers some tips on maintaining a healthy mouth.

If the patient doesn't wear dentures:

+ Brush the teeth, gums and tongue twice a day
+ Use a toothbrush with a small head and of medium texture
+ Use a pea-sized amount of fluoride toothpaste
+ Spend at least two minutes brushing to remove plaque
+ Gums should be brushed close to where they meet the teeth
+ The gums may bleed if plaque remains, but this usually lessens with more effective brushing
+ Dental floss can be used between the teeth to remove plaque from areas that difficult to reach with a toothbrush

If the patient wears dentures:

+ Brush the mouth and gums using a small-headed, soft toothbrush
+ Brush the dentures using a mild soap solution and/or running water
+ Toothpaste may scratch the polished surface of the denture
+ Soak non-metal dentures weekly for about 20 minutes in a solution recommended by a dentist or pharmacist
+ If the dentures are taken out at night, leave them in water
+ Have a dental check-up at least once a year

Exhibit 4.2 Care of the mouth

The nurse may have to help patients with mouth care, whether simply by ensuring that the patient has access to their toothbrush and other oral hygiene equipment or by giving full assistance with mouth care. It is very important that regular mouth care is given to patients who are unconscious or very ill. Mouth care packs are available in most hospitals; these packs usually comprise two small containers and some gauze or covered sticks, which are used to moisten or clean the mouth. If such packs are not available, it is easy enough to make one.

Most PCTs have policies and procedures regarding mouth care. Some practitioners use diluted mouthwash tablets to clean the mouth, but others use simply cooled boiled water. If the patient's lips are dry and cracked, a small film of petroleum jelly can be applied to them. If a patient is not taking any food or drink, they should be offered or assisted with mouth care every few hours.

Mouth cancer

The incidence of mouth cancer has increased in the UK over the past couple of decades. Nurses need to be able to recognise the signs of mouth cancer, as early detection is essential for successful treatment. The nurse should refer the patient to dental services if they detect any changes in a patient's mouth. Things to look out for include white or red patches in the mouth, lumps or painful ulcers that last for more than 2 weeks, sore patches, swelling or tightness in the mouth, and difficulty in opening the mouth fully. Wearing ill-fitting dentures can hide some of these changes. The risk of mouth cancer developing is increased by smoking tobacco, chewing betel quid or tobacco, and drinking more than a safe amount of alcohol. The combination of smoking and drinking increases the risk: three-quarters of mouth cancers are a result of this. Betel quid is traditionally chewed in some Asian countries. The risk of mouth cancer increases greatly if the betel contains tobacco. Patients should be encouraged to reduce the amount of betel they chew, to chew for shorter periods, and to rinse out the mouth after each chew.

Recap Questions

1. How can you keep your mouth healthy?
2. What are the early signs of mouth cancer?

Infection control

Infection control is the minimisation of the risk of infection by taking some simple precautions. These general principles were formally known as 'universal precautions'. Routine or everyday practice is made safe by applying these general principles of infection control. These general principles underpin all practice. The aim of infection control is to give protection to staff and patients from infection. Infection control nurses have been employed since the 1960s to help control outbreaks of antibiotic-sensitive strains of the bacterium *Staphylococcus aureus* (methicillin-sensitive *Staphylococcus aureus*, MSSA). In more recent years, methicillin-resistant *Staphylococcus aureus* (MRSA) has been high on the government's agenda (Royal College of Nursing, 2005). By applying standard precautions at all times, to all patients, best practice is internalised and the risks of infection are minimised (Royal College of Nursing, 2004). The principles of infection control are listed in Exhibit 4.3.

+ Achieving optimum hand hygiene
+ Using personal protective equipment
+ Managing sharps
+ Safely disposing of clinical waste
+ Managing blood and bodily fluids
+ Decontaminating equipment
+ Achieving and maintaining a clean clinical environment
+ Managing accidents

Exhibit 4.3 Principles of infection control
Source: Royal College of Nursing (2004)

Effective handwashing

Handwashing is the single most important activity for reducing the spread of disease. This has been acknowledged since Florence Nightingale was a nurse. Evidence suggests, however, that health professionals still do not wash their hands effectively (Royal College of Nursing, 2005). Soap and water remove 99% of transient bacteria and should always be used for soiled hands. Alcohol hand-rub kills 99.9% of transient bacteria and can be used on 'clean' hands. Washing with soap and water first and then applying alcohol gel gives the best protection; this system should always be used following care of infected patients. Hands should be cleaned before and after contact with patients and after any activity or contact that contaminates the hands. Alcohol gel is a practical alternative to soap and water; however, it must be remembered that alcohol is not a cleansing agent, which is why it should be used on clean hands whenever possible (Royal College of Nursing, 2005). Hands that are visibly dirty or potentially grossly contaminated must always be washed and dried thoroughly. Improper hand-drying can recontaminate hands that have been washed: wet surfaces transfer organisms more effectively than dry surfaces, and inadequately dried hands are prone to skin damage.

A handwashing technique should be followed, such as the RCN six-step technique illustrated in Figure 4.5.

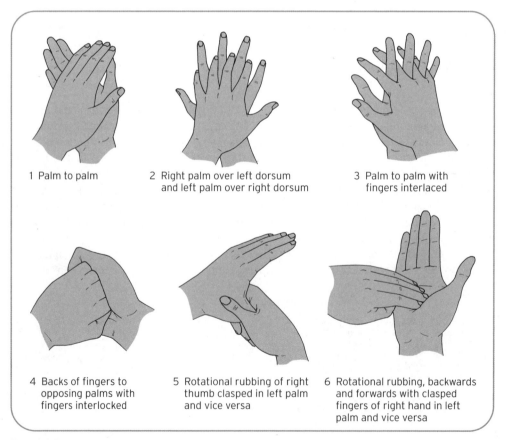

1 Palm to palm

2 Right palm over left dorsum and left palm over right dorsum

3 Palm to palm with fingers interlaced

4 Backs of fingers to opposing palms with fingers interlocked

5 Rotational rubbing of right thumb clasped in left palm and vice versa

6 Rotational rubbing, backwards and forwards with clasped fingers of right hand in left palm and vice versa

Figure 4.5 Handwashing technique
Source: Royal College of Nursing

Nurses should keep their fingernails short, clean and free from nail polish. Hand and wrist jewellery, especially rings with stones, wristwatches and bracelets, should not be worn. Artificial nails should not be worn. Any cuts or abrasions should be kept covered with water-proof plasters. Long sleeves should be rolled up before handwashing takes place.

Using personal protective equipment

The purpose of personal protective equipment is to protect the health worker and the patient from the risk of cross-infection. Examples of personal protective equipment are gloves, aprons, masks, goggles and visors. This equipment must be available and used when giving direct care at times when hands or clothing may be at risk of becoming contaminated. Disposable gloves and plastic aprons are single use-items and must be discarded after each patient contact. The technique for putting on disposable gloves is shown in Figure 4.6. Wearing gloves does not pre-clude washing hands: the hands should always be washed following the removal of the gloves. Polythene gloves are not suitable for use when dealing with body fluids.

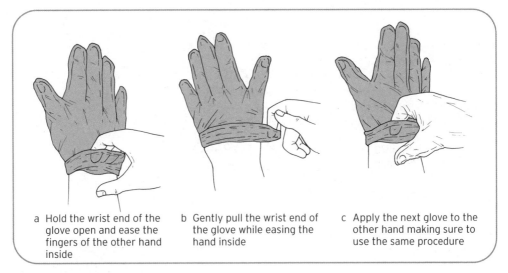

a Hold the wrist end of the glove open and ease the fingers of the other hand inside

b Gently pull the wrist end of the glove while easing the hand inside

c Apply the next glove to the other hand making sure to use the same procedure

Figure 4.6 Putting on surgical gloves
Source: Nursing Times, 2005

Sharps and waste management

There are specific legal requirements for sharps and other waste to be handled, safeguarded and disposed of properly. All workplaces have agreed policies and procedures on this, and these should be consulted and adhered to by all staff.

To think about

Which procedures do you think have a higher than average risk of causing injury?

Such procedures include handling:

+ Cannulae (needles) used for intravenous infusions
+ Winged (butterfly) needles
+ Needles and syringes
+ Phlebotomy needles
+ Infected linen
+ Faeces
+ Bodily fluids

Care must always be taken when handling any of the above. In addition, the points listed in Exhibit 4.4 should always be adhered to when handling sharps. Sharps include needles, scalpels, stitch cutters, glass ampoules and any sharp instrument. The main hazard of a sharps injury is the risk of contracting hepatitis B, hepatitis C or human immunodeficiency virus (HIV). Blood-borne viruses are the second most common cause (after back injuries) of occupational injuries to health workers (Royal College of Nursing, 2004). Consider Case study 4.7.

+ Keep handling to a minimum
+ Do not pass sharps directly from hand to hand
+ Do not break or bend needles before use or disposal
+ Do not dismantle syringes or needles before disposal
+ Never resheathe needles
+ Placed used sharps in a special container that conforms to UN Standard 3291 and British Standard 7320
+ Sharps containers should not be filled more than two-thirds and should be stored in an area away from the public

Exhibit 4.4 Safe handling of sharps

Case Study 4.7

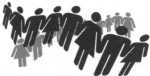

A 3-year-old girl is accompanying her mother to the local GP surgery. The mother is told to wait in a side room used for examinations and procedures. While the mother is getting undressed in preparation for an examination, her daughter sits on the floor. The mother discovers that her daughter is playing with a container for sharps. The container is full, and the little girl can easily reach the needles.

What immediate action needs to be taken?
How could this situation have been avoided?
Who is responsible for this happening?

Immediate action needs to be taken for any injuries. Bleeding should be encouraged by applying gentle pressure – but do not suck. The affected area should be washed under running water, dried and covered with a waterproof dressing. Treatment by a GP and/or specialist should be initiated; this may involve screening and treating of specific infections. The incident must be reported and a full risk assessment carried out. Advice should be sought from the trust's infection control team.

The situation in Case study 4.7 could have been avoided. The sharps box was over two-thirds full and therefore sharps could be reached. The box should have been kept out of reach of small children, and appropriate warning signs should have been displayed prominently so that staff and patients were aware of potential hazards. All the staff employed at the GP practice had some responsibility for the situation. All staff, including cleaning staff, should have regular health and safety training, and all employees should be made aware of the local policies and procedures regarding health and safety at work.

Waste disposal

All health and social care workplaces should have a written policy on disposing waste, providing guidance on all aspects of disposal, including for the disposal of pharmaceutical and cytotoxic waste. These guidelines are subject to continual updating. Waste disposal bags are colour-coded: yellow bags for clinical waste, black bags for household waste, and special cardboard boxes or bins for glass and aerosols. Changes in waste disposal procedures are made from time to time, and it is important that nurses are familiar with these.

Handling and processing linen

Used and soiled linen must be handled with care. Dirty linen should not be sorted in living or eating areas or placed on the furniture or floor. Fouled and infected linen should be placed in water-soluble bags, which can be put directly into a washing machine and cleaned without exposing staff to further risk of contamination. Staff should always wear protective clothing such as disposable plastic aprons and gloves when handling soiled and infected linen. Hands must always be washed following a six-step (or similar) technique, as described earlier.

Managing blood and bodily fluids

All health and social care settings have policies and procedures for dealing with spillages. These policies should always be consulted and used.

Decontaminating equipment

Decontamination is the combination of cleaning, disinfection and sterilisation (Royal College of Nursing, 2004) used to ensure that medical equipment is reusable. Reusable equipment must be decontaminated thoroughly after use on a patient. Safe decontamination is essential if the effective control of infection is to be achieved.

Thorough cleaning is required before disinfection and sterilisation. Cleaning with water and detergent removes visible contamination but does not necessarily destroy all micro-organisms. Disinfection using chemical agents or heat reduces the organisms' ability to infect but does not destroy all viruses and bacteria; therefore, disinfection should not be used as a substitute for sterilisation, which is a way of ensuring that all microorganisms are removed.

The use of disinfectants is governed by the Control of Substances Hazardous to Health (COSHH) regulations; employers have an obligation to employees to provide the necessary information and education about hazardous substances. Most Trusts have access to a central sterilising department where all reusable equipment can be sterilised. These local sterile services departments (SSDs) have to meet European standards of safety. If access to an SSD is not possible, pre-sterilised, single-use disposable items must be used. Some GP practices and private clinics use bench-top sterilisers; these must be maintained following the guidance given by the Medical Devices Agency (2000).

Healthcare-associated infection

Healthcare-associated infections (HCAIs) are often caused by bacteria that have developed a resistance to certain or even all antibiotics. These bacteria include MRSA and extended-spectrum beta-lactamases (ESBLs). Resistance to antibiotics is an inevitable consequence of antibiotic use. Penicillin resistance was first documented in the 1960s (Royal College of Nursing, 2005). Resistance does not mean necessarily that antibiotics have been used inappropriately or overused: it may be that there are now more vulnerable people with multiple medical problems and that there is an increased use of invasive procedures and devices. To control HCAIs, adherence to up-to-date, evidence-based infection control policies is essential. In 2000, the National Audit Office estimated that hospital infection is a primary factor in a significant number (possibly as many as 5000) of deaths per year (National Audit Office, 2000). This problem is escalating: death rates from MRSA increased 15-fold between 1993 and 2002. MRSA infection has serious consequences and is life-threatening. Treatment is limited because MRSA is sensitive to only a restricted range of antibiotics.

Recap Questions

1. What are the general principles of infection control?
2. How should you wash your hands in order to minimise the spread of infection?
3. How should you dispose of sharps?

Summary

Helping a patient to maintain their personal hygiene is one of the most important roles in nursing. All nurses are involved with this, whether they are giving the direct care themselves or supervising and/or monitoring others to do so. Unlike other staff, nursing staff are often with patients 24 hours a day, and therefore nurses are in a unique position to continually assess and monitor a patient's condition. To promote and/or maintain a person's hygiene requires skilled nursing practice and involves many aspects of holistic care. Lack of attention to this most fundamental aspect of care can and does have disastrous effects, as can be seen by the case studies in this chapter and in recent media reports. Nurses can work in partnership with other health and social care professionals to place the patient at the centre of care. Patients can be enabled to have some control over their life, disease, condition or disability, giving them dignity and independence. As seen in this chapter, aids and equipment are available for patients; it is essential that those assisting a patient to maintain their personal hygiene can access such aids and/or help the patient and their carers to obtain them.

We have known since the time of Florence Nightingale that dirt spreads disease. Handwashing and keeping patients and the environment clean and free from germs are simple tasks and the responsibility of all health and social care practitioners. Research from Bristol University has shown that plastic aprons attract over 80% more bacteria than aprons that carry a static charge (Hoban, 2005), proving the importance of changing aprons between patients and between procedures. However, protective clothing, including gloves, can never replace the need for basic hygiene procedures.

Waste must be disposed of appropriately: general waste in general waste bags and clinical waste in clinical waste bags. Bins must be emptied before they overflow. Clinical waste must be disposed of correctly.

Key Points

1. Assisting and overseeing washing and dressing of patients is a key nursing skill. The effect of helping a patient with their personal hygiene should never be underestimated.

2. All health and social care professionals can contribute so that patients can achieve their maximum levels of independence in meeting their hygiene requirements.

3. Paying attention to a patient's oral health and being able to recognise the signs of oral cancer are important.

4. Control of infection is paramount to the patient's recovery. Nurses play a vital role in ensuring infection is not transmitted.

5. All clinical waste and dirty linen must be disposed of in a safe way. Health and social care practitioners have a duty to be familiar with and to follow the appropriate policies and procedures of their workplace.

Points for debate

Now that you have come to the end of this chapter here are a few points that you may wish to think about when you are in practice. You may wish to discuss these with your work colleagues or fellow students.

Washing and dressing patients is not a part of a qualified nurse's role. This should be left to health care assistants.

I'm not clearing up vomit: I'm a nurse, not a cleaner.

Relatives should help patients to wash and dress themselves.

Links to Other Chapters

Chapter 1   What is caring?
Chapter 2   Dignity and privacy
Chapter 6   Fluid balance and continence care
Chapter 8   Pressure ulcers
Chapter 9   Rehabilitation and self-care

Further reading

Gilchrist, C (1999) *Turning Your Back on Us*. London: Age Concern.

Health Advisory Service 2000 (1999) *Not Because They Are Old*. London: Health Advisory Service.

References

Bates, S (1971) *Practical Paediatric Nursing*. Oxford: Blackwell.

Channel 4 (2005) *Dispatches: Undercover Angels*. 21 January 2005.

Department of Health (2001) *National Service Framework for Older People*. London: The Stationery Office.

Department of Health (2003a) *Essence of Care: Patient-Focused Benchmarks for Clinical Governance*. London: The Stationery Office.

Department of Health (2003b) *A Practical Guide for Disabled People or Carers*. London: The Stationery Office.

Dilks, A, Green, J and Brown, S (2005) The use and benefits of compression stocking aids. *Nursing Times* **101**, 32–33.

Gilchrist, C (1999) *Turning Your Back on Us*. London: Age Concern.

Health Advisory Service 2000 (1999) *Not Because They Are Old*. London: Health Advisory Service.

Hoban, V (2005) In short supply. *Nursing Times* **101**, 24–30.

Lewin, J and Reed, C (1998) *Creative Problem Solving in Occupational Therapy*. New York: Lippincott-Raven.

Medical Devices Agency (2000) *Guidance on the Purchase, Operation and Maintenance of Vacuum Bench Top Sterilisers*. London: The Stationery Office.

National Audit Office (2000) *The Management and Control of Hospital Acquired Infection in Acute NHS Trusts in England*. London: The Stationery Office.

Orem, D (1991) *Nursing: Concepts of Practice*, 4th edn. St Louis, MO: Mosby.

Roper, N, Logan, W and Tierney, A (2000) *The Roper Logan Tierney Model of Nursing*. Edinburgh: Churchill Livingstone.

Royal College of Nursing (2004) *Good Practice in Infection Control*. London: Royal College of Nursing.

Royal College of Nursing (2005) *Methicillin-Resistant Staphylococcus aureus (MRSA).* London: Royal College of Nursing.

Sergeant, H (2003) The truth about NHS hospitals. *Daily Telegraph*, 1 December 2003.

Sloane, P, Hoeffer, B, Mitchell, M *et al.* (2004) Effect of person-centred showering and the towel bath on bathing associated aggression, agitation and discomfort in nursing home residents with dementia: a randomised controlled trial. *Journal of the American Geriatrics Society* **52**, 1795–1804.

Strachan-Bennett, S (2004) Bedbathing can reduce aggressive incidents. *Nursing Times* **100**, 9.

Weller, B (1971) *Baillière's Nursing Dictionary*. London: Baillière Tindall.

Chapter 5
Nutrition

Case Study

Mrs Emily Jones, a 76-year-old woman, was admitted to hospital after breaking her hip. She has had surgery and is now to undergo rehabilitation to get her mobilising so she can return to her sheltered accommodation. On admission, Mrs Jones' nutritional state is poor: she is undernourished and underweight. The dietician has suggested giving Mrs Jones a high-protein diet with nutritional supplements. The nurse is responsible for ensuring that Mrs Jones receives this diet.

The dietician returns after a week to assess Mrs Jones' nutritional status. The dietician observes that Mrs Jones has not been weighed and that her nutritional chart has not been completed. There are several entries on the chart indicating that Mrs Jones has been refusing her diet; in other areas, nothing is noted on the chart. There are few recordings on the fluid balance chart to show that the patient had any of the prescribed nutritional supplements.

The dietician consults the nurse who is caring for Mrs Jones. The nurse states that they have not had time to weigh the patient and then proceeds to carry out this request. Findings reveal that Mrs Jones has actually lost weight. When asked about the patient refusing her diet, the nurse says: 'Her tray is placed in front of her, but she rarely eats much of it.' With regard to the patient taking her nutritional supplements, the nurse states that this is variable, depending on whether Mrs Jones likes the flavour. After chatting with Mrs Jones, the dietician finds out the main reason for her not eating her meal: she cannot see the tray very well because her eyesight is poor. When she asked for help with feeding, the nurse was too busy.

Introduction

Consider the scenario above and reflect on your reactions to it. It does not paint a good picture regarding the role of the nurse in ensuring the patient receives adequate nutrition in hospital. Good nutrition in hospital is essential to helping patients recover from illness and surgery. How can this example of poor nutritional care be improved? This chapter considers the important aspects of good nutrition. We identify essential nutrients, define what is meant by a 'balanced diet 'and explain how body weight can be measured. The important role of nutritional screening is discussed, and some of the problems associated with hospital food and how these can be overcome are addressed. Personal preferences can also affect what we eat, and such issues are covered in this chapter. The process of feeding a patient is outlined in order to ensure that incidents like that of Mrs Jones are not repeated. Finally, some patients have difficulty swallowing (dysphagia), usually following a cerebral vascular accident, and we consider this problem in this chapter.

LEARNING OBJECTIVES

By the end of this chapter you will be able to:

1. Identify essential nutrients and their dietary sources and explain what is meant by the term 'balanced diet' with reference to the concept of energy balance
2. Outline the factors that can influence what we choose to eat
3. Recognise the importance of nutritional assessment and screening and discuss what factors should be included in a nutritional assessment tool
4. Discuss the problems associated with hospital food and summarise how these problems may be overcome
5. Describe the process of feeding a patient and indicate other methods of feeding
6. Show an awareness of the problem of dysphagia and how the nurse can deal with this problem

The importance of good nutrition

Nutrition refers to the process of taking in food, which is then broken down in the body to produce the energy required by all living cells to maintain their structure and function. These living cells require a constant supply of nutrients to survive. In other words, if we do not eat we will not survive.

Consequently, good nutrition is essential to promote health and wellbeing. It also plays a major part in assisting patients to recover from trauma, surgery and disease. Paradoxically, there is growing evidence that malnutrition among hospital patients is on the increase. Malnutrition can be defined as a state of nutrition in which a deficiency, excess or imbalance of energy, protein or other nutrients, including minerals and vitamins, causes measurable adverse effects on a person's body function and clinical outcome (Royal College of Physicians, 2002). An individual's quality of life can be adversely affected by malnutrition: lack of nutrients leads eventually to malfunction of all body systems, as the body cells rely on the fuel and energy that is derived from food.

Malnutrition in patients has been documented as being a problem in hospitals. Several research studies have found that patients do not receive enough food, and in some wards up to 60% of patients do not eat enough calories or protein (Bond, 1997). Poor nutritional status is linked to delayed recovery and adverse outcomes of illness and injury. For example, Horan and Coad (2000) found that lack of nutrition can increase patients' physical and psychological stress, which affects almost every body system. Healing rates can be slowed down, leading to a lengthened hospital stay – with concomitant financial implications. The need for appropriate nutritional screening is essential to reduce the growing problem of many patients, particularly older people, being undernourished.

> Revision
>
> Before reading the next section, you need to revise the essential nutrients of the body and the dietary sources of each.

Essential nutrients

Nutrients are needed by the body for fuel and energy. Some nutrients are considered to be essential and must be ingested in adequate amounts to meet the body's needs. These essential nutrients fall into three main food categories: carbohydrates, fats and proteins. The body also requires certain vitamins and minerals. We will now consider these essential nutrients in more detail.

Carbohydrates

Carbohydrates consist of simple (sugars) and complex (starches and fibre) carbohydrates. The two types of carbohydrate are metabolised (broken down) slightly differently within the body.

Sugars are the simplest carbohydrates. They are water-soluble and are produced naturally by both animals and plants. Depending on their chemical structure, sugars can be monosaccharides (single molecules) or disaccharides (double molecules). Monosaccharides include fructose, galactose and glucose, the latter being the most plentiful.

Most sugars occur naturally in plants, especially fruits, sugar cane and sugar beet. Lactose (a combination of glucose and galactose) is also found in milk. Sugars such as table sugar, molasses and corn syrup can be processed or refined; this means that they have been extracted and concentrated from natural sources. These processed sugars are added to foods such as biscuits, cakes, sweets, ice-cream, soft drinks and breakfast cereals.

Starches are insoluble, non-sweet carbohydrates. They are polysaccharides composed of branched chains of up to hundreds of glucose molecules. Most starches occur in plants, such as grains, legumes (such as peas and beans) and potatoes. Like sugars, starches can be processed to make foods such as bread, flour, puddings and cereals.

Fibre is a complex carbohydrate derived from plants. Humans are unable to digest fibre, although it provides important roughage, or bulk, in the diet. This roughage helps to satisfy the appetite and assists the digestive tract to function well and eliminate waste products. Fibre occurs in the skin, seeds and pulp of many fruits and vegetables and in the outer layer of grains and bran.

By eating carbohydrates derived from natural sources, you are more likely to ingest other vital nutrients such as vitamins and minerals not found in processed food; for example, oranges contain vitamin C and bananas contain potassium. Processed carbohydrates are relatively low in nutrients in relation to the large number of calories they contain. Consequently, they are often referred to as 'empty calories'. Similarly, alcoholic drinks contain significant amounts of carbohydrates but are another source of empty calories.

Proteins

Every body cell contains protein, and about three-quarters of our body solids are protein (Kozier et al., 2004). Proteins are organic substances consisting of amino acids, the chemical subunits of proteins. There are 20 different amino acids; eight of these cannot be produced in the body and are therefore an essential aspect of the diet – they are known as *essential amino acids*. Non-essential amino acids can be produced in the body from amino acids derived from the diet.

Proteins may be complete or incomplete. Complete proteins contain all the essential amino acids and also some non-essential amino acids. Examples of complete proteins include meat, poultry, fish, dairy products and eggs. Some animal proteins are described as partially complete proteins, as they contain less than the required amount of essential amino acids and thus cannot support continued body growth. Examples of partially complete proteins include gelatine and the milk protein casein. Incomplete proteins contain one or more essential amino acids and are usually found in vegetables. It is important that patients are given complete proteins in their diet, especially if a high-protein diet is ordered, as in the case study of Mrs Jones at the start of this chapter.

To think about

Before you read the next section, consider your own diet, and that of your family, particularly in relation to your fat intake. You may like to record the amount and type of fat you consume in a typical week.

Lipids

Lipids are organic substances that appear greasy and are insoluble in water but are soluble in alcohol and ether (Kozier et al., 2004). Fats are lipids that are solid at room temperature, while oils are lipids that are in liquid form at room temperature. The terms 'fat' and 'lipid' tend to be used interchangeably, but the correct term is 'lipid'.

The basic structure of most lipids is three fatty acids consisting of carbon chains and hydrogen plus glycerol. The end product is called a triglyceride (Figure 5.1).

Glycerol consists of carbon, hydrogen and oxygen atoms. Fatty acids can be saturated or unsaturated, depending on the number of hydrogen atoms they contain. Saturated fatty acids are those in which all carbon atoms are filled to capacity (hence the term 'saturated') with hydrogen; an example is butyric acid found in butter. An unsaturated fatty acid can accommodate more hydrogen atoms than it currently does. It has at least two carbon atoms that are not attached to a hydrogen atom; instead, there is a double bond between the two carbon atoms. Fatty acids with one double bond are called monounsaturated fatty acids, and those with more than one double bond are called polyunsaturated fatty acids. Linoleic acid is an example of a polyunsaturated fatty acid found in vegetable oil.

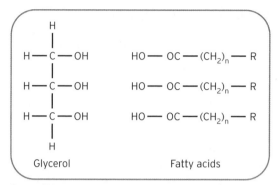

Figure 5.1 Basic structure of a triglyceride

Table 5.1 summarises the different lipid types.

Table 5.1 Types of lipid and food examples

Lipid	Examples
Saturated triglyceride	Butter, meat, full-fat dairy products
Unsaturated triglycerides	
Monounsaturated	Olive oil, nuts, avocados
Polyunsaturated	Vegetable oil, salmon, trout

There is a lot of talk nowadays about 'good' and 'bad' fats. So how do these fit into the above description of fats/lipids? Foods can contain four types of lipid: saturated, polyunsaturated, monounsaturated and hydrogenated. (Hydrogenated fats are also known as 'trans-fats'; they are made by processing vegetable oil into a solid fat through heating.) The percentage of these different fats varies between different foods. For example, meat is higher in saturated fat than polyunsaturated fat, whereas oily fish is high in monounsaturated fat.

Saturated fats and hydrogenated fats are considered to be 'bad' fats. Saturated fat comes from animal sources such as meat, butter and cream. Eating a lot of saturated fat increases the blood cholesterol level, which in turn contributes to damage to the cardiovascular system. Nutritionists recommend that 30% of our total daily calories should come from fat and that less than one-third of that amount (i.e. 10% of daily calorie intake) should come from saturated fats.

The 'good' fats are the monounsaturated and polyunsaturated fats. These fats do not raise the blood cholesterol level. The lipids found in avocados, olive oil, rapeseed oil, peanuts and almonds are examples of monounsaturated fats. Nutritionists advise that 10–15% of our total calorie daily intake should come from monounsaturated fats.

Examples of foods containing polyunsaturated fats are corn oil, mayonnaise and margarine. These fats should form less than 10% of our total daily calorie intake.

Some examples of 'good' and 'bad' fats are given in Exhibit 5.1.

'Good' fats	'Bad' fats
Monounsaturated fats	**Saturated fats**
✦ Olives	✦ Butter
✦ Nuts	✦ Meat
✦ Seeds	✦ Full-fat dairy products
✦ Avocado	
✦ Oils from the above	**Trans-fats**
	✦ Hard margarines
Polyunsaturated fats	✦ Packaged cakes and biscuits
✦ Trout	
✦ Salmon	
✦ Mackerel	
✦ Herring	

Exhibit 5.1 Food examples of 'good' and 'bad' fats

Cholesterol is a fat-like substance found in foods of animal origin. It also occurs naturally in the body. Large quantities of cholesterol are present in cell membranes (Kozier *et al.*, 2004). Most of the body's cholesterol is made in the liver, but some is also absorbed from the diet from milk, egg yolk and offal such as liver. The main function of cholesterol is to create **bile acids** and to synthesise steroid hormones. Too much cholesterol in the diet contributes to various health problems, such as heart disease and diabetes. The recommendation is that no more than 300 milligrams a day of fat should come from cholesterol.

Vitamins

Vitamins are organic substances needed in small amounts to **catalyse** metabolic processes. Vitamins cannot be produced in the body and therefore have to be ingested. A lack of vitamins in the diet causes metabolic deficits. An example of a vitamin deficiency is scurvy: historically, sailors developed this disorder as a result of a lack of fresh fruit and vegetables, and therefore, vitamin C, in their diet.

Vitamins are classified as water-soluble or fat-soluble (Exhibit 5.2). The body cannot store water-soluble vitamins; therefore, a daily supply of these is required from the diet. The body can store fat-soluble vitamins, but there is a limit to the amounts of vitamins E and K that can be stored; therefore, again a steady intake of these vitamins is necessary. Vitamins are affected by food processing, storage and preparation and thus vitamin content is highest in fresh foods that are eaten as soon as possible after harvest.

Bile acids are the digestive components of bile. Bile acids aid digestion by emulsifying fats, thus lowering their surface tension and breaking them into tiny droplets.

Catalysis is the speeding up of a chemical reaction with a catalyst, a substance that is chemically unchanged at the end of the reaction.

Water-soluble vitamins	Fat-soluble vitamins
+ Vitamin C	**+** Vitamin A
+ Vitamin B complex	**+** Vitamin D
+ B1 (thiamine)	**+** Vitamin E
+ B2 (riboflavin)	**+** Vitamin K
+ B3 (niacin)	
+ B6 (pyridoxine)	
+ B9 (folic acid)	
+ B12 (cobalamin)	

Exhibit 5.2 Essential vitamins

Minerals

Minerals are inorganic compounds that exist in the body as free **ions**. A good example is sodium chloride. When sodium chloride enters the body and dissolves in water, it dissociates (splits) into its constituent ions:

Sodium chloride	Sodium + chloride
NaCl	$Na^+ + Cl^-$

The plus and minus signs show that the sodium ion (Na^+) carries a positive charge and the chloride ion (Cl^-) carries a negative charge.

There are two categories of minerals: macrominerals and microminerals. Macrominerals are required daily in amounts over 100 mg and include calcium, phosphorus, sodium, potassium, magnesium, chloride and sulphur. Microminerals are needed in daily amounts of less than 100 mg and include iron, zinc, manganese, iodine, fluoride, copper, cobalt, chromium and selenium (Kozier *et al.*, 2004).

Recap Questions

1. What are the essential nutrients that we require to provide fuel and energy for our body?
2. What are meant by the terms 'good fats' and 'bad fats'?
3. Why are vitamins and minerals important in our diet?

Nutritional requirements

To obtain the essential nutrients required for a healthy body, a person must consume a daily diet composed of a variety of foods containing the nutrients outlined above. The term 'balanced diet' denotes the need to eat different types of food containing carbohydrates, proteins and fats, such as milk, meat, fish, fruit, vegetables and grains. If a variety of intake from each of the food groups is consumed, this should ensure the daily requirements of vitamins and minerals.

An **ion** is an atom or molecule that carries an electrical charge – either positive or negative.

A person is compelled by hunger to eat enough energy-providing nutrients to satisfy their energy needs. However, in order to be able to eat, other factors are also important, such as the availability, quantity, presentation and quality of food. These factors either encourage or reduce the desire and opportunity to eat. During rapid periods of growth, such as in infancy and adolescence, nutritional needs increase. Conversely, older people need fewer calories and may make or require dietary changes in order to reduce the risk of coronary heart disease, osteoporosis and hypertension. Food requirements differ between males and females due to their body composition and reproductive functions. Males have a larger muscle mass and hence require more calories and protein than females. Females, on the other hand, require more iron due to blood loss during menstruation, while pregnancy and lactation prompt the need for more calories and fluids, respectively.

The Balance of Good Health Plate model

Several models have been developed to help determine the quantity of each type of food that should be eaten on a daily basis. The Balance of Good Health Plate model is one such example (Figure 5.2). This model denotes the quantities and types of carbohydrate, protein and fat that should be consumed to help maintain a healthy, balanced diet.

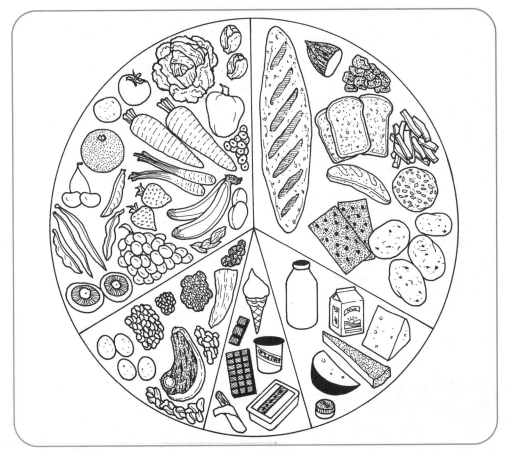

Figure 5.2 Balance of Good Heath Plate model
Source: Food Standards Agency

To think about

Next time you are giving a meal to a patient, try to identify whether you think the quantity of different food types is similar to, or based on, the Balance of Good Health Plate model. If not, why not? You may wish to discuss your findings with your work colleagues.

Energy requirements are met chiefly by carbohydrates (55%) and fats (30%); about 15% comes from proteins. Energy needs for an individual are determined by:

+ The amount of energy needed to maintain involuntary body functions at rest, for example breathing production and secretion of hormones (this is known as the basal metabolic rate – BMR)
+ The amount of energy needed to metabolise food
+ The person's physical activity

The amount of energy that nutrients supply to the body is termed their calorific value, which is measured in calories. A calorie (variously abbreviated to c, cal and kcal) can be described as a unit of heat energy. Different food types provide different amounts of calories. For example, a gram of either carbohydrate or protein provides 4 kcal, while a gram of fat provides 9 kcal and a gram of alcohol provides 7 kcal. Energy values can also be measured in the metric measurement kilojoules (kJ). Although most nutritionists tend to describe foods in terms of their calorific value, it is worth knowing that 1 calorie equals 4.18 kJ.

In order to maintain a suitable body weight, there needs to be an equal balance between the energy derived from food and the amount of energy used by the body. This is referred to as the person's energy balance. If food intake exceeds energy expenditure, then the body weight tends to increase. This is becoming an increasingly bad problem in developed countries due to the sedentary lifestyle many people employ, leading to an increase in overweight and obese individuals and the associated health problems.

Conversely, if food intake is not exceeded by energy expenditure, then the person is likely to lose weight.

Recap Questions

1. What is the Good Health Plate model?
2. What factors determine the energy needs of an individual?
3. What is a calorie?

Factors affecting nutritional choice

To think about

When you are next planning or eating a meal, try to identify the factors that influence your choice of foods. You may like to list them and compare them with the factors outlined below.

The nutritional content of food is important when planning a diet. However, individual food preferences and habits can have a major impact on what a person eats. These habits may be influenced by some or all of the following (Kozier *et al.*, 2004):

+ *Culture:* traditional foods such as rice in Asian countries and pasta in Italy and Italian-influenced regions continue to be eaten long after other customs are abandoned. However, it should be remembered that food preferences are not always related to culture and can differ greatly between individuals.

+ *Knowledge:* a person's knowledge about food may affect what they choose to eat. For example, many people have reduced their intake of animal fat as this is thought to be a major risk factor in cardiovascular disease.

+ *Personal preferences:* most people like and dislike certain foods, whether simply because they do or don't like the taste or based on associations with that food. For example, a child whose favourite grandparent always gives them apple crumble and custard is likely to enjoy this pudding, whereas another child whose strict neighbour occasionally offers a certain type of biscuit is likely to avoid such food.

+ *Religion:* the nurse should be sensitive to patients' religious dietary practices. For example, certain faiths prohibit the consumption of meat, tea, coffee or alcohol.

+ *Lifestyle:* people who work long hours tend to eat convenience foods, and those working shifts have to adapt mealtimes accordingly. Socioeconomic factors also affect what a person eats; for example, people on a low income may not be able to afford good-quality meat and fresh vegetables. Conversely, people on a higher income may eat more protein and fat.

+ *Health:* this can greatly affect a person's eating habits. Difficulty in swallowing (dysphagia) can prevent a person eating adequately. Diseases of the digestive tract can adversely affect appetite and nutritional status. Disorders affecting food metabolism such as diabetes mellitus can also influence food intake.

+ *Alcohol consumption:* drinking alcohol can contribute to weight gain through the addition of extra calories and the effect of alcohol on fat metabolism. A small amount of alcohol is converted directly into fat, and the remainder is converted into **acetate** by the liver. This acetate, when released into the bloodstream, is used instead of fat for energy; the fat is then stored. Excessive alcohol can also lead to nutritional deficiencies by replacing food in a person's diet and depressing the appetite.

+ *Psychological factors:* extreme weight loss and weight gain are associated with depression, stress and loneliness. Severe psychophysiological conditions such as anorexia nervosa and bulimia can lead to severe weight loss, particularly in teenage girls.

Acetate is the salt of acetic acid.

Consider Case study 5.1.

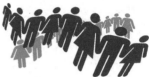

> ## Case Study 5.1
>
> Shirley Jones is a 15-year-old school girl admitted to the ward with weight loss. The cause of the weight loss is to be investigated, although anorexia nervosa is suspected. She looks pale and very thin. Her nutritional intake is being monitored strictly to identify her daily food intake. You note that Shirley has not eaten any food for breakfast, lunch or dinner. When you ask Shirley about her food intake, she says she did not like the food that she was given, and yet she had been involved in ordering it the day before.
>
> What would you do next?

You would need to report your findings to the nurse in charge. It is important to ask Shirley what her food preferences are and then to order these for her. If Shirley has not yet seen a dietician, then she must be referred urgently for dietary advice. It is important to do regular nutritional assessments with Shirley to ascertain her dietary intake and any weight gain or loss. Shirley's psychological state also needs to be observed. She will probably be referred to a psychiatrist or psychologist who specialises in eating disorders.

It is important for the nurse to be aware of how the factors outlined above may influence a patient's choice of food. For example, it is important to identify what the patient normally eats and to ensure cultural and religious preferences are taken into consideration when offering food in hospital. Patients with depression may need encouragement with their diet in terms of the type and amount of food consumed.

> ## Recap Questions
>
> 1. What factors affect nutrition?
> 2. Why is it important for the nurse to know about these factors?

Nutritional assessment

The main aim of carrying out a nutritional assessment is to identify patients who are at risk of developing malnutrition and those who already have a poor nutritional status. The responsibility of carrying out this assessment is usually shared between the doctor, dietician and nurse. A nutritional assessment involves nutritional screening, which is usually done by the nurse; if deemed necessary, a comprehensive nutritional assessment is then performed by the dietician, sometimes with involvement from the doctor.

Nutritional screening

The process of nutritional screening involves identifying patients at risk of malnutrition and patients who are already malnourished. Patients who are identified as being at moderate to high risk are generally referred to the dietician for a more detailed assessment.

The nutritional assessment can by carried out by the nurse during the admission process of history-taking and then when monitoring and recording vital signs. However, it is important not to bombard the patient with too many questions in the first instance.

Nutritional assessment should be an ongoing procedure, as changes can occur in the patient's physical and psychological state that can impinge on the patient's nutritional status. For example, a patient undergoing major surgery may require more high-calorific foods to aid the healing process. Likewise, a patient who has liver disease will probably be given a diet low in protein, as liver disease can impair the body's ability to break down protein. The Audit Commission's (2001) survey of hospitals in England and Wales revealed that 77% of trusts have a nutritional screening protocol in place and that screening is carried out by nurses. The survey also found, however, that less than half of these trusts review patients' nutrition weekly to check that any adjustments to the patients' changing needs are recognised and acted upon (Bradley and Rees, 2003).

To think about

Have you seen nutritional screening taking place when you are in practice, and are at-risk patients reviewed weekly? If not, why not? You may wish to discuss your findings with your work colleagues.

Measuring body weight

Generally nutritionists and other health professionals talk about an ideal body weight for an individual to achieve optimal health. There are many standardised percentile/ideal weight charts that can be used to help determine a person's ideal weight. The nurse needs to remember, however, that these charts are only a guide.

The body mass index (BMI) is used regularly as a weight monitoring tool and is thought to be a reliable indicator of a person's healthy weight. The BMI is used as part of the nutritional assessment process. The BMI applies to people over 18 years of age and is an indicator of changes in body fat stores and whether a person's weight is appropriate for their height. The BMI can also provide a useful estimate of malnutrition. The BMI is calculated by dividing the person's weight in kilograms (kg) by the square of the height in metres:

BMI = weight/height^2

For example, to calculate the BMI of a person who weighs 60 kg and is 1.69 m tall:

60/(1.69 × 1.69) = 21

A person with a BMI of less than 18 is considered to have a level of nutrition that is inadequate to provide the essential nutrients discussed earlier (Perry, 2004). A person with a BMI of less than 20 is considered to be thin. A BMI of 20-25 is considered normal. A person with a

BMI of 25-29.9 is overweight, and a person with a BMI over 30 is classed as obese. Using this definition, more than half the people in the UK are overweight or obese (Jarvis and Rubin, 2003). A person with a BMI over 40 is considered to be grossly or morbidly obese.

The BMI must be used with caution in patients with fluid retention, athletes and elderly people (Kozier *et al.*, 2004). Furthermore, it is important to remember that weight can have limitations as a nutritional index. Equipment may not be available to weigh immobile patients, and many scales are not regularly serviced and calibrated. Weighing cannot differentiate muscle from fat and does not take account of overall body size. Measuring the waist circumference is considered by some to be a more reliable indicator of body fat, particularly in relation to central obesity, where the majority of body fat occurs around the waist and central abdomen. This measurement is increasingly being used to assess weight in patients with diabetes mellitus and other metabolic disorders, where central obesity has a detrimental impact on the condition.

To think about

Obesity is increasing in today's society. Why do you think this is? What factors are contributing to this increasing problem? Discuss this with your work colleagues, family and friends.

In addition to the BMI, the nutritional assessment tool includes factors that are associated with the risk of malnutrition. These are considered below.

Factors affecting the physical ability to eat

+ *Dexterity:* it is important to assess whether the person has the ability to actually feed themselves.
+ *Difficulty swallowing (dysphagia):* this condition may be caused by a stroke or carcinoma of the mouth or throat.
+ *Dental problems:* patients with dental problems or wearing ill-fitting dentures may have difficulty with chewing.

Disease and illness

+ *Mental condition:* any deterioration in mental state or conscious level may affect the person's ability to eat and drink.
+ *Digestive tract functioning:* nausea, vomiting, diarrhoea and constipation interfere with a person's nutritional intake. Patients who have undergone surgery on the gastrointestinal tract may experience problems with eating. Conditions affecting the gastrointestinal tract, such as intestinal obstruction and Crohn's disease, also impair nutritional intake.
+ *Malignant disease:* there is an association of cancer with weight loss, particularly if the cancer is in a part of the digestive tract, such as the stomach or the intestine, which ultimately affects the intake and digestion of food.

+ *Neurological conditions:* disorders affecting mental state and coordination, such as Parkinson's disease and multiple sclerosis, may affect the patient's food intake.

+ *Major trauma:* patients who have undergone surgery following major trauma are at high risk of malnutrition and usually require a high-protein diet to help repair the body.

Other factors

+ *Weight:* the patient's current weight should be recorded, and any changes to weight should be noted. In particular, recent weight loss should be discussed with the patient in order to identify the amount of weight lost. Patients who are thin or look emaciated are at a greater risk of malnutrition. Weight loss of less than 5% in the previous 6 months is not usually significant; however, weight loss of 5-9% is significant if the patient is already malnourished, that of 10-20% is clinically significant and needs immediate intervention, and more than 20% weight loss requires long-term support (Nicol *et al.*, 2004).

+ *Appetite:* it is important to identify any changes to appetite or whether eating habits have altered recently. Patients with poor appetite are at greater risk of malnutrition.

+ *Pressure ulcers:* poor nutritional status makes the patient more susceptible to developing and healing of pressure ulcers. If the patient's skin appears dry and scaling, this may be an indication of dehydration and related malnutrition.

+ *Medication history:* some drugs have effects on nutrition; for example, aspirin can cause nausea and gastritis, diuretics can cause diarrhoea, nausea and vomiting, some antihypertensive drugs cause mouth dryness, nausea, vomiting, diarrhoea and constipation, and some antidepressants cause nausea, vomiting, malabsorption and diarrhoea.

Most nutritional assessment tools involve a scoring system that allocates a score for each of the risk factors outlined above. The total score identifies whether the patient is at risk. Depending on the assessment tool used, a high score is generally associated with a higher risk of malnutrition.

High-risk patients should be referred to a dietician immediately. All patients must be assessed within 24 hours of admission (Nicol *et al.*, 2004; Perry, 2004), and the frequency of further assessments should be ascertained based on the outcome of the initial assessment. If the patient is considered to be at high risk, then the assessment may need to be repeated after 48 hours (Nicol *et al.*, 2004).

Consider Case study 5.2.

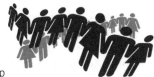

Case Study 5.2

Mrs Jessop is 79 years old. She is malnourished and has been prescribed nutritional supplement drinks by the dietician to help her gain weight. Mrs Jessop's daughters are concerned about her. They ask you whether their mother has been given any supplements over the day, as nothing has been recorded on her fluid or nutritional chart. Mrs Jessop cannot remember whether she has been given any nutritional supplements.

What do you do next?

You need to find out from the nursing staff who were caring for Mrs Jessop before you came on duty whether she has been given any supplements. If supplements have been given, you should identify why they have not been recorded on either the nutritional or the fluid balance chart and then record them on both charts immediately. If she has not been given the supplements, then you need to identify and discuss the reasons why with the nurse in charge. Mrs Jessop's dietary intake is poor, and therefore it is very important that she receives her food supplements. If her dietary intake is not recorded properly, this may lead to an inaccurate assessment of Mrs Jessop's dietary intake and will not contribute to any weight gain. You also need to inform the nurse in charge of Mrs Jessop's daughters' concerns as to whether Mrs Jessop has been given her food supplements.

Ongoing monitoring of nutritional status is important, as many patients experience nutritional deterioration during illness and treatment (Perry, 2004). At-risk patients should be weighed at least weekly. Accurate recording of food intake on the appropriate charts is essential in order to monitor nutritional stats on a daily basis. Liaison with colleagues such as dieticians, nutritional nurse specialists and hospital catering staff will help to ensure that patients receive the necessary nutritional support (Perry, 2004).

It is important to note that good nutritional support has been linked with shorter length of hospital stay and improvements in quality of life (Green, 1999).

Recap Questions

1. What is the main aim of a nutritional assessment?
2. What does the process of nutritional screening involve?
3. What is meant by body mass index?
4. What other factors need to be considered when carrying out a nutritional assessment?

Nutrition in hospital

There has been criticism of hospital food for the past 40 years. Girling (2002) suggests this ongoing problem of malnutrition in hospitals has been understood but effectively ignored. Perry (1997) describes the problem as a 'hard nut to crack'.

A number of factors can influence nutrition in hospital (Exhibit 5.3). Food in hospitals was a major target for improvement in the government's NHS Plan (Department of Health, 2000), and the NHS launched the Better Hospital Food project (NHS Estates, 2002) as a consequence. This initiative was introduced to consider ways of improving hospital food in terms of presentation, quality and food types. The project team included nurses, NHS and private sector dieticians, caterers, civil servants and the food critic and broadcaster Lloyd Grossman.

Improved nutrition has several positive benefits, as pointed out by the British Association for Parenteral and Enteral Nutrition (2001). These benefits include financial savings by reducing hospital-acquired infections, improving wound healing, improving rehabilitation and reducing length of hospital stay, all of which equate to a better quality of hospital stay for patients. This notion is endorsed further in a report on catering facilities in hospitals in Wales (Audit Commission, 2001) where great emphasis was placed on the need to serve nutritious appetising food to help patients' recovery.

Problems with the food

+ Poor quality
+ Poor quantity
+ Lack of variety
+ Poor general appearance (bland and unappetising)

System of supplying the food

+ Inadequate budget spent on patients' food
+ Poor monitoring of whether patients get appropriate food choices
+ Poor positioning of food, so patients cannot reach their meals
+ No system for monitoring and reporting whether food has been eaten
+ Lack of responsibility for taking action when patients do not eat their meals
+ Timing of food availability
+ Gaining access to special foods and meals that people enjoy eating when ill
+ Staff removing meals before patients have had a chance to eat

Exhibit 5.3 Factors influencing nutrition in hospital
Adapted from Bradley and Rees (2003)

To think about

Do you think patients always receive nutritious food when in hospital? Have you seen examples of any of the factors outlined in Exhibit 5.3? You may wish to discuss your findings with your work colleagues.

Improving nutrition in hospital

As a result of the Better Hospital Food project, essential targets were prescribed, which were to be implemented by the end of 2001. These included establishing a new menu framework and making food available to patients throughout the day and night. A Partnership Hospital Sites Club was established as a consequence, which currently has 51 members. This was set up by the NHS estates department and formed from hospitals that were associated with the Better Hospital Food programme as development sites. They have made considerable progress in implementing the 2001 Better Hospital Food targets. However, Lloyd Grossman implied at a national conference held by the Better Hospital Food group in May 2002 that other things needed to be changed as well as introducing better recipes to help make hospital food more appetising.

The Royal College of Physicians (2002) suggested that mealtimes are often the highlight of a patient's day in hospital and this should not be undermined by other ward routines. Furthermore, the College stipulated that patients who are not able to physically manage their own food should have staff available to assist them as required. Consequently, it has been suggested that there should be an increase in nursing presence during mealtimes to assist patients with feeding (Horan and Coad, 2000). There is also a need for better nutritional education to help staff recognise the signs of malnutrition (Bradley and Rees, 2003; Royal College of Physicians, 2002).

It is the responsibility of all healthcare professionals to ensure that patients eat their food. This is endorsed in the report by the Royal College of Physicians, which stated that clinical nutrition was a team responsibility. This provided the doctors with a wake-up call to their input in patient nutrition (Bradley and Rees, 2003). However, it is the nurse's role to ensure that the initial and continuing monitoring of nutrition is maintained for all patients under their care. This is achieved through helping patients to choose an appropriate diet from the menu and suggesting food supplements if required. It is important to ensure that patients eat their food and that it is not left on their locker, out of reach, and then taken away by hospital staff with no record being made of whether the patient has eaten the food.

Recent developments

An inpatient survey carried out by the Healthcare Commission in April 2006 revealed a worrying trend about hospital food. The survey found that although satisfaction with the food itself was relatively high, almost one-fifth of patients who needed help to eat never received such help, and a further 20% received help only occasionally (Vera-Jones, 2006). The findings of this report came a week after the news that the Department of Health decided to axe the Better Hospital Food programme outlined above and leave it to local hospital trusts to continue the good work. In the current hospital financial climate, this could lead to individual trusts trying to save on the cost of food in hospital. The average spend on each meal, including labour costs and services, is £2.60, but many nutrition nurses and caterers are concerned that catering budgets may be cut even further.

Similarly worrying findings from a major Food Watch survey by the Commission for Patient and Public Involvement in Health published in October 2006 revealed that (Hunt, 2007):

+ Over a third of patients (37%) left their meal because it looked, smelt or tasted unappetising.
+ Almost half of patients (40%) had their hospital meals supplemented by food brought in by visitors.
+ Over a quarter of patients (26%) did not receive the help they needed to eat their meals (this proportion was even greater – a third – in general hospitals).
+ Over a fifth of patients (22%) were given meals that were too small or too hot.
+ Almost a fifth of patients (18%) did not receive the meal they had chosen.

The National Institute for Health and Clinical Excellence (NICE) published guidelines on nutrition in February 2006. These guidelines recommend that each trust should employ at least one specialist nutrition nurse to ensure that all patients are screened for malnutrition on admission. They also state that nurses should receive training on nutrition.

Nutrition in hospital is still high on the agenda for the National Patient Safety Agency (NPSA), which is responsible for standards of hospital food. One idea being discussed to try and deal with the problem of patients not receiving their meals is for missed meals to be reported to the NPSA's National Reporting and Learning System in the same way that missed medication is reported. Food is also part of the Healthcare Commission's annual audit of trusts, which affects trusts' performance ratings. This should give some impetus to trust managers to continue to improve nutritional standards.

Some other good practice solutions have been introduced in order to improve patient nutrition, including introducing ward housekeepers or hostesses with the specific role of helping patients to eat. 'Red tray' systems have also been adopted widely, with the aim of alerting staff to patients who need extra help with feeding (Hunt, 2007). However, it is important to remember that, regardless of the systems in place, individual nurses should fulfil their important role in ensuring that their patients receive good nutrition.

Recap Questions

1. What factors can influence nutrition in hospital?
2. How can nutrition in hospital be improved?

Feeding patients

Ensuring that patients actually eat their food is an important part of the nurse's role in patient nutrition. It is important that the patient's ability to physically eat their food is assessed on admission. Failure to do this can result in patients not receiving adequate nutrition and could be viewed as neglect. Remember Emily Jones in the case study at the beginning of this chapter: her inability to see had not been identified on admission and had led to her not receiving adequate nutrition.

Procedure

Below is an outline of the process involved when feeding an adult patient (adapted from Nicol *et al.*, 2004):

1. Find out what the patient would like to eat and drink, and ensure there are no dietary restrictions.
2. Ensure the patient is comfortable: the patient should have an empty bladder, clean hands, clean mouth and, where relevant, clean dentures.
3. Ask or assist the patient to sit upright, if their condition allows.
4. Check that the patient is able to swallow: this will prevent choking and aspiration into the lungs.
5. Clear a space for the patient's tray.
6. Position a chair beside the bed.
7. Wash and dry your hands thoroughly before commencing feeding.
8. Wear an apron of the appropriate colour, according to local policy.
9. Protect the patient's clothing with a napkin or paper towel.
10. If the patient needs assistance, cut up their food.
11. Tailor the speed and manner in which food and drink are offered according to the patient's needs and wishes. Do not hurry the patient.
12. Allow the patient time to chew and swallow the food before presenting the next mouthful.
13. Avoid asking questions while the patient is eating.
14. Respect the patient's dignity and use a napkin to remove any dribbles of food or drink that may run down the chin.

15. Encourage the patient to eat and drink, but do not force the patient to eat once they have indicated they have had enough. Small amounts taken more frequently can be more successful.

16. After eating, assist the patient to meet their hygiene needs, such as cleaning their mouth, teeth and hands.

17. Remove the apron and wash your hands.

18. Ensure that any food and drink taken are recorded on the appropriate chart.

19. Report any food refusal or vomiting to the nurse in charge.

Other methods of feeding

Enteral feeding

If the patient is unable to eat, enteral feeding can be offered to ensure that the patient receives adequate nutrition. Enteral nutrition (EN) is prescribed if the patient is unable to ingest food in the normal way or there is impairment to the upper digestive tract, leading to an interruption to the transport of food to the small intestine (Kozier *et al.*, 2004). Nutrients are supplied to the gastrointestinal tract in fluid form via the nose (nasogastric feeding), stomach (gastrostomy) or jejunum (jejunostomy).

Nasogastric feeding

This involves the insertion of a nasogastric tube into one of the patient's nostrils. The tube is passed through the nasopharynx and oropharynx and into the alimentary tract to reach the stomach. Nasogastric feeding is used for patients who have intact cough and gag reflexes, who have adequate gastric emptying and who require short-term feeding (less than 6 weeks).

Gastrostomy and jejunostomy

Gastrostomy and jejunostomy are used for long-term nutritional support (usually more than 6–8 weeks). The tube is passed surgically by laparoscopy through the abdominal wall into the stomach (gastrostomy) or into the jejunum (jejunostomy). The surgical opening is sutured tightly around the tube or catheter to prevent leakage. This opening needs to be treated aseptically in order to ensure adequate healing of the stoma site. Once the incision has healed (usually after 10–14 days), the tube can be removed and reinserted for each feed. Sometimes, a prosthesis is used between feeds to close the ostomy opening (Kozier *et al.*, 2004).

A percutaneous endoscopic gastrostomy (PEG) or percutaneous endoscopic jejunostomy (PEJ) can be created by using an endoscope to show the inside of the stomach. A puncture is made through the skin and abdominal subcutaneous tissues, and the PEG or PEJ catheter inserted through this hole. The catheter has internal and external bumpers and an inflatable retention balloon to keep it in place. Once the opening has healed, replacement tubes can be inserted without using an endoscope. Before feeding, the correct tube placement position is confirmed by X-ray. Figure 5.3 shows the position of a PEG catheter in the stomach.

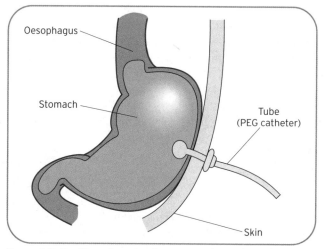

Figure 5.3 Position of a percutaneous endoscopic gastrostomy in the stomach

Parenteral feeding

Parenteral nutrition (PN), or total parenteral nutrition (TPN), is used when the gastrointestinal tract cannot be used due to an interruption in the continuity of the tract from an obstruction or tumour or due to absorption impairment. This form of feeding is administered intravenously through a central venous catheter that flows into the superior vena cava. Solutions of dextrose, water, fat, proteins, electrolytes, vitamins and trace elements are given to provide the patient with the required number of calories.

TPN is used for severely nutritionally compromised patients, such as those with severe malnutrition, severe burns, bowel disease disorders (e.g. ulcerative colitis), hepatic failure, acute renal failure or metastatic carcinoma, or following major surgery where the patient is unable to eat for more than 5 days (Kozier *et al.*, 2004).

All fluids administered must be recorded on the patient's fluid balance chart. Infection control is vital when caring for a patient receiving TPN. The nurse must change solutions, tubing and any dressings using an aseptic technique.

This section gives only a brief description of enteral and parenteral feeding, and you may like to read further on these areas.

Now that you have read about the nutritional needs of patients, consider Case studies 5.3 and 5.4.

Case Study 5.3

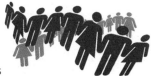

Mrs Ball is a 55-year-old woman with chronic bronchitis. She works as a personal assistant to a group of solicitors. She is married and has two teenage children. She is admitted to the ward suffering with shortness of breath. You are asked to admit Mrs Ball and collect the necessary information. The trained nurse carries out nutritional screening and finds that Mrs Ball has a BMI of 35. You notice several packets of biscuits and chocolate bars on Mrs Ball's locker.

What would you do next?

There are several things you can do. With a BMI of 35, Mrs Ball is considered to be obese and therefore requires dietary information on how to lose weight. She needs a referral to see a dietician as soon as possible. The dietician can then plan with Mrs Ball the most suitable diet to help her to lose weight. Ultimately, this will help to reduce Mrs Ball's shortness of breath. Mrs Ball's weight needs to be monitored on a weekly basis and recorded on her nutritional chart. Once her shortness of breath has improved, she will probably be discharged from the ward, but she will still need to have her weight and dietary intake checked regularly. If she is able, Mrs Ball should be encouraged to take some exercise daily, as this will help with her weight loss.

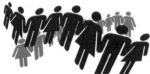

Case Study 5.4

Mr Jenkins is a 75-year-old man who has been treated for malnutrition. He has been in hospital for several weeks, and he has now made a complete recovery and is fit enough to return home. He lives alone in sheltered accommodation and has daily input from a home help. He has no relatives living close by. You are asked to give him some advice about his diet. He is a little hard of hearing, although he has a hearing aid he is reluctant to use it.

What will you do next?

Mr Jenkins needs to know what he should be eating. He could be given some literature on the Balance of Good Health Plate model and a full explanation of what it means. Try to identify what foods he likes to eat, and then plan accordingly. As Mr Jenkins has a hearing problem, make sure you speak clearly and that Mr Jenkins can see your face. This will enable him to watch your speech and help him to identify what you are saying. It would be useful to give Mr Jenkins some written information on essential dietary intake, which he can give to his home help. His food budget may be quite low, so he (and possibly his home help) needs to be advised that nutritious food does not have to be expensive. He also needs to monitor his weight regularly in order to ensure that he does not become malnourished again. Finally, Mr Jenkins should be encouraged to wear his hearing aid or, if he finds it difficult to use, to change to another model.

Recap Questions

1. What needs to be considered when feeding a patient?
2. What other methods of feeding are available when a patient is unable to eat in the normal way?

Dysphagia awareness

Introduction

Dysphagia, which literally means difficulty in swallowing, can result in a patient having problems achieving adequate nutrition. It is useful for the nurse to be aware of the potential problems associated with dysphagia.

> **Revision**
>
> Before reading the next section, you need to revise the anatomy and physiology of the mouth, pharynx and oropharynx, including the swallowing mechanism.

Normal swallowing

Swallowing is a muscular activity controlled by the ninth cranial glossopharyngeal nerve. There are four stages to the normal swallowing reflex:

1. *Anticipatory phase:* the person is thinking about eating food or has been presented with some food. The salivary glands start to produce saliva in order to moisten and soften the food.

2. *Oral phase:* food or liquid is placed in the mouth. The tongue squeezes this against the roof of the mouth and moves it backwards, ready to start the swallowing sequence. (This is sometimes called oral preparation time.)

3. *Pharyngeal phase:* as the swallow sequence starts, a series of things occur:
   - The soft palate moves up
   - The muscles of the throat move the bolus of food down
   - The larynx lifts, the vocal cords shut and the epiglottis moves over
   - The cricopharyngeal sphincter opens to allow the bolus to pass through.

4. *Oesophageal phase:* the bolus enters the oesophagus and passes down to the stomach.

Figure 5.4 shows the structures involved in the swallowing process.

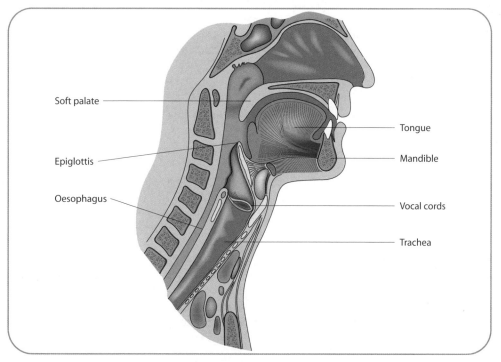

Figure 5.4   Structures involved in the swallowing process

> ### To think about
>
> How do you think a patient with dysphagia might feel? If you are nursing a patient with dysphagia when you are next in practice, ask how they feel and what problems they experience.

Dysphagia

Dysphagia is an abnormality in swallowing. It occurs in about 45% of patients admitted to hospital with cerebral vascular accident (CVA; stroke) (Royal College of Physicians, 2004). Due to an alteration in physiology, problems with the oral phase of swallowing are experienced. This can include difficulty with containing liquid in the oral cavity or difficulty chewing or initiating a swallow of solid food. Sometimes the pharyngeal clearance may be so severe that the patient is unable to ingest sufficient food to sustain life. In this instance, enteral feeding is used (Palmer *et al.*, 2000).

Rehabilitation can be impaired if the patient has dysphagia. Often, dysphagia is associated with dehydration, starvation, weight loss, malnutrition, silent aspiration (the patient is unable to clear the throat due to lack of the cough reflex), aspiration (this can cause a blockage in the bronchus, leading to aspiration pneumonia), chest infection and airway obstruction (Royal College of Physicians, 2004). Patients with dysphagia may experience emotional and psychological problems from the stigma of being unable to eat and the associated feelings of embarrassment, frustration or anger at needing assistance (Hamdy, 2004).

Causes of dysphagia

Dysphagia is a result of difficulty with any of the phases of the swallowing reflex. Such difficulties may be associated with various conditions, including the following:

+ Cerebral vascular accident
+ Severe head injury
+ Progressive neurological diseases, such as myasthenia gravis
+ Oral surgery
+ Cancer of the head, neck, mouth or tongue
+ Dementia
+ AIDS
+ Respiratory problems
+ Aspiration

If the patient is unable to swallow, they are at risk of aspiration. Aspiration occurs when there is entry of material (usually food or fluids) into the airway below the vocal cords. It is important to keep aspiration to a minimum. There are no clear guidelines as to the amount of aspiration that can be tolerated before complications arise. Any individual may occasionally experience a degree of aspiration and the feeling that food has 'gone down the wrong way'. However, if aspiration occurring continually, it can be a major problem for the patient.

Clinical signs of aspiration

Aspiration can present with acute (immediate) and chronic (ongoing) clinical signs. Acute signs include the following:

+ Coughing and choking
+ Change of patient colour (grey, cyanosed)
+ Sounds of respiratory wheezing or gurgling
+ Loss of voice
+ Rapid heart rate
+ Gurgly voice following swallowing
+ Drooling
+ Watering eyes

Chronic signs include the following:

+ Loss of weight
+ Hunger
+ Excessive oral secretions
+ Coughing and choking
+ Refusal to eat
+ Fatigue
+ Pallor
+ Pain

Disordered swallow

A swallow is classed as disordered when the following apply:

+ Aspiration is possible
+ The patient cannot take in enough food/drink due to:
  • Prolonged oral preparation time
  • Effortful swallowing
  • Poor chewing/oral movements
  • Delayed/absent initiation of a swallow
  • Reduced pharyngeal clearing
  • Poor respiratory status
  • Poor oral care or build up of oral secretions
  • Reflux/oesophagitis
  • Structural changes

The gag reflex

The **gag reflex** is highly variable among healthy people. A diminished gag reflex is probably significant only when found in patients showing evidence of weakened or paralysed pharyngeal musculature, asymmetrical gag reflexes or other signs of cranial nerve dysfunction. Historically, absence of the gag reflex was used as the main test for dysphagia; nowadays, the absence is seen as one of a number of things to consider when assessing a patient with dysphagia. It is better for the nurse to describe or note any problems when the patient attempts to swallow, rather than to rely on the presence or absence of a gag reflex. For example, noting whether the patient is unable to clear saliva, has difficulty chewing or struggles to initiate a swallow is important. The Royal College of Physicians (2004) and the Scottish Intercollegiate Guidelines Network (2004) agree that the swallowing assessment is a far more accurate way to identify dysphagia than relying on the gag reflex alone. Absence of the gag reflex does not necessarily indicate that the patient is unable to swallow safely. Conversely, some patients with dysphagia may have a normal gag reflex. Perry (2001) also found that the swallowing assessment produced a higher proportion of accurate results when detecting dysphagia than did the gag reflex.

To think about

Now you have read about dysphagia, its causes and some of the associated problems, what do you think the nurse can do to help a patient with dysphagia?

The nurse's role in dysphagia

The nurse is central to the management of the patient with dysphagia. It is often nurses who first recognise the initial signs of dysphagia and request that the doctor refers the patient to the speech and language therapist for a swallow assessment.

The nurse's role in dysphagia is wide ranging and includes the following:

+ Identifying and assessing patients with dysphagia
+ Working with the speech and language therapist to ensure the patient is managed appropriately
+ Supervising the patient with feeding and drinking
+ Observing the patient's eating and drinking habits
+ Management of tube feeding, if required
+ Ensuring adequate nutrition and hydration
+ Notifying the multidisciplinary team of any changes in the patient's status
+ Assisting with oral hygiene
+ Providing support and reassurance to the patient and their family

The **gag reflex** occurs when the back of the pharynx in the mouth is touched, causing 'gagging' to occur, with muscular movements associated with vomiting. The response is innervated by sensory neurons in the vagus nerve.

Swallowing assessment

Patients with CVA and other patients who are at risk of developing dysphagia should have their swallowing assessed by a dysphagia-trained nurse within 24 hours of admission. This is set out in the guidelines from the Royal College of Physicians (2004), the Scottish Intercollegiate Guidelines Network (2004), the National Service Framework for Older People (Department of Health, 2001) and the Collaborative Dysphagia Audit Study (1997). If a dysphagia-trained nurse is not available, the assessment must be carried out by a speech and language therapist (Mitchell and Finlayson, 2000).

Each stage of the swallowing process should be assessed, including the pre-oral (anticipatory), oral, pharyngeal and oesophageal phases.

It is important that a nutritional assessment is carried out at the same time in order to ascertain the patient's nutritional status, posture, breathing and cooperation levels. The clinical history should also include any **comorbidities** and other risk factors, such as smoking and respiratory disease, as these will identify whether the patient has an increased risk of developing aspiration pneumonia (Corcoran, 2005).

Modified diet

If the patient has a problem with swallowing, the diet can be modified accordingly. The dietician decides what type and texture of diet should be given. The nurse should liaise closely with the dietician and the speech and language therapist in order to ensure that the patient receives the correct diet. Although different hospitals use various systems, an example of a system of a modified consistency diet is as follows:

Stage 1: *cold and smooth*

Stage 2: *hot and cold and smooth*

Stage 3: *mashable with a fork*

Extra sauce may also be provided, to make the food easier to swallow.

It is important that dysphagic patients avoid certain foods, including:

+ Crumbly food, such as biscuits
+ Very dry foods
+ Skins on fruit and vegetables
+ Mixed-consistency food, such as thin soup containing vegetable pieces
+ Small vegetables, such as peas
+ Stringy bacon rind

Patients with dysphagia may also have problems with swallowing liquids. If necessary, liquids can be mixed with thickening agents to make them easier to swallow.

When assisting with feeding, it is important that the patient is in the optimum position (Figure 5.5 and Exhibit 5.4). The nurse should offer support if required but should aim to maintain the patient's independence as this will help with rehabilitation (Simpson, 2002).

Comorbidities are coexisting diseases in the same patient.

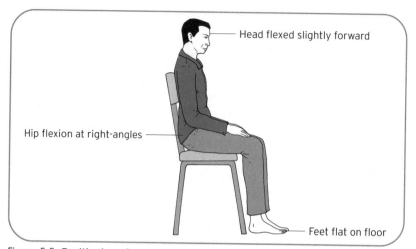

Head flexed slightly forward

Hip flexion at right-angles

Feet flat on floor

Figure 5.5 Positioning of a dysphagic patient for feeding

+ Sit the patient upright, with 90-degree flexion at the hips and knees, the feet supported flat on the floor, the trunk and head in midline, and the head flexed slightly forwards and the chin down (neck flexion)
+ Supports may be necessary for the head and neck
+ If the patient's head is unstable, support the forehead with the hand
+ If the patient is in bed, use Fowler's position: head and neck supported and neck slightly flexed
+ If there is hemiplegia, avoid neck extension and aspiration by tilting the patient's head slightly to the unaffected side and rotating the head towards the affected side, to help with detection of food
+ Advise the patient to hold their breath before swallowing in order to improve pharyngeal clearance of the bolus and reduce aspiration

Exhibit 5.4 Positioning of a dysphagic patient for feeding
Adapted from Mitchell and Finlayson (2000)

When the patient has finished eating, the nurse should check the patient's mouth for retained food and offer oral care. The patient may be unaware of 'pocketed' food due to reduced sensations in the mouth, and this can lead to aspiration (Mitchell and Finlayson, 2000). The nurse can teach the patient to check for pocketed food using the tongue. All food and drink taken should be recorded on the appropriate charts, in order to prevent dehydration and malnourishment (Simpson, 2002). It is important to check the patient's respirations regularly during feeding in order to avoid aspiration. Chest X-rays should be taken regularly to help detect the presence of infection arising from aspiration of fluids.

A stage 2 modified diet has been ordered by the dietician in liaison with the dysphagia-trained nurse. Therefore, it is very important that Mr Patel receives the type of diet ordered. A stage 2 modified diet consists of food that can be hot or cold but is smooth in consistency. Mr Patel's relatives need to speak with the dietician and the dysphagia-trained nurse in order to understand the type of diet Mr Patel should be eating. You need to inform the nurse in charge, who should then contact the appropriate healthcare professionals and arrange a meeting as soon as possible. It is very important to respect Mr Patel and his relatives' religious beliefs. Most Hindus are strictly vegetarian and will not eat any food containing meat, fish or egg products.

Now consider Case study 5.5.

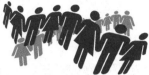

Case Study 5.5

Mr Patel is a 48-year-old man admitted following a cerebral vascular accident. He has left-sided weakness and problems with swallowing. Mr Patel's swallowing has been assessed by the dysphagia-trained nurse and a stage 2 modified diet has been ordered by the dietician. However, Mr Patel is a practising Hindu and his relatives insist on bringing him solid food from home, prepared and cooked according to their religion.

What would you do next?

When planning Mr Patel's modified diet, all of these factors must be considered. Once the patient's relatives are aware of the type and consistency of diet that Mr Patel needs, they can adapt the food they cook and prepare for him.

Recap Questions

1. What is dysphagia, and what can cause it?
2. What is aspiration, and what are the clinical signs?
3. What is the gag reflex?
4. What is the nurse's role in managing a patient with dysphagia?
5. What does a modified diet consist of?

Summary

This chapter has focused on the importance of nutrition to help promote health and well-being in patients. However, there is an evidence base that suggests that nutrition, particularly in hospital, is poor overall. The government has attempted to address this issue in the NHS Plan (Department of Health, 2002) with some degree of success. NICE has also published guidelines on how to improve nutrition in hospital through setting standards (National Institute for Health and Clinical Excellence, 2006).

Nutritional requirements have been considered and the Balance of Good Health Plate model has been proffered as an example of ensuring that a person receives their daily intake of essential nutrients, such as protein, fat and carbohydrates.

The nurse needs to be alert to the factors that can affect nutrition when assessing the patient's nutritional needs. A nutritional assessment tool such as the BMI status can help identify malnourished and at-risk patients.

Feeding a patient is a fundamental nursing role, but there is growing evidence that patients who need feeding do not always receive their food. Initiatives such as the Red Tray system have gone some way to addressing this issue.

Some patients are unable to eat in the normal way, and then other methods such as enteral and parental feeding may be employed. It is important that all nutrition given in this way is recorded on the patient's fluid balance and nutritional charts.

Finally, we have considered dysphagia, a serious problem that affects how and what a patient can eat. The nurse needs to be aware of dysphagia and ensure that patients with dysphagia receive adequate nutrition and food of the correct consistency.

Key Points

1. The body requires essential nutrients for fuel and energy. These nutrients are needed in different quantities in the form of a balanced diet, which helps to ensure that energy balance is maintained.

2. Many factors affect a patient's nutrition, and the nurse should be aware of these when assessing nutritional needs.

3. When carrying out a nutritional assessment, nutritional screening is essential to identify at-risk patients. The use of a nutritional assessment tool such as the BMI can assist with the screening process.

4. Improving food in hospitals has been on the government's agenda in recent years. Initiatives have been introduced in order to improve standards and the quality of hospital food. The measures have gone some way to improve matters, but issues still remain, particularly regarding patients who need help with feeding.

5. The process of feeding a patient is essential if patients who are unable to feed themselves are to receive adequate nutrition. Failure to do this could be viewed as neglect.

6. If a patient cannot eat in the normal way, nutrition can be provided by other routes, such as enteral and parenteral feeding.

7. Dysphagia affects patient nutrition. The nurse should be aware of this specific problem and how to deal with it.

Points for debate

Now that you have come to the end of this chapter here are a few points that you may wish to think about when you are in practice. You may wish to discuss these with your work colleagues or fellow students.

Many people prefer to eat food high in saturated fats, even though they know this is bad for them.

It is not surprising that patients lose weight when they are in hospital, as hospital food is not very appetising. Choices are minimal and the standard and quality of the food are poor.

Some patients who are unable to feed themselves often have their meal taken away before anyone has tried to feed them.

Links to Other Chapters

Chapter 2   Dignity and privacy
Chapter 3   Basic observations
Chapter 10 Record-keeping

Further reading

Shuttleworth, A (2003) *Nutrition: A Practical Guide*. London: EMAP Healthcare.

Thomas, B (2001) *Manual of Dietetic Practice*, 3rd edn. Oxford: Blackwell Science.

Wardlow, GM (1999) *Perspectives in Nutrition*, 4th edn. Boston, MA: McGraw-Hill

References

Audit Commission (2001) Acute Hospital Portfolio: Review of National Findings – Catering, Welsh Briefing. www.audit-commission.gov.uk/publications/brcateringwales.shtml.

Bond, S (ed) (1997) *Eating Matters*. Newcastle: Centre for Health Services Research, University of Newcastle.

Bradley, L and Rees, C (2003) Reducing nutritional risk in hospital: the red tray. *Nursing Standard* **17**, 33–37.

British Association for Parenteral and Enteral Nutrition (2001) The Better Hospital Food project. *In Touch: Newsletter of the British Association for Parenteral and Enteral Nutrition* **13**, 1.

Collaborative Dysphagia Audit Study (1997) *Guidelines for Screening and Management of Stoke Patients with Dysphagia*. London: Collaborative Dysphagia Audit Study.

Corcoran, L (2005) Nutrition and hydration tips for stroke patients with dysphagia. *Nursing Times* **101**, 24–29.

Department of Health (2001) *National Service Framework for Older People*. London: The Stationery Office.

Department of Health (2000) *The NHS Plan: A Plan for Investment, a Plan for Reform*. London: The Stationery Office.

Girling, R (2002) Government health warning: hospital food can make you ill (whether you eat it or not). *Sunday Times Magazine*, 9 June 2002, 43–50.

Green, CJ (1999) Existence, causes and consequences of disease-related malnutrition in the hospital and the community, and clinical and financial benefits of nutritional intervention. *Clinical Nutrition* **18** (suppl 2), 3–28.

Hamdy, S (2004) The diagnosis and management of adult neurogenic dysphagia. *Nursing Times* **100**, 52–54.

Horan, D and Coad, J (2000) Can nurses improve patient feeding? *Nursing Times* **96**, 33–34.

Hunt, L (2007) Rising to the nutrition challenge. *Nursing Times* **103**, 16–19.

Jarvis, S and Rubin, A (2003) *Diabetes for Dummies*. Chichester: John Wiley & Sons.

Kozier, B, Erb, A, Berman, A and Snyder, S (2004) *Fundamentals of Nursing: Concepts, Process and Practice*, 7th edn. Upper Saddle River, NJ: Prentice Hall.

Mitchell, A and Finlayson, K (2000) Identification and nursing management of dysphagia in adults with neurological impairment. *Best Practice* **4**, 1–6.

National Institute for Health and Clinical Excellence (2006) *Nutrition Support in Adults: Oral Supplements, Enteral and Parenteral Feeding*. London: National Institute for Health and Clinical Excellence.

NHS Estates (2002) *Partnership Club: At the Cutting Edge of Better Hospital Food.* www. patientexperience.nhsestates.gov.uk/bhf/bhf_content/whos_involved/partnership_club.asp

Nicol, M, Bavin, C, Bedford-Turner, S, Cronin, P and Rawlings-Anderson, K (2004) *Essential Nursing Skills.* London: Mosby.

Palmer, JB, Drennan, JC and Baba, M (2000) Evaluation and treatment of swallowing impairments. *American Family Physician* **61**, 2453-2462.

Perry, L (1997) Nutrition: a hard nut to crack. An exploration of knowledge, attitudes and activities of qualified nurses in relation to nutritional nursing care. *Journal of Clinical Nursing* **6**, 315-324.

Perry, L (2001) Screening swallowing function of patients with acute stroke: part two: detailed evaluation of the tool used by nurses. *Journal of Clinical Nursing* **10**, 474-481.

Perry, L (2004) Nutritional screening and assessment. In: Shuttleworth, A (ed) *Monitoring and Assessment.* London: Emap Healthcare.

Royal College of Physicians (2002) *Nutrition and Patients: A Doctor's Responsibility.* London: Royal College of Physicians.

Royal College of Physicians (2004) *The National Guidelines for Stroke.* London: Royal College of Physicians.

Scottish Intercollegiate Guidelines Network (2004) *Management of Patients with Stroke: Identification and Management of Dysphagia: A National Clinical Guideline.* Edinburgh: Scottish Intercollegiate Guidelines Network.

Simpson, P (2002) Eating and drinking. In: Hogston, R and Simpson, P (eds) *Foundations of Nursing Practice: Making a Difference.* Basingstoke: Palgrave Macmillan.

Vera-Jones, E (2006) Has food fallen off the NHS agenda? *Nursing Times* **102**, 11.

Chapter 6
Fluid balance and continence care

Case Study

Mrs Baker, an 83-year-old emergency admission, was found in a collapsed state at home. She is dehydrated and in a confused state. An intravenous infusion is commenced to help correct her dehydration. All fluid infused is recorded on Mrs Baker's fluid balance chart. Mrs Baker also appears to be incontinent of urine since admission. The continence nurse is contacted to assess Mrs Baker's incontinence and advise on what treatment should be ordered. The nurses are encouraging Mrs Baker to take some fluids by mouth in order to improve her dehydrated state. She is still quite confused at times, however, and needs supervision with her fluid intake.

Despite completing a detailed assessment of Mrs Baker, the continence nurse and the doctor cannot identify any physical cause for the patient's urinary incontinence and decide she probably has functional incontinence because of her confused state. Consequently, the nurses frequently remind Mrs Baker to visit the toilet. Her bed space is quite close to the bathroom so that she does not have to walk too far before reaching the toilet.

Introduction

Consider the case study above and reflect on your reactions to it. Mrs Baker is dehydrated and requires fluid to be given intravenously. She also has a continence problem, which needs to be assessed and the appropriate care ordered.

This chapter discusses fluid balance and how it is regulated and finely tuned to enable important body processes to occur. The factors that can affect fluid balance are examined, along with the causes and assessment of fluid overload and fluid loss. Finally, the accurate recording of a patient's fluid balance is addressed.

Urinary incontinence is considered, along with the physical and psychological effects that incontinence can have on an individual. The chapter emphasises person-centred continence care and describes the continence aids and appliances available to promote continence. A patient may need to be catheterised, but this is usually considered a last resort in the promotion of continence. Care of the patient with an indwelling catheter on continuous drainage is discussed.

The problems patients can have with the elimination of faeces are discussed, with particular reference to constipation and diarrhoea and the nursing interventions required to deal with these problems.

> ### LEARNING OBJECTIVES
>
> By the end of this chapter you will be able to:
>
> 1. Define fluid balance and explain how body fluids are regulated in the body to maintain fluid balance
> 2. Describe the causes and clinical assessment of hypervolaemia (fluid overload) and hypovolaemia (fluid loss)
> 3. Outline the factors that can affect micturition and summarise the abnormalities that can occur in urine production and elimination
> 4. Define incontinence, explain its possible causes and describe what should be considered when carrying out an assessment of incontinence
> 5. Consider the different types of incontinence and indicate how they can be treated
> 6. Be aware of the problems a patient may have with elimination of faeces, with particular reference to constipation and diarrhoea

Fluid balance

Introduction

In normal health there is a delicate balance of fluid and **electrolyte** levels in the body that is maintained through a physiological mechanism known as homeostasis. This biological process is dependent on many important physiological interactions that regulate fluid intake and output. Fluid balance literally means maintenance of the correct amount of fluid in the body. It is regulated by fluid intake, hormonal controls and fluid output (Potter and Perry, 2002).

Nearly every illness has the potential to disturb this fluid balance if adequate water and salt intake is not maintained. Therefore, it is important that an accurate fluid balance is maintained in any patient who exhibits signs of fluid imbalance or may have the potential to do so.

The recording of a patient's fluid balance is an important nursing role. This entails recording any fluids the patient takes into the body, whether in the form of drinks, intravenously, nasogastrically, directly into the stomach (via a gastrostomy) or via any other route; this is concordant with recording any fluids that exit from the patient, such as urine, vomit, sweat, water in the faeces and insensible losses from respiration. Fluid balance must be recorded in patients with the following problems, although note that this list is not exhaustive and there may be other reasons why fluid balance needs to be recorded:

> **Electrolytes** are charged ions capable of conducting electricity. They can carry a positive or a negative charge.

+ Gastrointestinal problems

+ Postoperatively

+ Heart failure

+ Diabetic ketoacidosis

+ Liver and kidney disease

+ Fever

+ Trauma

+ Haemorrhage

+ Critical illness

+ Brain injury

Revision

Before reading the next section, you need to revise the physiological mechanisms that regulate fluid balance in the body.

Anatomy and physiology

The body's fluid balance is maintained through various homeostatic mechanisms that are sensitive to any physiological changes occurring in the body. The proportion of the body composed of fluids is relatively large. The primary body fluid is water, accounting for 46–60% of the average adult's weight. In normal health, this proportion remains relatively constant with the person's weight, varying by less than 0.2 kg in 24 hours. This is irrespective of the amount of fluid ingested (Kozier *et al.*, 2004). Water is necessary to ensure optimal physical and chemical conditions for body cells to function. This is often referred to as maintaining a suitable 'internal environment' for normal cellular function. To achieve this, water serves as:

+ A medium in which various metabolic reactions occur within body cells

+ A transporter for nutrients, waste products and other substances, i.e. electrolytes

+ An insulator and shock absorber

+ A means of regulating and maintaining body temperature

+ A lubricant

A reduction in body fluids can have major effects on the body. For example, a reduction of 5% causes thirst, a reduction of 8% causes illness and a reduction of 10% can lead to death (Carroll, 2000). Total water content is affected by age, sex and body fat. For example, in infants water accounts for 70–80% of body weight, but this proportion of body water decreases with age to about 50%. Fat tissue does not contain any water, whereas lean tissue contains a significant amount of water. Consequently, water contributes to a greater percentage of a lean person's body weight than that in an obese person's body. Since women have more body fat than men, they have a lower percentage of body water (Kozier *et al.*, 2004): about 60% of body weight in males and 52% of body weight in females (Mooney, 2004).

The body's fluid is divided into two main compartments: intracellular and extracellular. Intracellular fluid is found within the body cells and constitutes about two-thirds of the total body fluid in adults. Extracellular fluid occurs outside the cells and accounts for the remaining third of total body fluid.

Regulation of body fluids

In a healthy person, the volumes and composition of the fluid compartments outlined above remain within narrow safe limits. Fluid intake and fluid output are finely balanced. Any illness or trauma to the body can disrupt this fine balance, resulting in the body having too little or too much fluid.

> ### To think about
>
> How much fluid should an average adult take in on a daily basis? It might be worth making a note of your own daily fluid intake and comparing this with the recommended daily intake. How do they compare?

Fluid intake

Under normal circumstances, the average adult drinks about 1500 mL of fluid per day. An additional 1000 mL is acquired from foods and **oxidation** of these foods during metabolic processes. The water content of food is relatively large, contributing to about 750 mL per day. For example, fresh vegetables contain about 90% water, fruit contains about 85% water and lean meats contain about 60% water (Kozier *et al.*, 2004). The remaining 250 mL of water is a by-product of food metabolism.

Fluid intake is regulated primarily by the thirst mechanism. The thirst centre is located in the **hypothalamus** of the brain.

Fluid output

Fluid losses from the body equate approximately to the average daily fluid intake of 2500 mL. There are four main routes whereby fluid is lost from the body:

+ Urine
+ Insensible loss (i.e. that which cannot be measured directly) through water vapour in expired air from the lungs and through the skin as perspiration

> **Oxidation,** or cellular respiration, is the breakdown of absorbed nutrients within the cell to produce energy.
>
> The **hypothalamus** is an important structure located in the hindbrain. It performs several functions, one of which is related to thirst.

+ Noticeable loss through the skin (sweating)

+ Through the intestines in faeces

The majority of fluid is lost in urine. The normal urine output for an adult is 1400-1500 mL in 24 hours; this may be expressed as at least 0.5 mL/kg/hour (Kozier *et al.*, 2004). However, urine output may vary from day to day in a healthy adult and is dependent on fluid intake; that is, urine volume automatically increases as fluid intake increases. If a lot of fluid is lost through per-spiration, then the urine volume decreases in order to compensate and maintain fluid balance.

Insensible loss occurs through the lungs and skin. It is called insensible as it cannot be measured directly. Water loss through exhaled air from the lungs is normally about 300-400 mL per day, and water loss via the skin by diffusion and perspiration is approximately 350 mL per day. Water loss from sweating and faeces is about 100-200 mL per day. Insensible loss should always be taken into account when calculating a patient's fluid balance. The total body fluid intake and output is shown in Table 6.1.

Table 6.1 Normal daily average fluid intake and output

	Fluid intake	**Fluid output**
Source/amount (ml)	Drink (1500)	Urine (1500)
	Food (750)	Insensible loss:
	Food metabolism (250)	Lungs (400)
		Skin (350)
		Sweat (100)
		Faeces (200)

Electrolytes

It is worth briefly considering electrolytes and their relationship with fluids. Any fluid imbal-ance in the body invariably leads to electrolyte imbalance, as water provides an important medium for the transport of electrolytes. Electrolytes are charged ions capable of conduct-ing electricity. They carry either a positive or a negative charge. They are present in all body fluids and fluid compartments. Maintaining electrolyte balance in the body is as important as maintaining fluid balance. There is an equal balance of positively charged ions (cations) and negatively charged ions (anions). This is needed to provide the correct internal environment for normal body functioning. Electrolytes perform several important functions, including:

+ Maintaining fluid balance

+ Contributing to acid-base regulation

+ Facilitating enzyme reactions

+ Transmitting neuromuscular reactions

There are several electrolytes in the body, and they perform many vital functions (Table 6.2).

Table 6.2 Electrolytes in the body and their main functions

Electrolyte	Function
Sodium (Na^+)	Regulates water balance
Potassium (K^+)	Regulates skeletal, cardiac and smooth muscle activity
Calcium (Ca^+)	Regulates neuromuscular and cardiac function
Magnesium (Mg^+)	Regulates intracellular metabolism
Chloride (Cl^-)	Regulates water balance with sodium, and acid-base balance
Phosphate (PO^-)	Regulates cellular and food metabolism, muscle, nerve and red blood cell function, and acid-base balance
Bicarbonate (HCO^-)	Major body buffer: regulates acid-base balance

Hormonal influences on fluid balance

Some hormones work together to maintain fluid balance. Antidiuretic hormone (ADH) is produced by the hypothalamus and released from the posterior **pituitary gland** situated at the base of the brain. ADH works by increasing the reabsorption of water via the kidneys, thus helping to maintain fluid balance. ADH is released when there is a reduction in circulating fluid (mainly blood volume) in the body, such as when a person bleeds profusely or loses a lot of fluid through vomiting, diarrhoea or excessive sweating.

If blood flow through the kidneys is reduced, cells called juxtaglomerular cells secrete the hormone renin into the bloodstream. Renin then converts the inactive angiotensinogen into angiotensin II via a complex cascade involving the liver and the lungs. Angiotensin II is a powerful **vasoconstrictor** that increases blood pressure and therefore raises the flow of blood through the kidneys.

Aldosterone plays a significant role in fluid balance. It is secreted by the **adrenal cortex** and helps to regulate the reabsorption of sodium and water.

Kidneys

The kidneys help to maintain the body's fluid balance by regulating the amount of water reabsorbed back into the body. For example, if the body loses 2% of its fluid, the kidneys will take steps to conserve water. The kidneys reabsorb more water from the filtration process, thereby helping to maintain the body's finely tuned fluid balance. Conversely, if the body is holding too much fluid, the kidneys reabsorb less water.

The **pituitary gland** is divided into the anterior lobe and the posterior lobe. It is a very important endocrine organ that secretes many hormones that regulate body activities.

Vasoconstrictors stimulate the lumen of blood vessels to narrow.

The **adrenal cortex** forms part of the adrenal glands situated above each kidney. The other part of the adrenal gland is made up of the adrenal medulla, which secretes different hormones, including adrenaline.

Factors affecting fluid and electrolyte balance

To think about

What factors might influence fluid and electrolyte balance?
In what way could such factors alter the finely tuned fluid balance of the body?

The ability of the body to adjust fluids and electrolytes is influenced by several factors, including the following:

+ *Age*: infants and children have a higher metabolic rate than adults and therefore a quicker fluid turnover due to increased fluid loss. Infants have immature kidneys and lose more fluid as a consequence. This more rapid turnover of fluid can create critical fluid imbalances more quickly in infants and children than in adults. The normal ageing process can affect fluid balance as the thirst response may be reduced and the kidneys may be less able to conserve water if required; this makes elderly people more susceptible to dehydration.

+ *Gender and body size*: total body water is affected by gender and body size. Women have more body fat and less body water than men, who have more lean tissue to hold water. An obese person has even less lean tissue, and water then accounts for just 30–40% of the person's weight.

+ *Environmental temperature*: fluid losses through sweating are increased in hot environments and during strenuous exercise. Salt and water must be replaced in order to prevent salt depletion and heat stroke.

+ *Lifestyle*: diet, exercise and stress can affect fluid and electrolyte balance. A person with an eating disorder or who is malnourished may be deficient in fluids and electrolytes. Exercise promotes calcium balance, reducing the risk of osteoporosis in older people. Stress can increase cellular metabolism, while stress hormones, such as adrenaline, decrease urine output and result in an overall increase in blood volume.

Fluid imbalances

Several factors affect the finely tuned mechanisms that maintain the body's fluid balance between fluid overload (hypervolaemia) and lack of fluid in the body (hypovolaemia) (Figure 6.1).

To think about

Do you know of any conditions that may lead to fluid overload/gain or to fluid loss in the body? You may wish to ask your work colleagues in practice to help you with this.

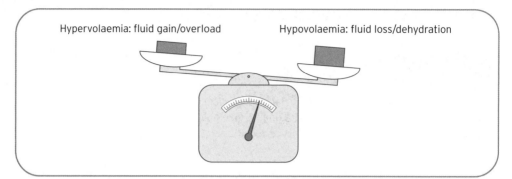

Figure 6.1 The balance between hypervolaemia and hypovolaemia

Hypervolaemia – fluid overload/gain

Hypervolaemia is the term used to describe fluid overload, when there is too much fluid in the body. There are three main causes for excess fluid volume:

+ Excessive fluid intake
+ Excessive sodium intake
+ Failure of regulatory mechanisms

A number of conditions can contribute to these causes, including the following:

+ Congestive cardiac failure
+ Renal failure
+ High sodium intake
+ Liver cirrhosis
+ Over-infusion of intravenous fluids
+ Pregnancy
+ Brain injury

There are many others causes, all of which may alter the fluid balance by increasing either the intracellular or the extracellular fluid and resulting in too much fluid in the body.

Hypovolaemia – fluid loss/dehydration

Hypovolaemia is lack of fluid in the body and is very often termed dehydration. Several factors can lead to hypovolaemia, including the following:

+ Diarrhoea
+ Vomiting
+ Gastrointestinal problems
+ Sweating/fever
+ Haemorrhage
+ Trauma

+ Diuretics

+ Excessive urination (polyuria)

+ Diabetic ketoacidosis

+ Reduced fluid intake, e.g. due to physical disability or stroke

All of these factors can be symptoms of disease. Reduced fluid intake can also be associated with a patient's physical mobility and abilities (Mooney, 2004).

Recap Questions

1. Why is it important that a stable fluid balance is maintained?
2. How are body fluids regulated, and which hormones help to maintain fluid balance?
3. What are the main factors that can affect fluid and electrolyte imbalance?
4. How do these factors influence fluid and electrolyte imbalance
5. What are hypervolaemia and hypovolaemia, and what are their main causes?

Recording fluid balance

To think about

When you are next in practice, look at your patients' fluid balance charts.

What do the charts tell you about the patients?

Has all the relevant/appropriate information been recorded on the fluid balance charts?

The accurate recording of a patient's fluid balance is a very important nursing role. It provides essential information about the patient that will influence any treatment or medication prescribed. When assessing a patient's fluid balance, the nurse should also consider the patient's history, including a physical examination, clinical observations and interpretation of laboratory results (Place and Field, 1997). A detailed account of the patient's fluid intake and output must be recorded.

When assessing the fluid balance, it is important to carry out a clinical assessment (Table 6.3). This includes recording the vital signs of blood pressure, pulse, respiration and temperature. The nurse should note the patient's physical state, in particular the skin, tongue and face. The patient's wellbeing is a good indication of fluid loss or gain. Table 6.3 outlines factors to consider when doing a clinical assessment. Patients with fluid imbalance usually present with more than one of these signs or symptoms.

Table 6.3 Clinical assessment of fluid balance

Observation	Fluid depletion	Fluid overload
Weight	Loss	Gain
Blood pressure	Lowered	Normal or raised
Respiration	Rapid and shallow	Rapid, moist cough
Pulse	Rapid, weak and thready	Rapid
Urine output	Reduced and concentrated	Increased or decreased
Skin	Dry, less elastic	Oedematous
Saliva	Thick and viscous	Copious and frothy
Tongue	Dry and coated	Moist
Thirst	Present	No disturbance
Face	Sunken eyes (severe depletion)	Per-orbital oedema
Temperature	May be raised	No disturbance

Adapted from Place and Field (1997)

A good indication of the amount of fluid in the body can be achieved by measuring the central venous pressure (CVP). This is pressure in the right atrium of the heart and is related to the amount of fluid circulating in the venous system (Mooney, 2004). CVP is usually recorded only in patients who are critically ill and require very close monitoring of their fluid levels. CVP monitoring is a complex task and thus is performed only by qualified nurses.

Fluid intake and output are recorded on fluid balance charts (Figure 6.2). Output is often recorded as 'passed urine ++' or 'up to toilet'. However, such notes are vague and do not contribute to an accurate fluid balance as there is no clear indication of the amount of urine passed. Therefore, the nurse should measure the urine output by collecting it in a bedpan, pouring the contents into a calibrated jug and recording the amount on the output section of the fluid balance chart.

All oral, intravenous and **nasogastric** intake should be recorded on the fluid intake section of the fluid balance chart. If the patient has continuous bladder drainage via an indwelling catheter, then this should be recorded on the output section. All urine voided should be measured and recorded in the output section, as should any diarrhoea or output from a **stoma**, nasogastric aspiration and vomit. Any drainage from a wound should also be noted on the output section. Finally, the nurse must consider insensible fluid losses when calculating the final fluid balance.

A new fluid balance chart is used for each 24-hour period. The fluid intake and output for the previous day are totalled and the balance calculated; this is usually done at midnight. The balance total may be positive or negative, depending on whether the input is greater or less than the output. For example, if the patient's input is 2575 mL and their output is 1760 mL, then the patient is in a positive balance of 815 mL. Conversely, if the patient's input is 1200 mL but their output is 2450 mL, then the patient is in a negative balance of 1250 mL.

The term **'nasogastric'** describes fluid taken via a tube inserted via the nostril and into the stomach.

A **stoma** is an opening on the surface of the skin, via the abdominal wall, through which the contents of the bowel are expelled.

Fluid balance chart							
Hospital/Ward: A1			Date: 13/6/06				
Hospital number: N317065 Surname: JONES Date of birth: 26/3/51			Forenames: Mary Sex: Female				
Fluid intake				Fluid output			
Time (hrs)	Oral	IV	Other (specify route)	Urine	Vomit	Other (specify)	
01.00	NBM	B/F 500				WOUND DRAIN	
02.00		N/SALINE 0.9%	N/SALINE 0.9%				
03.00							
04.00							
05.00							
06.00		5 % Dex		400		90	
07.00		1000					
08.00							
09.00							
10.00	30 H$_2$0						
11.00	30 H$_2$0						
12.00	30 H$_2$0			500			
13.00	30 H$_2$0						
14.00	30 H$_2$0						
15.00	30 H$_2$0						
16.00	30 H$_2$0						
17.00	30 H$_2$0						
18.00	60 H$_2$0	5 % Dex		450			
19.00	60 H$_2$0	1000					
20.00	60 H$_2$0						
21.00	60 H$_2$0						
22.00	100 TEA						
23.00							
24.00				350		50	
TOTAL	580mls	2000		1800		140	

KEY:
NBM = NIL BY MOUTH
B/F = BROUGHT FORWARD

ALL MEASUREMENTS IN MILLILITRES (MLS.)
TOTAL INPUT = 580 + 2000 = 2580 MLS.
TOTAL OUTPUT = 1800 + 140 = 1940 MLS.

Figure 6.2 Example of a completed fluid balance chart
Source: Nicol (2004)

To think about

In the fluid balance chart shown in Figure 6.2, does the patient have a positive or a negative fluid balance?

An imbalance of electrolytes can cause fluid imbalance. Laboratory blood tests such as urea and electrolytes (U&Es), glucose, magnesium and calcium can help to determine the cause and thus the treatment needed to correct the imbalance.

Recording fluid balance

Fluid balance should be recorded in any patient who shows signs and symptoms (see Table 6.3) of fluid imbalance. Any patient who is critically ill or has had surgery must have their fluid balance monitored strictly. Elderly patients with indwelling catheters with continuous drainage should be encouraged to drink plenty of fluids in order to ensure good **diuresis** and to prevent dehydration, to which elderly people are susceptible.

Importance of accurate fluid balance

It is important to remember that accurate recording of fluid balance is crucial to a patient's wellbeing and recovery. Any problems with fluid balance can then be detected early and treated appropriately. Any patient who is taking diuretic medication, which promotes the kidneys to excrete more urine, should have their fluid balance monitored closely.

Now consider Case studies 6.1 and 6.2.

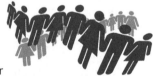

Case Study 6.1

Mrs Shields is a 63-year-old woman with congestive cardiac failure. She is a widow and lives alone. She has had 'heart problems' for many years. She takes medication for her heart, including diuretics to reduce fluid overload. Mrs Shields has her weight checked weekly. At the last weigh-in, she was 80 kg. You look at her fluid balance chart and find that she has had a fluid intake of 500 mL since midnight; it is now 5.30am and you notice she has passed only 10 mL of urine over a five-hour period.

What would you do next?

There are several things you should do in this instance. First, you need to alert the nurse in charge of your findings, as Mrs Shields requires immediate medical assistance. If a patient's urinary output falls below 30 mL an hour, this needs urgent attention. As this is a medical emergency, it is vital to continue to monitor Mrs Shield's fluid intake and output. The doctor

Diuresis is the secretion of urine.

may prescribe more diuretics to help promote diuresis. The patient's fluid intake is quite low, so you may need to encourage her to drink more fluids – but you must check with the nurse in charge first, as patients with congestive cardiac failure must have their fluid intake monitored closely in order to ensure that the circulatory system does not become overloaded. You should record any fluids given to Mrs Shields on her fluid balance chart. Fluid intake should normally be at least 1500 mL per day, which should promote diuresis and improve the patient's low urine output. Normal urine output should also be about 1500 mL per day. If Mrs Shields' urine output does not improve, you need to contact the doctor again and further clinical decisions will need to be made. It would also be useful to weigh Mrs Shields.

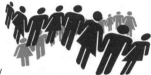

Case Study 6.2

Mrs Kaur is 28 years old. She is admitted to the ward with severe abdominal pain. She is vomiting large amounts of fluid. She is very anxious and informs you that her husband is working out of the country and her 3-year-old son needs to be picked up from nursery. You obtain the contact details of a neighbour, who might be able to collect her son. Following your assessment and recording of vital signs, Mrs Kaur's pulse is 120 bpm, her respirations are 26 breaths per minute and her temperature is 37.8 °C. It becomes clear that Miss Kaur is poorly and in a dehydrated state.

What would you do next?

You need to inform the nurse in charge immediately, as Mrs Kaur's dehydration needs correcting as soon as possible. You need to continue monitoring the patient's vital signs, as she is showing signs of shock due to fluid loss and she is pyrexial; therefore, you need to be able to quickly detect any deterioration in her condition. Mrs Kaur requires intravenous fluids; you need a doctor to **cannulate** and commence the intravenous infusion and prescribe the fluids to be given. All fluids infused must be recorded on a fluid balance chart, and the patient's fluid intake and output must be strictly monitored. Mrs Kaur should be given an **antiemetic** and analgesia to relieve her abdominal pain. The doctor requests an abdominal X-ray to help identify the cause of Mrs Kaur's pain. Continuous monitoring of her vital signs, fluid balance and pain relief are required to assess any changes in the patient's condition. You also need to contact the patient's neighbour as soon as you can in order to allay her anxiety and reduce her severe pain.

Recap Questions

1. Why is it important to record a patient's fluid balance accurately?
2. When carrying out a clinical assessment, what signs and symptoms may indicate fluid overload?
3. When carrying out a clinical assessment, what signs and symptoms may indicate fluid depletion/loss?

To **cannulate** means to insert a cannula into the vein to facilitate the giving of fluids via the bloodstream.

An **antiemetic** is a drug used to reduce vomiting.

Urinary continence

The ability to be continent of both urine and faeces is something most people take for granted. However, incontinence is a widespread and serious medical problem (Irwin *et al.*, 2001), and it has been estimated that more than five million people in the UK have some form of incontinence (Continence Foundation, 2000). Incontinence rates are especially high among patients in hospitals and nursing and residential homes, where over 50% of patients are thought to be affected (Sander, 1999). It is arguable whether these high numbers reflect the healthcare professionals failing to address the problem adequately (Bignell, 1999; Burgio and Goode, 1997; Irwin *et al.*, 2001).

Over the past two decades, there has been a considerable growth in knowledge regarding the promotion, assessment and treatment of continence (Irwin *et al.*, 2001). The introduction of specialist nurses and continence advisers has helped to improve continence care, but there is still room for improvement, as the study by Irwin and colleagues (2001) demonstrated. The aim of this study was to determine the adequacy of diagnosis for patients with a continence problem and the provision and appropriateness of treatment in a UK trust. The knowledge of healthcare staff on incontinence was also assessed. The results identified a range of deficiencies in the quality of incontinence care. For example, no diagnosis of the underlying cause of incontinence had been made in 53 of the 66 patients (80.3%) studied. Interventions such as bladder re-education and **anticholinergic** medication were rarely used. In 14 patients (21.2%), no treatment had been given. Response to treatment had not been recorded in the patients' notes. The study also found that the knowledge of nursing staff on incontinence and its management was inadequate. The authors concluded from their findings that urinary incontinence remains poorly managed in the particular trust involved in the study. There was evidence of inadequate standards of care, underuse of active interventions and insufficient nursing knowledge.

It is important to emphasise the vital role of the nurse in continence care. Incontinence is generally more common in older people, and nurses make a significant contribution to the healthcare of older people, particularly in relation to the provision of continence care (Billington, 2002), whether in hospital or nursing or residential homes. Unfortunately, ageism is sometimes related to continence issues; ageist attitudes can lead to inappropriate care based on incorrect assumptions, for example that all old people have continence problems or that all incontinence needs to be treated with pads. This can lead to discrimination in continence care in older people (De Laine *et al.*, 2002). This issue is addressed later in the chapter.

Revision

Before reading the next section, you need to revise the anatomy and physiology of the renal system, with particular reference to the bladder and the process of micturition.

Anticholinergic drugs inhibit the action of acetylcholine.

Anatomy and physiology

The urinary, or renal, system consists of two kidneys, two ureters, one bladder and one urethra. Urinary elimination is dependent on the effective functioning of these four urinary tract structures (Figure 6.3).

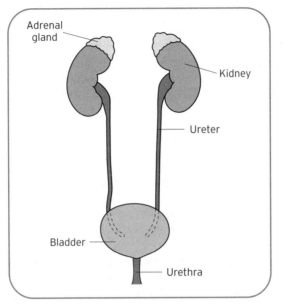

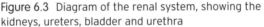

Figure 6.3 Diagram of the renal system, showing the kidneys, ureters, bladder and urethra

Kidneys

The kidneys are positioned against the posterior abdominal wall, lying close to the aorta and inferior vena cava, to which they are joined by blood vessels (see Figure 6.3). The most important function of the kidney is to maintain constant composition and volume of body fluids, primarily the blood, from which the other fluids are formed. The functional unit of the kidney is the nephron, which is responsible for filtering the blood and removing metabolic waste. In an average adult, 1200 mL of blood (about 21% of the cardiac output) passes through the kidneys every minute (Kozier *et al.*, 2004). Each kidney contains about one million nephrons. The filtration process through the nephrons results in the production of urine. Approximately 1500 mL of urine is produced and excreted daily.

Ureters

Once the urine is formed in the kidneys, it passes into either ureter. The ureters are hollow muscular tubes that actively convey urine from the kidneys to the bladder. Small volumes of urine are squeezed along the ureters by peristaltic waves. Urine arrives in the bladder at an average rate of four or five jets per minute.

Bladder

The bladder is a hollow muscular organ that stores urine. The bladder wall consists of several layers, including three layers of smooth involuntary muscle fibres known collectively as the detrusor muscle. The bladder is capable of considerable distension because of the elasticity of its walls, and it can hold up to 1000 mL of urine – although this would be extremely uncomfortable for the patient.

Urethra

The urethra extends from the bladder to the urinary meatus (opening). The urethra is shorter in females (3.7 cm), due to the anatomical position in which it lies. In males, it is 20 cm in length. The urethra serves as a passageway for the elimination of urine (micturition) and is comprised of smooth muscle.

Micturition

Micturition, also known as voiding or urination, refers to the process of emptying the urinary bladder. In the healthy adult, the process is under voluntary control. As the bladder fills, the pressure inside it rises. Contraction waves appear in the muscular coat, stimulating pressure receptors and sending nerve impulses to the brain, where the desire to urinate is registered. The next phase depends on whether it is convenient to micturate. The pressure receptors are stimulated when the bladder contains 250-450 mL of urine in adults or 50-200 mL in children.

If it is convenient to urinate, then impulses from the cerebral cortex in the brain are transmitted down the spinal cord, stimulating the detrusor muscle in the bladder to contract. This opens the internal sphincter. The perineal muscles and external sphincter relax voluntarily. This coincides with raised intra-abdominal pressure resulting from contraction of the diaphragm and abdominal muscles, and the bladder empties.

If it is not convenient to urinate, impulses from the cerebral cortex cause inhibition of the detrusor muscle, enlarging the bladder to accommodate the increasing volume of urine. The pressure in the bladder falls and the desire to urinate wears off for a time. The bladder can be trained to hold large volumes of urine, but eventually the pressure rise becomes painful and the bladder must be emptied.

Most people empty their bladder four to six times a day. If a person repeatedly empties their bladder when there is only a small amount of urine in it, the bladder shrinks and is not stretched properly; this can lead to weakness of the bladder muscles, resulting in possible problems with continence in later years.

Recap Questions

1. What are the structures of the urinary system?
2. In an average adult, how much blood flows through the kidneys in a minute?
3. How is the process of micturition controlled to ensure that urine is voided only when it is convenient to do so?

Factors affecting micturition

Many factors can affect the process of micturition, including the following:

+ *Age*: infants are born without voluntary control. Most children develop control between the ages of 2 and 5 years. Most preschool children have voluntary control but still have the occasional accident. The schoolchild's elimination system reaches maturity during this period, with the kidneys doubling in size between the ages of 5 and 10 years. Most 6-year-olds have total control of the bladder both day and night. Before this they may have the occasional accident - **enuresis** - which tends to occur more at night, i.e. nocturnal enuresis. Bladder changes occur in elderly people, resulting in problems with urinary urgency and frequency. Furthermore, the capacity of the bladder and its ability to empty diminishes with age and explains why many elderly people have to get up in the night to void; this is called nocturnal frequency. The retention of residual urine predisposes elderly people to bladder infections.

+ *Psychosocial factors*: the conditions have to be right for many people to be able to urinate. For example, privacy, normal position, sufficient time and sometimes the sound of running water can promote urine flow. If these factors are not present, this can lead to anxiety and muscle tension, which can interfere with the process of micturition, giving rise to an increased risk of urinary tract infections because urine remains in the bladder for longer than it should.

+ *Fluid and food intake*: certain fluids, such as alcohol, increase fluid output by inhibiting the production of ADH. Fluids such as coffee, tea and cola drinks that contain caffeine also increase urine output. Certain foods such as bacon and fluids that are high in sodium can cause fluid retention.

+ *Medications*: some drugs, such as those acting on the autonomic nervous system, interfere with the urinary process, causing urinary retention, while others, such as diuretics (e.g. furosemide), increase urine formation. Some medications alter the colour of urine; for example, the antibiotic nitrofurantoin can cause urine to be dark yellow, and metronidazole, another antibiotic, can turn the urine a reddish brown.

+ *Muscle tone*: good muscle control is needed to maintain the stretch and contractibility of the detrusor muscle so that the bladder can fill adequately and empty completely. Abdominal and pelvic muscles also contribute. A problem with any of these muscles can lead to problems with bladder control.

+ *Pathological conditions*: kidney disease can affect the formation of urine. Heart and circulatory disorders can also affect blood flow to the kidneys, thus interfering with urine production.

Enuresis is the involuntary passing of urine.

Abnormalities in urine production and elimination

Certain abnormalities occur in the production and the elimination of urine:

+ *Polyuria*: this is the production by the kidneys of abnormally high amounts of urine, sometimes as much as several litres per day. Polyuria is usually associated with diseases such as diabetes mellitus, diabetes insipidus and chronic nephritis (inflammation of the nephrons within the kidney).

+ *Oliguria*: this is decreased urine output, usually less than 500 mL a day or 30 mL an hour. Oliguria often indicates impaired blood flow to the kidneys or impending renal failure and should be dealt with immediately.

+ *Anuria*: this is the absence of urine production. Anuria is a serious medical condition that usually follows oliguria. It must be treated immediately in order to prevent death from renal failure. **Renal dialysis** is used when the kidneys are no longer able to filter blood.

Several problems are associated with urinary elimination; these are summarized in Table 6.4.

Table 6.4 Problems associated with altered urinary elimination

Problem	Symptom	Causes
Urinary frequency	Voiding frequently	Increased fluid intake, urinary tract infection, pregnancy
Nocturia	Voiding more than twice a night	Weakened bladder muscles
Urgency	Urgent need to void	Psychological distress, bladder irritation
Dysuria	Pain/difficulty in voiding	Urethral stricture, urinary infection
Enuresis	Involuntary voiding	May be associated with psychological and emotional insecurity; nocturnal enuresis tends to affect boys more than girls; diurnal (daytime) enuresis is pathological and affects females more frequently than males
Urinary incontinence	Involuntary urination	Urinary incontinence is usually a symptom rather than a disease (see later for examples)
Urinary retention	Impaired bladder emptying	Prostatic enlargement, surgery, some medications
Neurogenic bladder	Loss of sensation to the bladder	Impaired neurological function, e.g. due to paraplegia, tetraplegia or multiple sclerosis

In **renal dialysis**, the patient's blood is artificially fed through a dialysis machine, which acts like an artificial kidney and filters the blood.

Incontinence

Voluntary control of the bladder and bowel – continence – is a skill most of us take for granted. We use the toilet when we need to and seldom think about it. However, urinary incontinence affects one in four females and one in ten males. It has no respect for age, occupation or lifestyle. Incontinence is not a disease but a symptom of an underlying cause. Although urinary incontinence is not life-threatening, it can have a devastating impact on a person's life. Fortunately, most incontinence can be treated effectively; if a cure is not available, then good management is required (see later for details of treatments).

The International Continence Society (2000) defines incontinence as a 'condition in which involuntary loss of urine is a social or hygienic problem and is objectively demonstrable'.

Incontinence can cause great distress, particularly if the person has both urinary and faecal incontinence. Incontinence can have a devastating effect on body image (how the person sees themselves), self-esteem and sense of wellbeing. Incontinence can make the person feel dirty and unattractive. The nurse must always consider the patient's feelings when dealing with incontinence and be sensitive when helping the patient to cope with any problems of continence. To ensure continence, certain factors are essential.

To think about

What do you think these factors may be? Think about the processes involved when a person needs to go to the toilet to pass urine.

Continence depends on the following factors:

+ Knowledge to recognise the need to pass urine or faeces
+ Ability to identify the correct place in which to urinate or defecate
+ Ability to reach the appropriate place in a timely manner
+ Ability to not pass urine or faeces until the appropriate place is reached
+ Ability to pass urine when the appropriate place has been reached

If there are problems or deficits with any of these factors, the person may become incontinent. With this in mind, we can consider the possible causes of urinary incontinence, which include the following:

+ Infection
+ Constipation

+ Muscle damage
+ Nerve damage
+ Congenital problems
+ Immobilisation/problems with mobility
+ Inability to communicate appropriately
+ Stress incontinence after childbirth

A detailed assessment is necessary to determine the type and cause of the person's incontinence (Exhibit 6.1). This ensures that the appropriate treatment and management can be offered. To promote continence, the nurse needs to know why the individual is incontinent. Questions asked can relate to problems with any of the five factors necessary to maintain continence, as outlined above. Does the person have weak muscles? Is their bladder unable to hold urine? Does the person have mobility problems in trying to reach the toilet? When the person does get to the bathroom, does it take a long time to make the necessary adjustments to clothing, resulting in it being 'too late'?

+ Biographic data
+ Bladder symptoms as described by the patient
+ Onset of symptoms
+ Previous urinary tract investigations
+ Previous medical history
+ Lifestyle
+ Social data
+ Psychological data
+ Patterns of healthcare

Exhibit 6.1 Taking an oral history to help identify the causes of incontinence

To think about

Next time you go to the toilet, wear a pair of thick gloves to simulate stiff arthritic hands and see how much harder it is to undo buttons and zips. Imagine you have only a few seconds before it is too late. If you did have a accident, how would you feel? How would you react if the nurse told you off for getting in a mess?

The components of the assessment should include a baseline frequency/volume chart (Figure 6.4), which is kept for 3-5 days. This should consider the following:

+ Number and severity of incontinence episodes
+ Frequency of toilet visits
+ Fluid intake
+ Volume of urine passed

Weekly progress chart

Name _A.N. OTHER_   Week beginning _____

KEY ▣ NUMBER OF DRINKS   ☐ NUMBER OF TIMES URINE PASSED

SPECIAL INSTRUCTIONS

W = WET

	Sunday		Monday		Tuesday	Wednesday	Thursday	Friday	Saturday
6am				550ml					
7am	200 ml TEA	500ml	200 ml TEA						
8am	200 ml TEA		200 ml TEA						
9am									
10am	200 ml COFFEE		150 ml ORANGE	W					
11am	200 ml COFFEE								
Noon		250ml		300ml					
1pm	200 ml WATER		200 ml WATER						
2pm									
3pm	200 ml TEA		200 ml COFFEE						
4pm		300ml							
5pm		W		250ml					
6pm	200 ml WATER		200 ml WATER						
7pm		300ml							
8pm	150 ml COLA		500 ml BEER						
9pm									
10pm	200 ml MILK		500 ml BEER						
11pm		200ml		300ml					
Midnight									
1am									
2am									
3am	100 ml WATER			400ml					
4am									
5am									
Total	1850	1550	2150	1800					

Figure 6.4 Example of a completed weekly progress chart
Source: © Clinical Skills Ltd

A general history should also be taken, including the following:

✛ Onset of symptoms

✛ Previous urinary tract investigations

+ Any previous operations affecting the urinary tract

+ Details of medical, surgical, obstetric, gynaecological and urological history

+ Review of any prescribed and over-the-counter medications taken

Urinalysis

If the patient has urinary incontinence, **urinalysis** should be carried out. If the urine is obviously infected or blood-stained, a clean specimen that has not been contaminated should be sent to the laboratory for culture and sensitivity. If there is a positive test with a reagent strip for protein, blood, nitrates or leucocytes, then a clean specimen should also be sent.

An assessment of the person's cognitive ability also needs to be made. If the person has perceptual problems (agnosia), which are common in patients after stroke and in patients with senile dementia, they might be able to see the toilet but not recognise it as such (Sander, 1999).

A physical examination, usually done by a doctor, may be carried out to provide any extra information and to highlight any structural abnormalities, such as an enlarged prostate in male patients or a prolapsed uterus in female patients.

Identifying the cause of the incontinence

Once a detailed assessment has been done, it is possible to start to identify the cause of the incontinence. Identifying the cause is vital to continence promotion. The causes of incontinence can be divided into acute (transient) and chronic (persistent) problems.

Acute incontinence has a sudden onset and is often associated with an underlying medical condition, such as urinary tract infection, hyperglycaemia (high blood glucose levels in the blood) or vaginitis (inflammation of the vagina). Wyman (1991) used the mnemonic 'DRIP' to list the causes of acute incontinence:

+ *D*: delirium

+ *R*: restricted mobility, retention (acute)

+ *I*: infection, inflammation, impaction

+ *P*: pharmaceuticals, polyuria, psychological

Urinalysis is a test used to identify the presence of a variety of substances in the urine, such as protein, blood, glucose, leucocytes (white blood cells) and ketones, which should not normally be present.

Chronic incontinence usually develops gradually and persists over a period of time. It is commonly divided into four main groups:

+ Stress incontinence
+ Urge incontinence
+ Overflow incontinence
+ Functional incontinence

Stress incontinence

Stress incontinence (Table 6.5) is caused by a weak urethral sphincter mechanism. (Note that in this case the word 'stress' is not related to the everyday meaning of the word, such as 'I feel stressed'.) Stress incontinence results in urine leakage, usually occurring simultaneously with a rise in abdominal pressure such as during exercise. Contributing factors include childbirth, menopause, obesity, chronic cough and constipation. Stress incontinence mainly affects females, but it can occur in males after prostatectomy.

Table 6.5 Different types of incontinence

Types of incontinence	Cause	Contributory factors
Stress incontinence	Weak urethral sphincter mechanism	Childbirth, menopause, obesity, chronic cough, constipation
Urge incontinence	Detrusor muscle instability/hypersensitivity	Urinary tract infection, large intake of fluid, medication, menopause, anxiety
Overflow incontinence	Obstruction to the outflow of urine	Benign prostatic hyperplasia (males), faecal impaction, atonic/hypotonic bladder
Functional incontinence	Severe mobility, dexterity restrictions	Demetia, *iatrogenic* incontinence associated with some healthcare practices

Urge incontinence

Urge incontinence (Table 6.5) is due to detrusor muscle instability or detrusor hypersensitivity. Urine leakage is associated with a strong desire (urgency) to pass urine. Incontinence may be sudden and large in volume. Contributing factors include urinary tract infection, certain types and large quantities of fluid intake, medication, menopause and anxiety. Urge incontinence is also likely to occur if there is damage to the nervous system, such as in stroke, Parkinson's disease, Alzheimer's disease and multiple sclerosis (Sander, 1999).

Overflow incontinence

Overflow incontinence (Table 6.5) is caused by an outflow obstruction such as **benign prostatic hyperplasia** in males, faecal impaction, or an **atonic** or **hypotonic bladder**. Urine leakage is associated with incomplete bladder emptying, resulting in urinary retention (Marjoram, 1999); this accounts for less than 10% of incontinence in older people. Contributing factors include the side effects of some medications, constipation and sudden immobility.

Functional incontinence

Functional incontinence (Table 6.5) occurs as a result of severe mobility and dexterity restrictions that impair the person's ability to reach the toilet unaided. It can affect people with dementia or confusion when an inappropriate response to bladder signals occurs. This type of incontinence can also be associated with some practices carried out in healthcare facilities; this is called iatrogenic incontinence. The following are some examples (Stone, 1991):

+ The patient is unable to locate the toilet

+ There is no access to a urinal or commode and the patient is unable to reach the toilet

+ There is a delayed response to the nurse-call bell

+ The use of certain medication, such as diuretics, sedatives, anticholinergics and antiparkinson drugs, which can lead to increased diuresis

Accurate diagnosis of the cause of the incontinence is important to ensure that the correct treatment and care are prescribed. We now consider some of the treatment regimes available for the different types of incontinence.

Treating the cause of incontinence

To think about

We have discussed the different causes of urinary incontinence. Can you identify some of the ways in which urinary incontinence can be treated? You have probably seen some of these treatments in practice. Are some treatments used more commonly than others?

Benign prostatic hyperplasia is enlargement of the prostate gland.

Atonic or **hypotonic bladder** is 'slackening' of the bladder muscles that control micturition, such that they do not operate effectively.

Acute incontinence

Treatment of acute incontinence depends on the cause and can be relatively simple. For example, antibiotics can eradicate a urinary tract infection, while aperients/laxatives can deal with the problem of faecal impaction. Advice on lifestyle changes may be required to prevent any further problems; for example, an adequate daily fluid intake is necessary to reduce the risk of bladder infections and help to prevent constipation. Patients should be made aware of the importance of not restricting fluids for fear of bladder or bowel dysfunction.

Stress incontinence

Increasing the tone of the pelvic floor muscles is the main treatment for stress incontinence in women. This can be achieved by regularly performing pelvic floor exercises. The aim is to squeeze the muscles around the vagina, hold for a few seconds and then release. Repetition is the key to success, with the above procedure being carried out 20 times and repeated at least three times a day. Another helpful exercise for the patient is to try to stop and then restart the normal flow of urine during voiding. These exercises may need to be continued for 3–6 months before incontinence improves. Information should be given on an individual basis and supported with some written guidelines.

Stress incontinence can also be treated with drugs such as imipramine. This drug stimulates smooth muscle to contract, which helps to increase urethral pressure. Oestrogen preparations can also help by improving the tone of the pelvic floor muscles (McDowell and Burgio, 1992).

Urge incontinence

Reducing the intake of caffeine can help some people with urge incontinence, as caffeine increases detrusor instability. Adequate fluid intake is important to help reduce the concentration of irritants in the bladder. An intake of at least 1500–2000 mL per day should be recommended.

Bladder retraining can also help. This can be achieved by encouraging the patient to increase the amount of urine that the bladder can hold. This can be monitored by keeping a diary and gradually increasing the intervals between going to the toilet by 15 minutes each day. The patient may have to follow the programme for several weeks before they can visit the toilet at two- or three-hourly intervals, but eventually they will master some control over the problem. An antispasmodic drug, such as imipramine or oxybutynin, may be prescribed to inhibit detrusor contractions (McDowell and Burgio, 1992). Oestrogen preparations may also help to reduce inflammation, which can contribute to urinary urgency. This form of bladder training is effective, but it is quite labour-intensive and the patient has to be well motivated in order to succeed (McCreanor et al., 1998).

Overflow incontinence

If the cause is an obstruction, such as an enlarged prostate gland, it may be possible to remove the obstruction by surgery. If the cause is constipation, then the administration of aperients may help. If the cause of a partial obstruction cannot be removed, then the Crede manoeuvre can be employed. This manoeuvre involves expelling urine by applying gentle pressure on the **suprapubic area** (McDowell and Burgio, 1992). This technique should be used

The **suprapubic area** is located just above the pubic bone, in the area of the bladder.

with caution and by a healthcare professional trained in the technique in order to avoid any damage from excessive pressure. Intermittent catheterisation, in which a catheter is inserted into the bladder two or three times a day to empty any urine, may be used. If the problem is severe, a permanent catheter may be the best (and sometimes the only) solution. Care of the patient with a permanent catheter is addressed later in this chapter.

Functional incontinence

This involves diversity and depends greatly on the cause.

To think about

If a patient has some form of functional incontinence, what could you do to help promote their continence?
Think of a patient you have nursed with functional incontinence. Was a lot of thought given to the promotion of continence in this patient?
If not, how could it have been improved?

One of the main causes of functional incontinence is reduced mobility. In this case, continence can be promoted by considering the following:

+ Move the patient closer to the toilet so they do not have so far to travel.
+ Give regular and effective pain relief to help increase mobility.
+ Give the patient assistance to reach the toilet and then, if they are able, try to encourage them to make their own way back.
+ Consider the patient's medication, such as sedatives, which can interfere with mobility, and ensure that there are no obstacles such as trolleys and lockers that could impair the patient's progress to the toilet.
+ Ensure that the chair the patient is sitting in is the correct height so that the patient is able to get up.
+ The use of grab-rails and bars on the walls can give the patient support.
+ There should be adequate lighting and non-slip surfaces in the bathroom, and the toilet should be clearly signposted.
+ The toilet area should be warm and clean-smelling, with plenty of toilet paper available and handwashing facilities at the right height.

Adjustments such as enlarged openings, Velcro fastenings and elasticated waists can be made to the patient's clothing to help them use the toilet more easily. People with cognitive dysfunction need to be taken to the toilet regularly and reminded of why they are there.

Recap Questions

1. What are the possible causes of urinary incontinence?
2. Why is it necessary to carry out a detailed assessment of a person's incontinence?
3. What are the four main types of chronic urinary incontinence, and how are they treated?

Promoting continence

It is important to remember that continence care should be 'the total care package tailored to meet the individual needs of patients with bladder and bowel problems' (Department of Health, 2000). The ultimate aim is to promote continence wherever possible but to remember that in a few patients incontinence is intractable and continence promotion will not help. For these patients, it is important to ensure that their comfort and self-esteem are maintained at all times and to give them choices regarding the incontinence pads and pants they wish to use (Sander, 1999). The first two standards in the NSF For Older People (Department of Health, 2001), which are concerned with antidiscriminatory practice and person-centred care, imply that the older person should be at the centre of their treatment; consequently, the services provided should be needs-led and not service-led.

Consider Case study 6.3, which is a development of Case study 1.5 in Chapter 1.

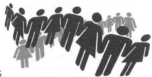

Case Study 6.3

Richard Brown is 9 years old. As a baby he had surgery to correct a congenital abnormality of his urinary system. The surgery was successful but resulted in some scar tissue forming around the urethra, which is causing stress incontinence. Richard has to attend a yearly outpatient appointment to monitor his progress. At school, due to his stress incontinence, he has to go to the toilet quickly and frequently. When he asked the teacher if he could do this, the teacher told him that he could go but that he would receive a detention for each extra time he left the classroom. This caused Richard to become more anxious about asking to go to the toilet, and consequently his stress incontinence worsened. His parents were not happy with the way the teacher was dealing with Richard, even though they had explained to her about Richard's stress incontinence. Richard's parents reported the issue to his consultant at the hospital, who wrote a letter to the school explaining about Richard's stress incontinence and the associated problems. As a result, the situation was resolved.

Reflect on your reactions to Case study 6.3. It clearly outlines a young child with stress incontinence and whose teacher does not fully understand the effects this has on the child. The teacher seems to think that Richard is playing up by visiting the toilet frequently. Imagine how this will influence Richard's behaviour and his stress incontinence. It is not surprising that his parents were unhappy. The teacher showed a lack of understanding and did not help in the promotion of Richard's continence.

To promote person-centred continence care, three factors must be considered (De Laine et al., 2002):

+ Eliminate any discrimination in continence care
+ Ensure staff have adequate knowledge of continence care
+ Contribute to the provision of a seamless continence service by providing single assessment (this means a patient-centred, interprofessional/interagency assessment of health and social care needs)

> ### To think about
>
> You are a student nurse working on a care of the elderly ward. You identify a patient who is experiencing incontinence and ask to be involved with the patient's continence assessment. You are told that there is no point in doing a continence assessment as the patient is old. Your supervisor tells you to 'just give her some pads'.
>
> What is your reaction to this statement?
> Do you think this is acceptable?
> What could you do?

This scenario is clearly an example of ageism. The implication is that incontinence is an accepted and expected consequence of ageing. Even though the incidence of incontinence does increase with age, the expressed attitude goes against the standard of the NSF for Older People (Department of Health, 2001). This standard relates to discrimination and states that no patient should be declined medical diagnosis and treatment because of their advanced age.

Continence aids and appliances

When it is not possible to achieve continence, there are a range of products to help the person manage their incontinence. Careful assessment is essential to ensure the products meet the patient's requirements. The use of absorbent pads is the most common method of managing incontinence and is the only option for women, other than catheterisation, as there is no satisfactory external device at present (Olsen-Vetland, 2003). Penile sheaths may be useful for men; these sheaths can be connected to a bed or leg-worn drainage bag, but they require a degree of manual dexterity to use. A long-term indwelling urinary catheter may be used, but this should always be seen as a last resort when other methods have failed (Simpson, 2001).

The emphasis should always be on the promotion of continence rather than on the containment of incontinence. Therapeutic strategies, such as bladder re-education, the use of anticholinergic medications and surgery, should also be considered before the so-called 'pad culture' is reached, in which pads are used for continent patients, a finding demonstrated clearly in a study by Irwin *et al.* (2001). This study considered a group of 200 patients with urinary incontinence. They found that in 80% of patients with incontinence, an accurate diagnosis had not been made. The study also found that there was a marked underuse of therapeutic strategies to promote continence and a significant overuse of containment strategies such as incontinence pads. The study showed that 60% of patients stated that they had not been given the opportunity to discuss their continence problem with medical or nursing staff. The knowledge of incontinence and its management was also inadequate in the nursing staff included in the study.

It is useful to remember that continence aids should have two main functions:

+ To promote continence by managing incontinence temporarily and thereby providing confidence, while regaining/achieving continence
+ To promote confidence, by managing irreversible incontinence effectively, when continence is not achievable

The relationship between continence and confidence is important to consider. The best continence aid is that which works effectively every time, is acceptable to the user and suits the person's lifestyle. In other words, it should enable the person to achieve social continence.

Incontinence aids can be divided into absorbent or containment aids, and collection or conduction aids. These are now considered in more detail.

Absorbent/containment aids

These include body-worn disposable pads, holding garments and incontinence garments. A large variety of different pad types are available. Disposable body-worn pads are the most commonly used to contain and absorb urine and faeces (Pomfret, 2000).

The cost to the NHS of supplying continence pads has been estimated at £80 million per annum (Euromonitor, 1999) and is a huge financial burden on local services. In the UK, disposable pads are generally supplied by NHS community continence services or hospital supplies departments (Gilbert, 2005). Although these products are supplied to patients free of charge, there is great disparity between the types of product available due to local and national contracts. To overcome these differences, the *Essence of Care* continence benchmark (Modernisation Agency, 2003) has included a factor that relates to patient access to continence supplies and to the Department of Health's formalised key principles for the supply of products (Department of Health, 2000). These include the remit that pads are issued only after an initial assessment, that a full range of products is available, that supply of products is governed by clinical need and that the patient's needs are reviewed on a regular basis.

The main aim of using absorbent pads is to absorb, contain, conceal and manage incontinence loss without leakage, thereby preserving the dignity and confidence of the user. The benchmark for continence and bladder and bowel care in the *Essence of Care* benchmark stipulates that practitioners must respect patient dignity. If the correct pad is not worn, the patient may experience many problems, as outlined in Exhibit 6.2. A detailed individual assessment is important to ensure that this is achieved. Offering patients body-worn pads prematurely can lead to them being unwilling to give them up and start a programme of treatment (Department of Health, 2000). Sadly, sometimes absorbent pads are used as an alternative to an individual toileting programme (Pomfret, 2000). No product should be supplied without a continence assessment (Department of Health, 2000). Several factors should be considered at assessment, including the following:

+ Patient preference

+ Level of disability

+ Physical and cognitive function

+ Gender

+ Type and severity of incontinence

+ Skin integrity

+ Products previously used

It is essential to select the correct type, size and absorbency of the product in order to maintain the patient's comfort and security. This ultimately improves the patient's quality of life, preserves dignity, encourages independence and helps promote continence (Gilbert, 2005).

> + Leakage
> + Skin integrity problems, such as sweat rash and skin sensitivity (caused by inappropriate use of pads)
> + Compromise of patient's dignity, such as pad dependency, leakage and odour (caused by not changing the pad often enough)
> + High cost associated with inappropriate use, overstocking, a culture of pad dependency and no consideration to alternatives or to treatment programmes

Exhibit 6.2 Problems associated with wearing disposable body-worn pads
Adapted from Gilbert (2005)

Two types of absorbent pad are available: a two-piece system and an all-in-one product.

The two-piece system is a pad (with or without an adhesive strip) shaped to fit the body. The pad is worn inside close-fitting underwear or underwear designed specifically to hold a pad. With this method, it is important to use the correct size pad and underwear. When applying a pad, several factors should be considered. Have you done the following:

+ Made the correct assessment?

+ Selected the correct pad?

+ Cupped the pad before putting it on?

+ Selected the correct pant size?

+ Checked that the seams of the pants are on the outside of the body?

+ Ensured the pad and pants are fitted closely into the groin?

+ Maintained regular toileting?

+ Used barrier creams sparingly?

All-in-one products are designed to be worn without additional underwear, similar to a nappy or pull-up pants. All-in-one pads tend to be more expensive and are used less frequently. However, they can be used very effectively to help promote continence, as the wearer is able to manipulate the product in the same way as normal underwear. This also helps promote independence (Gilbert, 2005).

Some nurses view the management of incontinence as low-status work, considering the use of disposable incontinence products as a menial job that does not require specific knowledge and skills. This assumption is incorrect, as disposable incontinence products are listed as medical devices (Medicines and Healthcare Products Regulatory Agency, 2001) and therefore nurses need to ensure that they are competent to use them (Gilbert, 2005).

Collection/conduction aids

These can be divided into internal and external devices. Internal devices include urinary catheters, which may be urethral, suprapubic, intermittent or self-containing. Although urinary catheters are an essential part of continence treatment and care, they should be the last method of choice for the management of incontinence, because they carry the risks of trauma and infection.

External devices include penile sheaths (Figure 6.5), and urinary and faecal collection appliances.

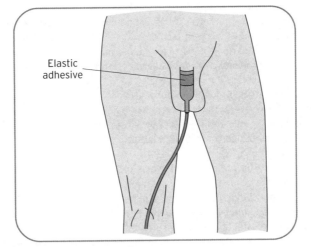

Figure 6.5 Penile sheath
Source: Nicol (2004)

This section has considered the importance of promoting continence and ensuring that a detailed assessment and diagnosis of the cause of the urinary incontinence is made before treatment. Emphasis should be on the use of therapeutic strategies to help promote continence rather than on the use of containment strategies.

Recap Questions

1. Why is it important to promote continence?
2. What continence aids and appliances are available to help promote continence?
3. What different types of absorbent/containment aids are available?

Catheter care

Catheters may be used for male and female patients. There are two main types of catheter – one for short-term use and the other for long-term use (Exhibit 6.3). They differ in the type of material used in the manufacture. Long-term catheters are more durable and can remain in situ for longer periods of time (up to 3 months). Urine drainage systems are used for the collection of urine from catheters and penile sheaths (Figure 6.6). Drainage bag may be drainable (i.e. they can be emptied) or non-drainable.

Maintaining a closed drainage system is very important, as disconnection of the bag from the catheter is associated with an increased risk of infection. The **non-ambulant** patient may use a 2-L drainable bag connected directly to the catheter; this bag can be emptied as required and changed every 5-7 days. More mobile patients can use body-worn drainage systems; the closed system can be maintained by using link-system bags, in which a body-worn bag of 350-750 mL capacity is connected to a larger 2000-mL bag for night-time use.

Non-ambulant patients are those who are not walking about.

+ Polyvinyl chlorine or plastic catheters (for short periods only e.g. one week or less, because they are inflexible).
+ Plain latex catheters (for periods of 2-3 weeks). Latex may be used for patients with no known latex allergy. However, because of these allergies, latex is being phased out of heathcare products.
+ Polytetrafluorothylene ((PTFE) for up to four weeks).
+ Silicone elastomer catheters (for long-term use e.g. 2-3 months because they create less encrustation at the urethral meatus. However, they are expensive).
+ Hydrogel catheters (for periods of up to 12 weeks).
+ Polymer hydromer (for up to 12 weeks).
+ Pure silicone catheters (for patients who have latex allergies and can be left in place for up to 12 weeks).
+ Determine appropriate catheter length by the patient's gender. For adult female patients, use a 22 cm catheter; for adult male patients, a 40 cm catheter.
+ Determine appropriate catheter size by the size of the urethral canal. Use sizes such as #8 or #10 for children, #14 or #16 for adults. Men frequently require a larger size than women, for example, 18.

Exhibit 6.3 Types of catheter

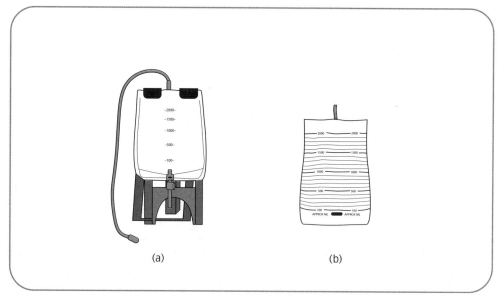

(a)   (b)

Figure 6.6 (a) Drainable 2-litre urine bag; (b) non-drainable 2-litre urine bag

A catheter may either be inserted intermittently, which means it is inserted to drain urine and then removed, or be there all the time, when it is referred to as a retention catheter. Whichever form of catheterisation is used, the assessment and care plan below must be followed in order to minimise the risk of infection and trauma.

Assessment and care of the catheterised patient

Nursing care of a patient with an indwelling catheter with continuous drainage is aimed largely at preventing infection of the urinary tract and encouraging urinary flow through the drainage system. Care includes the following:

+ Encouraging the intake of large amounts of fluids and recording them accurately on a fluid balance chart
+ Changing the retention catheter and tubing regularly, as required
+ Maintaining the patency of the drainage system
+ Preventing contamination of the drainage system
+ Preventing trauma to the drainage system
+ Teaching these measures to the patient and carer (if appropriate)

Fluid intake

The patient should be encouraged to drink up to 3000 mL a day if permitted. This ensures that the bladder is kept flushed out and reduces the likelihood of urinary stasis and subsequent infection. The large volumes of urine produced minimise the risk of sediment and other particles obstructing the drainage bag.

Changing the catheter and tubing

Routine changing of the catheter and tubing is not recommended. Special catheters are used for patients requiring long-term catheterisation, and these need changing only every 3-4 months. If there is sediment in the catheter or tubing, or urine drainage is impaired, these are good indicators that the system warrants changing. Taking out a used catheter and inserting a new catheter carries the risk of infection and therefore should be kept to a minimum. The nurse must follow strict handwashing protocol before and after any procedures involving the urinary drainage system. The perineal area should be cleansed regularly using soap and water, especially after defecation.

Maintaining the flow of the drainage system

It is very important to ensure the drainage system remains closed in order to reduce the risk of infection. The nurse needs to check that there are no obstructions in the drainage system: there must be no kinks in the tubing, the patient must not be lying on the tubing, and the tubing must not be clogged with mucus or blood. There should be no tension in the catheter or tubing; this can be prevented by securely taping the catheter to the patient's thigh or abdomen and fastening the tubing to the bedclothes. In order to prevent backflow of urine, gravity drainage should be maintained at all times by ensuring that the drainage bag is below the level of the patient's bladder. The flow of urine should be observed every 2-3 hours to monitor the patency of the drainage system.

Preventing contamination of the drainage system

The nurse must ensure that a sterile closed drainage system is maintained in order to prevent contamination from microorganisms that could give rise to urinary tract infection. Before the use of the closed drainage system, almost all catheterised patients developed urinary tract infections (Baillie, 2005; Laurent, 1998). The closed drainage system has been shown to reduce the rate of infection and is now accepted as good practice, but there is evidence that a significant number of hospital-acquired infections are still related to urinary catheterisation; these infections cause significant morbidity and sometimes mortality. It has been estimated that one in eight patients in hospital has an indwelling catheter, and problems with infection affect about 50 per cent of catheterised patients (Laurent, 1998); thus, prevention of infection is one of the main aims when caring for a patient with a catheter. The catheter and drainage tubing should not be disconnected unless absolutely necessary. Good handwashing techniques should be employed at all times when dealing with the catheter or drainage system or emptying the drainage bag. When the drainage bag is connected to a stand, it is important to ensure that the bag does not drag on the floor, which could lead to contamination, as any infection has the potential to travel up the tubing to the catheter site.

When emptying the drainage bag, the nurse should follow local hospital policy concerning the wearing of gloves and apron. Strict handwashing techniques must be followed before and after the procedure.

Teaching the patient

If the patient is to return home and resume a normal lifestyle, then they need to be aware of the care that is needed with regard to their catheter. The patient, and their carer if necessary, must be taught the catheter care outlined above. Written information can be very helpful for the patient and their carer after discharge from hospital.

Hygiene of the perineum and the penile meatus must be maintained at all times in order to reduce the risk of infection and to promote self-care and dignity. The area should be washed with soap and water (National Institute for Health and Clinical Excellence, 2003) as part of routine daily hygiene.

Now you have read about the care of a patient with an indwelling catheter and continuous bladder drainage, consider Case study 6.4.

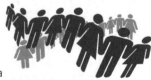

Case Study 6.4

Mrs Talbot is 68 years old. She has had an indwelling catheter for several months. She has been admitted to your ward with a urinary tract infection. You are serving lunch. On reaching Mrs Talbot, you observe that the drainage bag connected to her catheter is on the floor. You can see no evidence of a bag stand. On closer inspection, you find that her catheter is pulling due to the tubing being wrapped around her leg. You observe blood in the catheter. Mrs Talbot is complaining of pain around the perineum site. What would you do next?

This scenario is an example of poor nursing care and could be viewed as neglect. The trauma experienced by the patient is due to inadequate care from the nursing staff. There is a great risk of further infection, because the drainage bag is on the floor. The first thing to do is to ensure Mrs Talbot's comfort by unwrapping the catheter drainage tubing from around her leg. You must then tell the nurse in charge about the incident. You should find a drainage bag stand and attach the drainage bag, so that it is no longer on the floor. This must be done quickly in order to reduce the risk of infection. However, you are in the middle of serving lunch and do not want them to get cold. You could ask a colleague to take over the task of serving food while you attend to Mrs Talbot. You should not tell Mrs Talbot that you will 'sort her out' when you have a minute and then carry on serving lunch.

Recap Questions

1. What are the different types of urinary drainage system?
2. What is the main aim of care when dealing with a patient with continuous bladder drainage?
3. How is this aim achieved?

Problems with elimination of faeces

Defecation, or the passage of faeces, is a natural process whereby the waste products of digestion are eliminated from the body via the rectum and anus. This process is essential to health. The frequency of defecation is individual, varying from several times a day to two or three times a week (Kozier *et al.*, 2004).

The characteristics of faeces are affected by factors such as diet, lifestyle, health and mental state. Any abnormalities can be assessed by considering the following:

✢ Colour

✢ Smell

✢ Abnormal content

✢ Shape

✢ Solidity

Figure 6.7 shows the seven types of stool, according to the Bristol stool chart.

Assessment

A lot of information can be gleaned from observing the faeces or stool specimen. The colour and consistency can provide data that can assist in the diagnosis of a patient's condition. Any persistent alteration to a patient's bowel habits must be investigated thoroughly, as it could be indicative of a serious disorder such as carcinoma of the bowel or inflammatory bowel disease.

The nursing assessment should include a record of the patient's normal pattern of defecation. Any abnormal findings should be recorded accurately and reported. Faecal abnormalities and their possible causes are outlined in Exhibit 6.4.

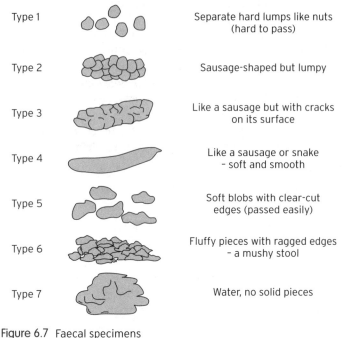

Figure 6.7 Faecal specimens
Source: BMJ, Bristol Stool Chart

+ *Black and tarry stools (malaena)*: may indicate bleeding from the gastrointestinal tract caused by a bleeding duodenal or peptic ulcer or oesophageal ulceration
+ *Maroon-coloured stool*: may indicate bleeding from the lower gastrointestinal tract due to inflammatory bowel disease or malignancy
+ *Bright-red (blood)*: usually associated with haemorrhoids or fissures, but may also indicate colonic cancer or inflammatory bowel disease
+ *Putty-coloured stool*: may indicate obstruction to the flow of bile. The faeces are also foul-smelling, bulky and difficult to flush away
+ *Black stool*: often a side effect of treatment with iron
+ *Hard, compact stool*: indicates constipation
+ *Loose, watery stool*: indicates diarrhoea

Exhibit 6.4 Faecal abnormalities that may be found on assessment

To think about

Imagine you are a patient in hospital and you need to open your bowels. What factors would you like the nurse to consider when assisting you with this process? Try to keep this in mind when you next assist a patient with their elimination needs.

Assisting a patient with elimination needs

Assisting someone with their elimination needs should be a therapeutic action given by the nurse. The patient should feel as relaxed as possible in order to complete a bowel action successfully. Defecation is a very private experience, and privacy and dignity must be maintained at all times. Exhibit 6.5 outlines the important principles that the nurse should adhere to when assisting with elimination.

+ Approachability and communication
+ Privacy and dignity
+ Promptness
+ Prevention of infection
+ Observation
+ Prevention of accidents
+ Promotion of independence
+ Promotion of hygiene and comfort

Exhibit 6.5 Principles to consider when assisting with elimination
Source: Baillie (2005)

Constipation

Consider Case study 6.5 and reflect on your reactions to it.

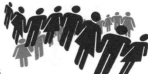

Case Study 6.5

Mr Beck is 79 years old. He has just returned from the operating theatre following evacuation of his bowels, because he was severely constipated.

Mr Beck had been a patient on the medical ward for several weeks, where he had been complaining of abdominal pain. He was regularly given codeine-based analgesia for the pain, but the codeine had contributed to his constipation. The nurses failed to monitor his bowel actions on a daily basis and consequently did not detect that Mr Beck had not opened his bowels properly for 4 weeks. He suffered with faecal overflow incontinence, which was noted as a proper bowel action on his chart. Consequently, all laxatives were withheld and Mr Beck became even more constipated. Eventually it was detected that Mr Beck had not opened his bowels for several days, and he was given suppositories and enemas, but with little success. Finally, it was decided that surgery was the only way to deal with Mr Beck's constipation.

Case study 6.5 highlights a situation that should never have happened. If Mr Beck's bowel actions had been monitored daily, then the problem would have been identified and dealt with quickly, thus avoiding the surgical intervention with its added costs to both Mr Beck, in terms of pain and discomfort, and the NHS, in financial terms.

Constipation may be defined as the passage of three or fewer bowel movements per week (Kozier *et al.*, 2004). However, bowel emptying varies widely between individuals, as does the perception of constipation. A more useful definition may therefore be 'the passage of hard stools less frequently than the patient's own normal pattern' (British National Formulary, 1998).

It has been estimated that the management of constipation costs the NHS up to £810 000 per year in nursing time in the community alone (Poulton and Thomas, 1999). Heading (1987) suggested that the NHS spends £8 million a year on laxatives, while a more recent study implies this amount is actually more than £43 million per year (Petticrew, 1997).

Causes of constipation

Constipation has a variety of causes. The patient needs a comprehensive assessment of their bowel function in order to ensure that the correct plan of care is ordered. The main causes of constipation are outlined in Table 6.6.

Table 6.6 Causes of constipation

Causes of constipation	Contributory factors/medical conditions
Diet	Inadequate fibre
Lack of exercise	Immobility, bedrest
Psychological factors	Using bedpans and commodes, lack of privacy
Psychiatric conditions	Dementia, depression
Neurological conditions	Paraplegia, multiple sclerosis
Metabolic abnormalities	Hypothyroidism, hypercalcaemia
Gastrointestinal tract abnormalities	Obstruction, chrohn's disease, diverticular disease, neoplasm
Drug therapy	Opiates, anticholinergics, laxative abuse

Constipation can result from faeces being lodged in any part of the large bowel, but it is most frequently experienced in the sigmoid colon and rectum (Richmond, 2003). The sigmoid colon and rectum can be identified in Figure 6.11.

The diagnosis is made by the presence of symptoms such as straining to defecate, hard stools, a feeling of abdominal fullness, pain or bloating, a feeling of incomplete evacuation, a sensation of blockage, or difficulty in relaxing the muscles to have a bowel movement (Stewart *et al.*, 1999). On examination, the abdomen appears distended and bowel sounds are reduced. On digital examination, which must be carried out only by a qualified nurse or doctor, the rectum may be impacted (full) with faeces. An abdominal X-ray may reveal a full colon (Richmond, 2003).

Constipation is a common problem among residents in nursing and residential homes and in the community setting. A study conducted in the UK revealed that 3% of young adults and 20% of older people are regularly constipated (Thompson and Heaton, 1980). There should be greater emphasis on the prevention rather than the treatment of constipation, as several of the causes can be addressed, for example by changing the diet, increasing fluid intake and doing more exercise.

Prevention of constipation

Constipation can lead to discomfort and distress for the individual and should be avoided where possible. There is also the potential for the development of serious complications, such as bowel perforation and confusion in elderly people. Therefore, prevention of constipation is of prime importance. Initially, an assessment of the patient's lifestyle should be made. This should include environmental factors, drug history and dietary intake. The constipated individual may not be eating enough dietary fibre, which comes mainly from fresh fruit and vegetables. Lack of exercise can contribute to constipation, and so more exercise such as walking should be encouraged. If the patient is taking a medication that can contribute to constipation, such as an opiate, antidepressant or anticholinergics, a laxative may need to be prescribed. Reduced fluid intake can contribute to constipation, so the patient should be encouraged to take at least 1500 mL of fluid daily.

Treatment of constipation

Once the cause of the constipation has been identified, advice and treatment should be given in order to promote regular opening of the bowels without strain or discomfort. Medication may be prescribed initially, but for the long-term treatment of simple constipation, a change in dietary habits, increased fluid intake and improvements in mobility may be all that are needed.

When constipation is related to pathological problems, use of prescribed drugs (such as opiates for pain relief) or abuse of laxatives, bowel medication may have to be prescribed. Abdominal massage can be effective in the promotion of regular bowel movements for some patients.

If the patient has **faecal impaction**, spurious (false) diarrhoea can occur, which may be treated, wrongly, with an anti-diarrhoea agent. This spurious diarrhoea may give the false impression that constipation is no longer a problem, but in reality the problem is getting worse. This can commonly lead to constipation being missed, as we saw in Case study 6.5.

Laxatives can be prescribed for constipation, but their effects should be monitored closely. Common laxatives fall into the following types:

+ Stimulants, e.g. senna, bisacodyl
+ Bulk-forming laxatives, e.g. ispaghula husk (note that adequate fluid intake must be maintained when using this)
+ Osmotic laxatives, e.g. lactulose
+ Iso-osmotic laxatives, e.g. macrogols

Faecal impaction is a mass of hardened faeces in the rectum.

All laxatives can cause unpleasant side effects such as abdominal cramps, flatulence, hypersensitivity, abdominal discomfort, pain and nausea. Prolonged use can result in an **atonic colon**. Therefore, care must be taken when prescribing and taking laxatives.

If the faeces are thought to be impacted in the colon or rectum, an enema may be prescribed. This involves the administration of liquid designed to soften and move the faeces so they can be evacuated. The enema tube is inserted directly into the rectum and the contents expelled. Usually the patient is asked to retain the enema for as long as they can, as this helps to ensure better evacuation of faeces. If the patient is severely constipated, they may require several enemas.

Suppositories, usually glycerine, may also be given. Suppositories are a medicated solid formulation that dissolves at body temperature. They are inserted into the rectum, where they dissolve.

Recap Questions

1. What are the causes of constipation?
2. How can constipation be prevented?
3. What is the treatment of constipation?

Diarrhoea

Diarrhoea is the passage of liquid faeces and an increased frequency of defecation (Kozier *et al.*, 2004). Diarrhoea is the opposite of constipation and results from the rapid movement of faecal contents through the colon. Spasmodic cramps often accompany the increased defecation, and irritation of the anal region usually results. If diarrhoea continues for several days, the patient becomes weak and fatigued, with general malaise and emaciation.

Causes of diarrhoea

There are several causes of diarrhoea, including:

+ Infection
+ Inflammatory bowel disease, e.g. ulcerative colitis
+ Drug-induced, e.g. antibiotics
+ Cancer of the rectum
+ Exposure to radiotherapy

Atonic colon is the loss of all normal muscular tone in the colon.

Effects of diarrhoea

If diarrhoea is continuous, the following consequences may arise:

+ Dehydration
+ Electrolyte imbalance
+ Malnutrition due to malabsorption
+ Vitamin deficiency
+ The skin around the anus, perineum and buttocks becomes broken and excoriated
+ Risk of spread of infection

Nursing interventions

The patient needs to be positioned close to a toilet to enable them to visit frequently if required. Privacy and dignity should be maintained at all times; a side room should be used if possible. The patient's diet should be low-residue (reduced fibre) to reduce **peristalsis** and cramping. To correct fluid and electrolyte imbalance, an intravenous infusion may be ordered if the patient is severely dehydrated; otherwise, extra fluids can be given. A fluid balance chart must be maintained in order to ascertain fluid loss. If the skin is sore and broken, care should be taken when washing around the anal, perineal and buttock areas.

If diarrhoea is the result of an infection, then universal precautions should be applied in the form of barrier nursing, handwashing and the wearing of gowns and gloves when dealing with the patient.

Finally, medication to reduce the diarrhoea may be prescribed, such as loperamide. Care should be taken when giving constipating agents to ensure that constipation does not develop.

Now consider Case study 6.6.

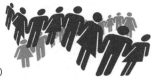

Case Study 6.6

Amy is a 6-month old baby admitted to the ward during the night suffering with severe diarrhoea. Her vital signs are: pulse, 170 bpm; respirations, 40 breaths per minute; temperature, 39 °C. She is in a febrile state and looks dehydrated and pale. When you change her nappy, the faeces are very runny and have a foul, offensive smell. Her distressed mother is very tearful, but she wishes to be involved in caring for Amy.

What would you do next?

Amy is very poorly and needs immediate medical attention. Her vital signs must be monitored and the findings reported immediately to the nurse in charge. Amy's diarrhoea may be infected, so she will require barrier nursing in a side room. A specimen of the faeces should be collected and sent to the laboratory to isolate the causative organism. All barrier nursing

Peristalsis is the muscular contraction of the intestinal walls that propels the contents of the bowel through the body.

precautions need to be explained fully to Amy's mother and any other family members. Infants are extremely susceptible to dehydration, and so Amy will need an intravenous/subcutaneous infusion to replace fluid loss. This will be commenced quickly by the doctor, who will prescribe the intravenous fluids to be infused. The infusion must be monitored closely to ensure that fluid is given at the correct rate and in the correct amount. Fluid imbalances in babies and young children can have more devastating effects than in adults. Similarly temperature control is not so finely tuned in babies, and they are susceptible to convulsions if the body temperature becomes very high. Therefore, Amy's temperature must be monitored strictly and any increase in temperature reported immediately. Other measures such as tepid sponging can be used to help reduce Amy's temperature. Finally, Amy's mother will require constant reassurance and support to allay her distress and to explain to her about barrier nursing procedures.

Faecal incontinence

Sometimes healthcare professionals mistakenly treat the faecal overflow incontinence caused by constipation by giving bulking agents or antimotility drugs such as loperamide. This aggravates the constipation and may cause obstruction, with severe consequences for the patient, as indicated in Case study 6.5.

The patient with faecal incontinence must be monitored for the following:

+ Frequency
+ Consistency
+ Quantity

In many patients with faecal incontinence, the problem can be improved if the correct cause is identified. This needs to be achieved sooner rather than later in order to avoid the incorrect use of incontinence/absorbent pads, which can lead to problems with privacy and dignity.

Recap Questions

1. What are the causes of diarrhoea?
2. What effect can severe diarrhoea have on an individual?
3. What nursing interventions are required for a patient with diarrhoea?
4. What is faecal incontinence, and how would you recognise it?

Summary

The first part of this chapter considered the importance of fluid balance and the role the nurse plays in ensuring that an accurate record is maintained for patients who present with fluid imbalance. The physiological mechanisms involved in the balance of body fluids and electrolytes are complex and finely tuned and need to be understood in order to appreciate the problems a patient with a fluid imbalance can experience. Any disturbance to fluid balance can have severe effects on the patient's physiological state if it is not detected and monitored on an ongoing basis. We considered the many factors that affect fluid and electrolyte balance, along with the effects of fluid imbalances, with particular reference to hypervolaemia (fluid overload) and hypovolaemia (fluid loss/dehydration). Finally, the importance of accurately recording a patient's fluid balance was discussed, with particular reference to the clinical assessment of fluid balance.

The second part of this chapter considered the care required by patients with bladder problems. It is important to preserve the patient's privacy and dignity, as urinary and faecal elimination problems may be embarrassing for the patient. When attending to patients' bladder and bowel needs, it is worth considering the following factors when assessing, planning and evaluating care given:

+ Ensure that evidence-based information is available for all patients and carers (if appropriate)
+ Patients should have access to professional advice and treatment
+ Each patient should be assessed fully
+ All treatment should be planned, implemented and evaluated
+ Staff working with patients should receive appropriate education and training
+ Patients should be able to access continence supplies and to choose the type they wish to use
+ Users should be involved in planning and evaluating services

If these factors are considered when caring for a patient with a continence problem, this should ensure they have a comprehensive assessment, which must include the patient; consequently, the correct care and treatment will be prescribed. The importance of promoting continence at all costs should not be overlooked. Age should never be viewed as a barrier to receiving the necessary care.

The final part of this chapter focused on the problems patients can experience with elimination of faeces, with particular reference to constipation and diarrhoea. Throughout this chapter, the need to preserve the patient's privacy and dignity has been emphasised. The nurse must be aware of and be able to recognise the sensitive issues that can arise regarding elimination. These issues should be remembered at all times when caring for patients with or urinary and faecal problems.

Key Points

1. Fluid balance must be recorded accurately, otherwise inaccurate care and treatment could be given.
2. It is important to preserve the dignity and privacy of any patient who has bladder or bowel problems.
3. The nurse needs to be aware of the causes of urinary incontinence and how to treat them effectively.
4. An accurate assessment of the patient's continence issue should be carried out with the patient and (if appropriate) the carer.
5. Promotion of person-centred continence care is imperative to ensure that the correct management is prescribed and that it is needs-led rather than service-led.
6. The nurse needs to be able to detect and treat any elimination problems, with particular reference to constipation and diarrhoea.

Points for debate

Now that you have come to the end of this chapter here are a few points that you may wish to think about when you are in practice. You may wish to discuss these with your work colleagues or fellow students.

The accurate recording of a patient's fluid balance is vital to ensure that a comprehensive picture of the patient is established.

Urinary incontinence is generally managed poorly. This is due mainly to inaccurate diagnosis and treatment of the continence problem.

The daily recording of a patient's bowel action is not seen as important and is rarely carried out nowadays.

Links to Other Chapters

Chapter 1   What is caring?
Chapter 2   Dignity and privacy
Chapter 3   Basic observations
Chapter 4   Personal hygiene
Chapter 10   Record-keeping

Further reading

Brandis, K (2007) *Fluid Physiology: An On-line Text*. www.anaesthesiamcq.com/FluidBook/index.php

Chester, R (1998) *Towards Continence*. London: Counsel and Care.

Getliffe, K and Dolman, M (eds) (2003) *Promoting Continence: A Clinical Research Resource*, 2nd edn. London: Baillière Tindall.

References

Baillie, L (ed) (2005) *Developing Practical Nursing Skills*. London: Hodder Education.

Bignell, V (1999) Alleviating the distress in urinary incontinence. *Community Nurse* **10**, 19-22.

Billington, A (2002) Managing incontinence. *Primary Health Care* **12**, 41-48.

British National Formulary (1998) *British National Formulary*. London: British Medical Association and Royal Pharmaceutical Society of Great Britain.

Burgio, K and Goode, P (1997) Behavioural interventions for incontinence in ambulatory geriatric patients. *American Journal of Medical Science* **314**, 257-261.

Carroll, H (2000) Fluid and electrolytes. In: Sheppard, M and Wright, M (eds) *Principles and Practice of High Dependency Nursing*. Edinburgh: Baillière Tindall.

Continence Foundation (2000) *Making the Case for Investment in an Integrated Continence Service*. London: Continence Foundation.

De Laine, C, Scammell, J and Heaslip, V (2002) Continence care and policy initiatives. *Nursing Standard* **17**, 45-51.

Department of Health (2000) *Good Practice in Continence Services*. London: The Stationery Office.

Department of Health (2001) *National Service Framework for Older People*. London: The Stationery Office.

Euromonitor (1999) *Disposable Paper Products: The International Market*. London: Euromonitor.

Gilbert, R (2005) Choosing and using disposable body-worn continence pads. *Nursing Times* **101**, 50-51.

Heading, C (1987) Nursing assessment and management of constipation. *Nursing* **21**, 778-790.

International Continence Society (2000) Continence assessment: quick reference guide. *Nursing Standard* **14** (suppl), 1-2.

Irwin, B, Patterson, A, Boag, P and Power, M (2001) Management of urinary incontinence in a UK trust. *Nursing Standard* **16**, 13-15.

Kozier, B, Erb, A, Berman, A and Snyder, S (2004) *Fundamentals of Nursing: Concepts, Process and Practice*, 7th edn. Upper Saddle River, NJ: Prentice Hall.

Laurent, C (1998) Preventing infection from indwelling catheters. *Nursing Times* **94**, 60-66.

Marjoram, B (1999) Elimination. In: Hogston, R and Simpson, P (eds) *Foundations of Nursing Practice*. Basingstoke: Macmillan.

McCreanor, J, Aitchison, M and Woods, M (1998) Comparing therapies for incontinence. *Professional Nurse* **13**, 215-219.

McDowell, BJ and Burgio, KL (1992) Urinary elimination. In: Burke, MM and Walsh, MB (eds) *Gerontologic Nursing of the Frail Elderly*. St Louis, MO: Mosby.

Medicines and Healthcare Products Regulatory Agency (2001) *Devices in Practice: A Guide for Health and Social Care Professionals*. London: Medicines and Healthcare Products Regulatory Agency.

Modernisation Agency (2003) *Essence of Care: Patient-Focused Benchmarks for Clinical Governance*. London: The Stationery Office.

Mooney, G (2004) Fluid balance. In: Shuttleworth, A (ed) *Monitoring and Assessment*. London: Emap Healthcare.

National Institute for Health and Clinical Excellence (2003) *Infection Control: Prevention of Healthcare-Associated Infection in Primary and Community Settings. No. 2: Care of Patients with Long-Term Urinary Catheters*. London: National Institute for Health and Clinical Excellence.

Olsen-Vetland, P (2003) Urinary incontinence after a cerebral vascular accident. *Nursing Standard* **17**, 37-41.

Petticrew, M (1997) Treatment of constipation in older people. *Nursing Times* **93**, 55-56.

Place, B and Field, D (1997) The management of fluid balance. *Nursing Times* **93**, 46-48.

Pomfret, I (2000) Catheter care in the community. *Nursing Standard* **14**, 46-51.

Potter, PA and Perry, AG (eds) (2002) *Fundamentals of Nursing*, 5th edn. St Louis, MO: Mosby.

Poulton, B and Thomas, S (1999) The nursing cost of constipation. *Primary Health Care* **9**, 17-22.

Richmond, J (2003) Prevention of constipation through risk management. *Nursing Standard* **17**, 39-46.

Sander, R (1999) Promoting urinary continence in residential care. *Nursing Standard* **14**, 49-53.

Simpson, L (2001) Indwelling urethral catheters. *Primary Health Care* **11**, 57-64.

Stewart, W, Liberman, JN, Sandler, RS *et al.* (1999) Epidemiology of constipation (EPOC) in the United States: relation of clinical subtypes to sociodemographic features. *American Journal of Gastroenterology* **94**, 3530-3540.

Stone, JT (1991) Preventing physical iatrogenic problems. In: Chenitz, WC, Stone, JT and Salisbury, SA (eds) *Clinical Gerontological Nursing*. Philadelphia, PA: Saunders.

Thompson, W and Heaton, K (1980) Functional bowel disorders in apparently healthy people. *Gastroenterology* 79, 283-288.

Wyman, J (1991) Incontinence and related problems. In: Chenitz, WC, Stone, JT and Salisbury, SA (eds) *Clinical Gerontological Nursing*. Philadelphia, PA: Saunders.

Chapter 7
Pain management

Mrs Carol Parker, a 46-year-old university lecturer, is admitted to the emergency assessment unit (EAU) complaining of severe pain. She is accompanied by her husband. Both are extremely anxious, as Mrs Parker's pain developed quite suddenly that evening.

On arrival at the EAU, Mrs Parker is placed in a bed. Her observations are recorded by the nurse, who does not ask the patient anything about her pain, even though she is clutching her abdomen, her knees are bent up and she is almost crying. The EAU is very busy and Mrs Parker is not seen by a doctor for an hour. During this time, the nurse does not return to assess the patient's pain, which is getting worse.

Eventually, the doctor examines Mrs Parker and orders an abdominal X-ray. The doctor prescribes two tablets of paracetamol (a mild analgesic) to relieve the pain. Mrs Parker then waits a further 45 minutes before the analgesia is given. By this time, her pain is severe and she is pale, anxious and clammy. Her husband is in despair and tries to find a nurse. After giving the analgesia, the nurse has not returned to see whether the patient's pain has been relieved.

Four hours after her arrival at the EAU, Mrs Parker is seen again by the doctor, because, according to the nurse, who has done no further observations or assessment of the patient's condition, 'she is still complaining of severe pain despite having had two paracetamol tablets'. The X-ray confirms that Mrs Parker has an obstruction in her bowel and requires immediate emergency surgery. She is prepared hurriedly for the operating theatre and is eventually given some stronger analgesia (morphine) to help relieve her pain.

Introduction

Consider the scenario above and reflect on your own reactions to it. Does it show that the patient's pain was assessed and managed effectively? If not, what could have been done better? If you were Mrs Parker's husband, how would you have felt seeing her in severe pain and not receiving adequate pain relief?

This chapter explores the essential aspects of pain assessment and management, from defining what pain is to discussing various ways in which pain can be relieved. Emphasis is placed on the individuality of the pain experience. Each person's pain is unique to them and cannot be felt by another. Because of the subjective nature of pain, it is crucial that each patient's pain is assessed correctly and consequently managed in an effective and humane way. This should ensure that scenarios such as that described above are not repeated.

LEARNING OBJECTIVES

By the end of this chapter you will be able to:

1. Define pain and explain how pain is felt, recognising the complexities of the pain experience
2. Outline how pain is assessed and indicate the factors that can influence both the perception of and the response to pain
3. Recognise the factors that can influence the nurse's perception of patients' pain
4. Indicate the types of analgesia used to relieve pain, and explain how these drugs work
5. Outline the methods of administration of analgesia and consider the advantages and disadvantages of each method
6. Show an understanding of other methods used to relieve pain

What is pain?

To think about

Try to define pain. Ask your friends and family to tell you what pain is.

What did they say?
How would you explain it to them?

Pain and its meaning have always fascinated humans. In Ancient Greece, the philosopher Aristotle considered pain to be an emotion opposite to pleasure. In the seventeenth century, Descartes conceived pain to have a physiological basis in the form of a channel running from the skin to the brain (Figure 7.1). He proposed that a flame held near the foot would set particles in motion. This movement would then be transmitted via the leg to the head, and the individual would then feel pain. Although this theory is very simple, it does form the basis of more recent complex theories of how pain is felt.

Other philosophers and psychologists have focused on the emotional and subjective nature of pain. They have considered the importance of trying to define pain and noted how difficult it is to reach a consensus because of its complex nature.

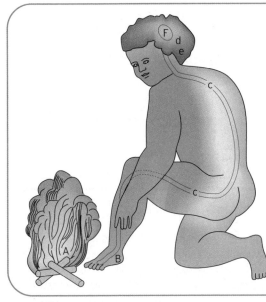

Descartes' (1664) concept of the pain pathway: 'If for example fire (A) comes near the foot (B), the minute particles of this fire, which as you know move with great velocity, have the power to set in motion the spot of the skin of the foot which they touch, and by this means pulling upon the delicate thread (c) which is attached to the spot of the skin, they open up at the same instant the pore (d e) against which the delicate thread ends, just as by pulling at one end of a rope one makes to strike at the same instant a bell which hangs at the other end (F).'

Figure 7.1 Descartes' theory of pain
Source: Melzack and Wall (1982)

The International Association for the Study of Pain (IASP) use the following definition:

Pain is an unpleasant sensory and emotional experience associated with actual or potential tissue damage or described in terms of such damage.
(International Association for the Study of Pain, 1986)

This definition considers both the sensory and emotional aspects of pain and its association with damage to the body. For example, a small cut to the finger can appear to be more painful than a bullet wound to a soldier's limb during battle: the soldier may see the injury as a means of being removed from the battlefield and being spared his life.

More recent definitions by psychologists and healthcare professionals have emphasised the personal experience of pain and how factors such as culture and the situation in which pain occurs can affect the outcome.

Margo McCaffery's definition of pain focuses on the patient's perspective of pain: 'Pain is what the patient says it is' (McCaffery, 1968). This definition considers the subjectivity of the pain experience in that no two people's pain will feel exactly the same.

The definition given by Melzack and Wall (1982) outlines the effect of how each individual perceives (or sees) their pain: '[Pain is] a highly personal experience, depending on cultural learning, the meaning of the situation and other factors that are unique to each individual.'

Pain involves several entities, including the individuality and subjectivity of pain, the physiological aspects of pain in terms of what is happening in the body, and the meaning of the pain to the individual. Other factors such as culture can affect how a person perceives pain and how they respond to it in a given situation. We consider these factors later in this chapter.

Ultimately, the consensus on the definition of pain is highly complex, and it is difficult to produce a concise, clear-cut meaning of pain. Pain is individual to the person in pain, which helps to explain why we find it so difficult to define.

1. What are the main themes that philosophers, psychologists and healthcare professionals have considered when trying to define pain?
2 Why is pain difficult to define?
3 Can you now explain to your friends and family what pain is?

How is pain felt?

Revision

Before reading the next section, you need to revise the anatomy and physiology of the central nervous system (CNS) and peripheral nervous system, focusing on nociceptors (pain receptors), sensory/afferent neurons, motor/efferent neurons, the dorsal horn of the spinal cord, and the parts of the brain, including the thalamus, limbic system and cerebral cortex.

In order to understand how a person feels pain, it is important to appreciate the complex processes that occur when pain is experienced, including the sensory (sensation), emotional (feeling), and cognitive (thinking) aspects. Philosophers and scientists have attempted to explain how pain is felt. As early as 1664, a theory known as the specificity theory suggested that pain was felt and transmitted along specific pain pathways. This notion arose from Descartes' definition of pain, which suggested that particles, set in motion, travelled via these specific pathways from the site of pain to the head, where the pain was then felt by the individual.

From the end of the nineteenth century until the start of the 1960s, the pattern theory was in vogue, mainly because no other theory was proposed. The pattern theory comprised a number of closely related suggestions that explored the balance of activity between different pain pathways. These theories focused primarily on the physiological aspects of pain (i.e. those related to bodily functions). No consideration was given to the psychological or emotional components. The pattern theory could not explain how a soldier losing his leg on a battlefield seemed to feel less pain than a person cutting a finger in the kitchen.

The answer came in 1965, when Melzack and Wall introduced the gate control theory. This ground-breaking theory seemed to explain both the physiological and the psychological dimensions of pain. The theory proposes:

> ... a neural mechanism in the dorsal horn of the spinal cord acts like a gate which can open or close thus increasing or decreasing the flow of nerve impulses from peripheral nerve fibres to the central nervous system (CNS). The degree to which the gate increases or decreases sensory transmission is determined by the relative activity in large diameter (A beta) and small diameter (A delta and C) nerve fibres and by descending influences from the brain.
> (Melzack and Wall, 1965)

This proposed gating mechanism is thought to occur in specific dorsal horn cells within the spinal cord called substantia gelatinosa. The theory helped to clarify the variation in perception of pain in relation to identical pain stimulation – in other words, the same pain stimulation can lead to different perceptions of that pain in individuals and the experience of pain is not related directly to the level of pain input. This can be highlighted in cases where pain is disproportionate to the severity of injury, such as the soldier in the battlefield, or when pain occurs long after an injury has healed, such as chronic lower back pain or phantom limb pain. In phantom limb pain, the person feels pain even though the limb has been amputated.

The gate control theory can be explained in simple terms. The 'gate' in the spinal cord allows certain pain impulses to pass through and to be felt (interpreted by the brain). This means that not all pain impulses will be felt. When the gate is 'open' the pain impulses can flow through easily, but when the gate is 'closed' none can pass through. The 'gating process' that allows the gate to be open or closed is influenced by two modifying factors:

+ Balance of activity of pain fibres/afferent neurons
+ Descending control from higher centres in the brain

Afferent neurons/pain fibres

There are three types of pain fibres/afferent neurons: small A delta (fast) and C (slow) fibres, and large A beta (very fast) fibres. The different types of fibre respond to different types of pain (Table 7.1). The small A delta and C neurons release substance P, an excitatory neurotransmitter that opens the gate. The larger A beta neurons release inhibitory neurotransmitters that close the gate. The gating mechanism is influenced by the dominant input of neurons. Therefore, if the main input to the gate is via the larger, faster A beta neurons, then the gate will close because of the inhibitory transmitters. This explains why massaging a painful area can help to reduce pain, as the A beta neurons are stimulated by touch and pressure. Transcutaneous electrical nerve stimulation (TENS) is also thought to evoke activity in the A beta neurons (Melzack and Wall, 1988). However, if the dominant input is from the relatively slower A delta and C neurons, then the gate is open and more pain is perceived (Figure 7.2).

Table 7.1 Types of pain fibre

Pain fibre	Classification	Pain response
Small A delta	Fast pain fibres (4–30 m/s)	Sharp, localised distinct pain
Small C	Slow pain fibres (0.4–1.6 m/s)	Dull, burning, poorly localised, visceral, persistent pain
Large A beta	Mechanoreceptors (very fast transmission, (30–100 m/s)	Touch, pressure, muscle contraction

To think about

Take note of what you or other people do if they experience pain due to trauma or injury. You can now explain why the automatic reaction to rub the area is therapeutic and helps to ease pain.

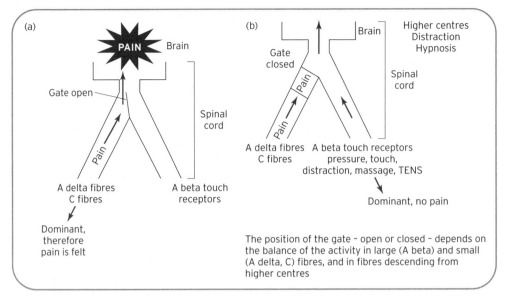

Figure 7.2 Gate control theory (a) pain is felt (b) no pain is felt

Descending control from higher centres in the brain

Even if the input from these pain afferent neurons is opening the gate, it may be closed by influences from the higher centres in the brain, such as the thalamus, cortex and limbic system. These centres can modify the gating mechanism by releasing a variety of endogenous opiates (encephalins and endorphins), which close the gate by inhibiting the release of substance P. This form of pain control influences the higher centres in the brain and can be exemplified through the use of distraction, diversion therapy, counselling and placebo techniques (Melzack and Wall, 1996).

Whipple (1990) suggested that TENS machines operate by stimulating the release of endogenous opiates. This theory opposes Melzack and Wall's (1988) theory that TENS initiates stimulation of A beta neurons.

Endorphins are endogenous morphine-like opiates produced in the higher centres in the brain, such as the thalamus and cerebral cortex. Endorphins are released from specific sites called opiate receptors in response to tissue damage and injury and act as the body's own analgesic system. Endorphins act by helping to close the gate, hence inhibiting the release of substance P. Endorphin levels are increased in states of stress, such as during childbirth, and are decreased following long-term administration of morphine. Acupuncture and TENS also increase endorphin release. It has been suggested that the production of endorphins develops after birth and declines with age.

In summary, several processes occur that affect the overall pain experience. Our present understanding of this mechanism has been greatly enhanced by the gate control theory proposed by Melzack and Wall, which states that a gating mechanism within the spinal cord modulates the amount of input from pain receptors/fibres. Put simply, this gate can be either open or closed, and this process is influenced by input from different pain fibres/afferent neurons (A beta, A delta and C fibres) and from the higher centres in the brain, such as the thalamus and limbic system. The body produces opiate-like substances called endorphins, which help to reduce pain. Figure 7.3 summarises the neural pain pathways.

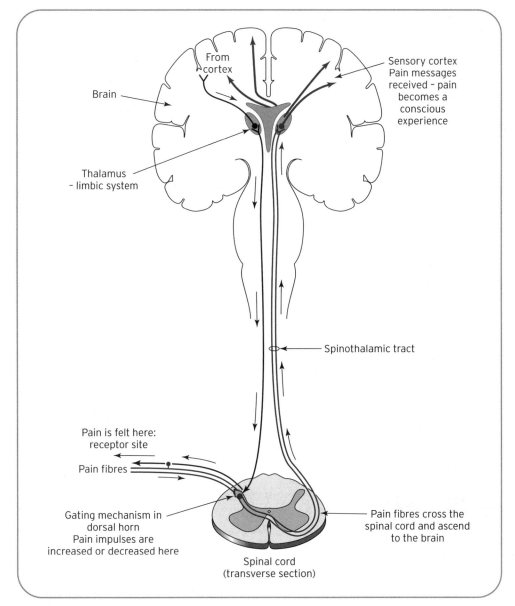

From cortex

Brain

Sensory cortex
Pain messages
received - pain
becomes a
conscious
experience

Thalamus
- limbic system

Spinothalamic tract

Pain is felt here:
receptor site

Pain fibres

Gating mechanism in
dorsal horn
Pain impulses are
increased or decreased here

Pain fibres cross the
spinal cord and ascend
to the brain

Spinal cord
(transverse section)

Figure 7.3 Neural pain pathways

Recap Questions

1. How does the gate control theory contribute to a fuller understanding of how pain is felt?
2. What is the main difference between the A beta, A delta and C pain fibres/afferent neurons?
3. What is substance P, and what effect does it have on the gating process?
4. What are endorphins, and how do they influence how pain is felt?

Government policy developments in pain management

In January 2003, the Nursing and Midwifery Practice Development Unit became part of the NHS Quality Improvement Scotland. This was established as a special health board bringing together Scotland's five clinical effectiveness organisations. Its aim is to improve the quality of healthcare provided in Scotland by setting standards and monitoring performance. Best practice statements have been issued, including one on postoperative pain relief.

The Welsh Assembly has also launched a document, which can be viewed as the Welsh equivalent to the Department of Health's (2003) *Essence of Care* document. The Welsh Assembly's document *Fundamentals of Care* has a section on pain management that considers 12 aspects of care, including alleviating pain identified by patients and carers.

In March 2005, the DH launched a document entitled *Integrated Services to Treat People with Long-Term Conditions*. This document has a detailed section on palliative care, with great emphasis placed on the importance of adequate pain relief (Department of Health, 2005).

The DH has also launched a National Service Framework considering the management of pain. This government initiative, as with other National Service Frameworks, has vast implications for how pain is managed in the future and includes all the aspects of pain considered in this chapter.

Pain assessment

We now consider how pain can be assessed and how important it is to get it right. Think about the case study at the beginning of this chapter, in which the patient's pain was not assessed and consequently was not managed in a satisfactory way. It is important to remember to re-assess pain after analgesia has been given in order to identify whether the analgesia is appropriate or whether a larger dose is required to alleviate the patient's pain.

> ### To think about
>
> How is pain assessed in your workplace?
> Is it done well?
> What factors might influence how patients' pain is assessed?

Methods of pain assessment

There are four main ways to assess pain:

+ Talking to the patient
+ Observing the patient's behaviour
+ Recording the patient's physiological signs
+ Using pain assessment tools

Talking to the patient

The most fundamental way to assess a patient's pain is to ask the patient about it. Pain should be assessed with the patient rather than on the patient; this means that the nurse should not assess the patient's pain in isolation from the patient. This is important, as the patient's own estimate of pain must be used as the basis for treatment. The nurse must not be influenced by their own beliefs, attitudes, values or personal experiences of pain when carrying out the assessment of a patient's pain. Personal influences can lead to biases in the nurse's assessment of the pain, which carries the possibility of underestimating such pain. Several factors can influence nurses' biases, and these are considered later in this chapter.

It is useful to find out how the patient usually deals with pain. The nurse should listen to the patient empathetically and accept that only the patient can really know what hurts, when it hurts and how much it hurts. Think again about McCaffery's (1968) definition of pain: 'Pain is what the patient says it is.' Some patients deny having pain because they do not want to bother the 'busy' nurse. The patient may expect to have some degree of pain and therefore not report fully the degree of pain that they do have. Many factors contribute to variations between patients in how much pain they report and how they perceive and view their pain. These factors are discussed in more detail later in this chapter. Consider Case study 7.1.

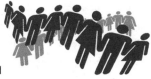

Case Study 7.1

Mr Mason has advanced cancer and complains of pain. However, he does not appear to be in pain, as he is sitting quietly and reading a book. You ask him how bad his pain is, and he replies that it is very bad. You have been caring for Mr Mason for only a few days and are unsure how to proceed.

Should you believe what the patient says?
What aspects of pain should be assessed?
How do you know how bad someone's pain is?

Think about the responses to these questions. You may like to discuss them with a colleague or qualified nurse in your clinical placement.

Observing the patient's behaviour

Pain can be assessed by observing the patient's behaviour and non-verbal cues. If a person is in a lot of pain, they may show signs of facial grimacing, hold the painful area, groan or cry, and display a certain degree of anxiety, especially if the cause of the pain is unknown. However, the patient's behaviour is influenced by factors such as their culture, gender, age and pathology, and these play a part in the patient's perceptions and outward displays of pain.

Recording the patient's physiological signs

If the patient is unconscious or unable to communicate verbally, it is difficult to observe their behaviour or ask them about their pain. In this case, the nurse can use physiological signs and clinical observations to assess pain. Accurate recording of the pulse and blood pressure can help to indicate the patient's pain levels. When a person is in pain, the **autonomic nervous system** causes the body to exhibit signs of stress, which usually result in an increase in the pulse and blood pressure if pain is mild or moderate. When pain is very severe, the patient exhibits signs of neurogenic shock, whereby the blood pressure is low and the pulse is rapid, weak and thready.

Sometimes nurses find it easier to assess pain by observing behaviours and recording physiological signs rather than relying on patients' verbal reports of pain, mainly because behaviours and signs can be measured objectively. Asking the patient to tell you about their pain gives a far more subjective assessment and relies on the patient telling the truth and the nurse believing the patient.

Pain assessment tools

Measurable pain assessment tools (PATs) have been developed as a means of assessing patients' pain in a more objective way. These tools provide a written record of a patient's pain at any given time, similar to the record made of the patient's temperature, pulse and respiration. The use of a pain assessment chart gives the nurse a more accurate measure of the patient's pain in terms of the site, intensity and level of pain, what makes the pain worse, and whether any analgesia given has relieved the pain. When asking the patient about their pain, questions can be focused on these issues.

Various PATs have been devised to assess different types of pain. For example, pain rating scales, which include verbal, graphical and numerical rating scales, are generally used to assess acute postoperative pain, while more detailed pain questionnaires are used to assess chronic pain associated with cancer and terminal illness. Figure 7.4 shows several PATs.

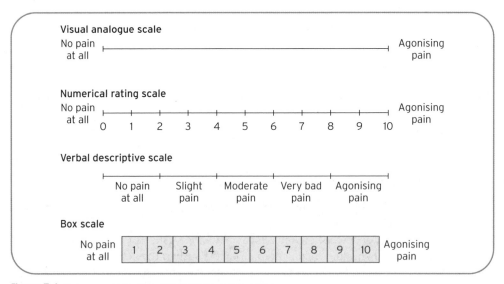

Figure 7.4 Pain assessment tools: (a) pain rating scales

The **autonomic nervous system** is the part of the nervous system that is not under voluntary control.

McGill-Melzack Pain Questionnaire

Patient's name _____ Date _____ Time _____ a.m./p.m.

Analgesic(s) _____ Dose regimen _____ Time given _____ a.m./p.m.

_____ Dose regimen _____ Time given _____ a.m./p.m.

Analgesic time difference (hours): +4 +1 +2 +3

Pain rating index (PRI)[1]: S_____ A_____ E_____ M(S)_____ M(AE)_____ M(T)_____ PRI(T)_____

(1-10) (11-15) (16) (17-19) (20) (17-20) (1-20)

		Present pain intensity (PPI)
1 Flickering _ Quivering _ Pulsing _ Throbbing _ Beating _ Pounding _	11 Tiring _ Exhausting _ 12 Sickening _ Suffocating _	Comments:

1 Flickering _
  Quivering _
  Pulsing _
  Throbbing _
  Beating _
  Pounding _

2 Jumping _
  Flashing _
  Shooting _

3 Pricking _
  Boring _
  Drilling _
  Stabbing _
  Lancinating _

4 Sharp _
  Cutting _
  Lacerating _

5 Pinching _
  Pressing _
  Gnawing _
  Cramping _
  Crushing _

6 Tugging _
  Pulling _
  Wrenching _

7 Hot _
  Burning _
  Scalding _
  Searing _

8 Tingling _
  Itchy _
  Smarting _
  Stinging _

9 Dull _
  Sore _
  Hurting _
  Aching _
  Heavy _

10 Tender _
   Taut _
   Rasping _
   Splitting _

11 Tiring _
   Exhausting _

12 Sickening _
   Suffocating _

13 Fearful _
   Frightful _
   Terrifying _

14 Punishing _
   Gruelling _
   Cruel _
   Vicious _
   Killing _

15 Wretching _
   Blinding _

16 Annoying _
   Troublesome _
   Miserable _
   Intense _
   Unbearable _

17 Spreading _
   Radiating _
   Penetrating _
   Piercing _

18 Tight _
   Numb _
   Drawing _
   Squeezing _
   Tearing _

19 Cool _
   Cold _
   Freezing _

20 Nagging _
   Nauseating _
   Agonizing _
   Dreadful _
   Torturing _

PPI
0 No pain _
1 Mild _
2 Discomforting _
3 Distressing _
4 Horrible _
5 Excruciating _

Present pain intensity (PPI)
Comments:

Constant _
Periodic _
Brief _

Accompanying Symptoms:
Nausea _
Headache _
Dizziness _
Constipation _
Diarrhoea _

Comments:

Sleep:
Good _
Fitful _
Can't sleep _

Comments:

Activity:
Good _
Some _
Little _
None _

Food intake:
Good _
Some _
Little _
None _

Comments:

Comments:

[1]S = Sensory; A = Autonomic; E = Emotional

Figure 7.4 Pain assessment tools: (b) McGill-Melzack Pain Questionnaire

The Royal Marsden Hospital

Pain assessment chart

Surname: Hospital no.

First name: Date:

Initial assessment

Patient's own description of the pain(s):

What helps relieve the pain?

What makes the pain worse?

Do you have pain
i)   at night?   Yes/No (comment if required).

ii) at rest?   Yes/No (comment if required).

iii) on movement?   Yes/No (comment if required).

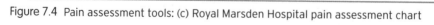

Figure 7.4 Pain assessment tools: (c) Royal Marsden Hospital pain assessment chart

The London Hospital

Pain observation chart

This chart records where a patient's pain is and how bad it is, by the nurse asking the patient at regular intervals. If analgesics are being given regularly, make an observation with each dose and another half-way between each dose. If analgesics are given only 'as required', observe two-hourly. When the observations are stable and the patient is comfortable, any regular time interval between observations may be chosen.

To use this chart, ask the patient to mark all his or her pains in the body diagram below. Label each site of pain with a letter (i.e. A, B, C etc). Then at each observation time ask the patient to assess:

1. The pain in each separate site since the last observation. Use the scale above the body diagram, and enter the number or letter in the appropriate column.
2. The pain overall since the last observation. Use the same scale and enter in the column marked overall.

Next, record what has been done to relieve pain. In particular:

3. Note any analgesic given since the last observation, stating name, dose, route and time given.
4. Tick any other nursing care or action taken to ease pain.

Finally note any comment on pain from patient or nurse (use the back of the chart as well, if necessary) and initial the record.

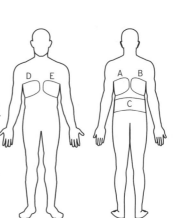

Date _____ Sheet number _____   Patient identification label

Time	Pain rating By sites								Overall	Measures to relieve pain (specify where starred)								Initials
	A	B	C	D	E	F	G	H		Analgesic given (Name, dose, route, time)	Lifting	Turning	Massage	Distracting activities	Position change	Additional aids	Other	Comments from patients and/or staff

Figure 7.4 Pain assessment tools: (d) London Hospital pain observation chart

Assessing different types of pain

Pain can present in different ways. Pain that is sudden in onset, associated with an injury or postoperative is considered to be acute pain and needs to be assessed in a different way from chronic pain associated with longer-term conditions such as arthritis or low back pain, where pain occurs on a daily basis and has been present for several months. Different pain types need different PATs to accurately assess pain levels.

Acute pain

Acute pain can be defined as pain that subsides as healing takes place and has a predictable end (McCaffery and Beebe, 1989). The duration of acute pain is generally brief and is usually defined as lasting less than 3 months. Pain intensity can vary from mild to severe, and the onset may be sudden or gradual (such as with a headache). Acute pain is usually accompanied by fight or flight features, as the body exhibits signs of stress, resulting from activation of the sympathetic (autonomic) nervous system. This causes dilation of the pupils, increased sweating, and raised pulse, respiratory rate and blood pressure. Nurses encounter patients in acute pain mainly in accident and emergency departments, surgical wards and intensive care units.

In order to assess acute pain, nurses need to use a PAT that is quick and easy to complete with the patient, such as a visual analogue scale, numerical rating scale or verbal/descriptive rating scale (see Figure 7.4). These PATs are used to assess pain and to monitor the effects of analgesia given.

Chronic pain

Chronic pain can be defined as 'pain that has lasted 3 months or longer, is ongoing on a daily basis or recurs on a regular basis, is due to non-life-threatening causes, has not responded to currently available treatment methods and may continue for the remainder of the patient's life' (McCaffery and Beebe, 1989). The above definition can be applied to chronic pain of a non-malignant origin. This means that the pain is not due to cancer but may include conditions such as low back pain, rheumatoid arthritis, neuralgia, irritable bowel syndrome, neuropathic pain, chronic pancreatitis and osteoarthritis.

Chronic pain can be constant or intermittent. Examples of conditions where the pain is recurrent and acute are sickle cell crisis and migraine.

The pain associated with cancer is considered to be chronic in nature as it is generally present for at least 3–6 months. However, unlike with chronic non-malignant pain, there is a foreseeable end: either the patient is cured of the cancer, with a consequent loss of pain, or they die.

The cause of chronic pain is not always fully understood, as there may be no evidence of disease or tissue damage. In this instance, pain may continue after the original injury shows every indication of having healed. It is believed that this is due to a process called sensitisation, which occurs in the pain pathways. Pain messages become amplified and distorted, similar to turning up the volume on the radio. This results in a painful condition that is out of proportion to the original injury. In the spinal cord, sensitisation can result from chemical reactions that increase pain messages being sent to the brain. In the peripheral nervous system, sensitisation can result from inflammation, which causes the nociceptors (pain receptors) to fire with greater intensity; this can cause emotional and psychological suffering.

Chronic pain is often associated with certain psychological factors such as behavioural changes, and adjustment in motivation, mood and cognition (thinking). The nurse needs to be aware of the effect of such psychological factors on the pain experience and how they can exacerbate pain problems and influence pain behaviour.

The different classifications of chronic pain require different PATs in order to assess pain adequately. For example, chronic non-malignant pain can be associated with sleep disturbances, loss of appetite and libido, constipation, preoccupation with the illness, depression, personality changes and inability to work; these aspects of the patient's overall condition should be included on the PAT. Consequently, a detailed PAT is required. A good example is the McGill-Melzack pain questionnaire (see Figure 7.4b), which uses sets of words to quantify and describe how the pain feels for the patient. This helps to provide a comprehensive analysis of the pain and how it might be alleviated.

The type of PAT needed to assess cancer pain should include an assessment of a variety of different pains associated with malignancy. Cancer is a process of progressive change, whereby pain sites and pain relief need to be reviewed regularly as the pattern of pain changes. The Royal Marsden Hospital pain assessment chart and the London Hospital pain observation chart have been devised specifically to assess cancer pain (see Figure 7.4c,d).

Recap Questions

1. Why do we need to assess pain?
2. What methods do we use to assess pain?
3. Are all of these pain assessment methods always used? If not, why not?
4. Why is acute pain assessed differently from chronic pain?

Pain perception

The experience of pain is unique, subjective and reliant on the individual's perception of their own pain. Melzack and Wall's (1982) definition of pain perception implies that pain perception involves more than the physical effects of pain from an injury; rather, pain perception also includes psychological and social factors, which vary greatly between individuals. This section considers these factors in more detail.

Factors that influence patients' perceptions and responses to pain

You may recall that pain is not related to bodily damage alone. The amount and quality of pain are also determined by the meaning of the pain, which in turn can be linked to the patient's previous experiences of pain, how well they are recalled, and the ability to understand the cause of pain and its consequences. Moreover, social and cultural factors play an essential role in how a person feels and responds to pain. Thus, the pain experience is linked to how we perceive pain, which varies greatly from one person to the next. Consider Case study 7.2.

Case Study 7.2

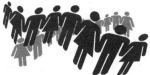

Two patients, Miss Shields and Mr O'Mara, are to undergo similar operations on the same day. Both are having hernia repairs. Miss Shields is a 34-year-old Afro-Caribbean woman. This is her first experience of having surgery – and of being in hospital – and she is very anxious. Mr O'Mara is a 68-year-old Irish man who has had many hospital admissions following heart surgery last year.

After the surgery, both patients are given pain control. However, Miss Shields complains of pain more frequently and requests more analgesia than Mr O'Mara.

Why do you think this is?
What factors may be influencing both patients' perceptions of pain?
What might influence how they cope with pain?

Case study 7.2 highlights some of the differences between individual patients. Although these two patients underwent the same type of surgery, they perceived and coped with their pain in different ways. Why is this? What factors affect how we deal with pain? We consider these factors in more detail in the following sections.

Reluctance to request analgesia or complain of pain

Some patients do not like to ask for pain relief or even complain of pain as it may be seen as a sign of weakness. They may not want to bother the busy nurses. Some patients may be afraid to take strong analgesia as they fear the sedative or addictive effects of opioids. Others may have a needle phobia and fear the injection, if this is the route of administration of their analgesia. Sometimes patients are not aware of the analgesia that has been prescribed for them and how often they can receive it. As a consequence, they are not able to make an informed choice about when to have pain relief and may suffer in silence when analgesia could be given.

Gender

Are there differences between the way males and females deal with or complain of pain? The evidence base is variable. In one study, pain levels in 90 male patients and 90 female patients aged between 5 and 17 years were assessed following **venepuncture**. The study found that males tended to report less pain than the females (Fowler-Kerry and Lander, 1991). Erickson (1992) argues that males and females have similar pain thresholds but exhibit different pain-related behaviour: males often display a 'stiff upper lip' image while females complain more readily of pain. Think about Case study 7.2: could gender differences related to pain help to explain why Miss Shields complained of pain more frequently than Mr O'Mara?

An interesting laboratory study in the USA revealed that men, when asked to assess the pain they experienced while their hand was immersed in very cold water, reported significantly lower levels of pain to female experimenters than they did to male experimenters (Levine and De Simone, 1991). This finding implies that males may underreport their pain to females.

McCaffery (1983) and Davitz and Davitz (1985) found that female patients received more analgesia and tended to ask for analgesia more frequently than male patients, who often displayed a 'macho' image when asked about pain. Could this notion also apply to Miss Shields and Mr O'Mara in Case study 7.2?

However, Seers (1987) and Field (1996a) found no significant effect of patient gender on pain assessment.

Age

Our perceptions of pain may alter as we age. As sensory changes occur with normal ageing, it seems reasonable to assume that changes in pain perception should also occur. However, both Harkin (1988) and Ferrell (1991) found little evidence regarding differences in pain perception when comparing younger and older people. More recent experimental evidence suggests that older people have a lower **pain tolerance**, which means they feel pain sooner and at a greater intensity (Briggs, 2003). The experimenters concluded that this may be due

Venepuncture involves insertion of a cannula into the vein and is quite a painful procedure.
Pain tolerance is the amount of pain that a person is willing to tolerate.

to the physiological and neurological changes associated with ageing. However, older adults are more likely to experience multiple pathology and consequently suffer more pain than younger people. Very often, pain in older adults is inadequately reported, recognised and treated (Davies *et al.*, 2004).

There appear to be many misconceptions surrounding pain in the older person. Many healthcare professionals believe that pain is a normal aspect of ageing and that the older person should expect to suffer pain (Briggs, 2003). Pasero and colleagues (1999) highlighted this notion with the following example: A 101-year-old man visited his GP and complained of pain in his left leg. When the doctor suggested this was to be expected at his age, the man retorted that his right leg was the same age as his left but did not hurt at all. Schofield (2006a) found significantly higher levels of depression and lower levels of wellbeing in nursing-home residents, whose pain was often undetected by carers, compared with people whose pain was noted. In a qualitative study, Schofield (2006b) looked at barriers to reporting pain held by residents living in a number of care homes within one district. Age-related perceptions of pain were identified. People in the older age group (over 80 years) were reluctant to take analgesics and were also reluctant to admit they had pain. Residents under 74 years of ages were more willing to voice their pain and consequently take analgesics.

When considering very young patients, it is often wrongly assumed that neonates are incapable of feeling pain and healthcare professionals interpret a baby's distress following birth as being due to separation from the mother. However, Johnson and Strada produced experimental evidence to support the notion that babies do feel pain and exhibited intense reactions to pain in their behaviours, such as crying and body movement.

Emotional state

The emotional state of the patient in pain can impact on their perception and expression of pain. Think about Case study 7.2: Miss Shields was very anxious about her admission to hospital and subsequent operation. Did her raised anxiety levels contribute to her increased pain levels? Most patients experience some degree of emotional distress, the most common being anxiety or depression. Various factors contribute to the extent of emotional distress in a patient, such as the nature and prognosis of their condition, the patient's coping abilities and social support network, the attitudes and behaviours of health professionals, and the patient's own beliefs about the meaning of pain (Adams and Field, 2001). Evidence suggests that there is a direct causal relationship between pain and anxiety in the clinical setting, indicating that increased anxiety levels contribute to increased levels of pain and higher requests for analgesia (Adams and Field, 2001; Cottle, 1997; Hayward, 1975; Thomas *et al.*, 1990, 1995).

Culture

It is recognised that people from different cultures display different pain behaviours. For example, people of Anglo-Saxon and Irish origin tend to show minimal outward displays of pain compared with people of Mediterranean origin, who may express their pain more outwardly (Adams and Field, 2001). These reactions may be related to early childhood experiences and how a child is taught to cope and react to pain. Consider the mother who fusses over an injured child and another mother who tells the child they will 'get over it'. These parental reactions to pain affect how the child deals with pain in the future. Therefore, perceptions of pain are linked to both cultural and socialisation processes. Could this help to explain why, in Case study 7.2, Miss Shields appeared to complain of more pain than Mr O'Mara?

One of the most striking examples of the impact of cultural values on pain is the hook-swinging ritual, which is still practised in parts of India. In this ritual, a member of the community is chosen to represent the gods. He is swung from a steel rope attached to a cart. The rope is attached to the man by hooks embedded in his back under the skin and muscle, and yet apparently he feels no pain.

With reference to the gate control theory of pain, what would the man swinging from the steel hooks feel if he were to stub his toe on descent from the hook? Would he feel pain physiologically in the normal way?

This example adds further credence to the gate control theory of pain, implying that pain is an individual experience influenced by cultural factors.

Past experience of pain

A patient's earlier experiences of pain can affect how they perceive and deal with pain in a new situation. For example, if the pain experienced previously was controlled well with appropriate analgesia, then the patient will have had a more positive experience than a patient whose pain was not controlled well. Consider Mr O'Mara in Case study 7.2. He previously underwent heart surgery and is not requesting frequent analgesia for his current operation. Perhaps his pain control was good when he had his previous surgery, which may help to explain why his pain seems to be well controlled this time. It would appear that previous bad and good experiences of pain and pain control can either increase or allay anxiety, which in turn affects pain perception.

Self-efficacy and coping

This is concerned with the patient's confidence to cope and the conviction that the patient is competent to perform successfully, irrespective of having pain. Coping has a lot to do with feeling in control of pain in order to perform daily activities such as shopping and going to work. Therefore, controllability and coping are influential factors in how a person perceives and deals with pain on a long-term basis. Studies looking at patients' abilities to cope with pain have considered such aspects as memory, coping style, **self-efficacy**, **locus of control** (LOC), fear, anxiety and depression. Findings of these studies have indicated that the ability to cope is linked to whether positive coping strategies are adopted, whereby pain is viewed as something that can be dealt with in a positive way, or whether more maladaptive, passive coping strategies are used, such as: catastrophising, having low self-esteem and becoming depressed (Adams and Field, 2001).

Self-efficacy is associated with confidence, i.e. the conviction or expectation that one can perform certain behaviours successfully. It is not static but can change in relation to different situations.

Locus of control is related to self-efficacy. A person has an internal LOC if they believe success or failure is due to internal events – a consequence of their own effort to achieve something. If a person has an external LOC, they attribute success or failure to chance, and their own actions make little difference to what happens.

Personality

A patient's personality can affect how they perceive pain. Personality is linked to behaviour and emotions, both of which play a part in the expression of pain. For example, an extroverted person may readily let the nurse know they have pain, expressing the pain and asking for pain relief. A quieter, more introverted person may suffer in silence, feeling too shy to ask for pain relief or exhibit outward signs of pain. Perhaps in Case study 7.2 Miss Shields complains about her pain more because she has a more extroverted personality than Mr O'Mara.

Psychoanalytical studies focusing on personality and pain have deduced that there is a certain type of personality described as a 'pain-prone personality'. People with this personality type seem to have many of the following traits: excessive guilt, and a need to atone for the guilt, a strong unfulfilled aggressive drive, a history of suffering and defeat, intolerance of success, use of pain as a replacement for loss when a relationship is threatened, and a tendency to masochistic sexual practices.

This section has considered some of the factors that influence how patients perceive and ultimately cope with their pain. Considering all of these factors and their potential impact on pain helps to explain why pain is difficult to assess accurately.

The next section looks at the factors that can influence nurses when assessing a patient's pain.

To think about

What factors do you think might influence the nurse when assessing a patient's pain? Could these factors be linked to the case of Miss Shields and Mr O'Mara? Consider these factors when you are next in practice. Talk to other health professionals about pain assessment.

Factors influencing nurses' assessment of patients' pain

Nurses can be influenced by their own attitudes and beliefs when assessing and managing patients' pain. It is important to remember that nurses are not unbiased measuring tools but have a raft of previous experiences and biases that can have an important effect when assessing and managing pain. Some of these factors are outlined below.

Patient's operation or illness

This can influence the nurse's judgement when assessing pain. Nurses tend to associate certain types of operation and illness with preconceived ideas about how much pain the patient should have and how much analgesia the patient needs (Melzack and Wall, 1982; Walsh and Ford, 1989). For example, nurses tend to assume that a patient who has a minor operation should have less pain and therefore need less analgesia compared with a patient who has had major surgery. However, think about the factors we have considered above that could influence patients and how they deal with the pain. Furthermore, sometimes nurses compare pain levels between patients who have had similar operations or illnesses. Think about Miss Shields and Mr O'Mara in Case study 7.2. They had the same type of operation, and yet they had different pain levels. Were the nurses comparing pain levels here?

Fear of addiction

Some nurses have a fear of causing addiction in their patients and tend to withhold analgesia. Addiction in patients receiving opiates for pain control is minimal: the risk of addiction is less than 1% when opiates are given to relieve pain (Cohen, 1980; Weis et al., 1983). However, most nurses overestimate the risk and as a result do not give enough opioid analgesia to relieve pain effectively. Closs (1990) found that 68.4% of nurses in her study estimated the risk of addiction as greater than 1%, resulting in only 20-30% of maximum doses of opioid analgesia being given postoperatively. Weis and colleagues (1983) found that an even higher percentage of doctors and nurses in their study (84.1% and 81.3%, respectively) overestimated the risk as more than 1%. The evidence base also seems to suggest that nurses have a poor knowledge of the pharmacology of opioid analgesia, which contributes to the unrealistic fear of addiction (Dalton, 1989; Field, 1996b; Seers, 1987).

Nurse's attitude

The nurse's belief that the patient is or is not in pain can influence the assessment process. The evidence base suggests that when assessing postoperative pain, some nurses believe that patients should not expect complete pain relief (Balfour, 1989; Carr, 1990; Cohen, 1980). For example, 38.3% of nurses in one study believed that the aim of postoperative analgesia was to relieve pain just enough for the patient to function; 57.3% said they aimed to relieve pain as much as possible; but only 3.5% believed the aim was to completely eradicate pain (Cohen, 1980).

Sometimes nurses may not believe a patient is in pain as they do not 'look like they are in pain' – but it is important to remember that the patient may be coping privately with the pain. Think about the patient's personality and outward displays of pain. Revisit McCaffery's definition of pain, which tells us that we should always believe the patient. There is the potential that nurses may assess and manage pain according to their own attitudes and beliefs about suffering and pain. Poor coping by the patient when in pain can be viewed negatively by nurses, with the suggestion that analgesic intake is related to the patient's coping ability rather than to the pain intensity (Adams and Field, 2001). In Case study 7.2, is Mr O'Mara to be congratulated because he appears to be coping better with his pain than Miss Shields is with hers?

Nurse's culture

The evidence suggests that the culture of the nurse can affect how they assess pain. A large international study that considered culture and its effects on nurses' inferences of suffering found that British nurses assessed the amount of pain suffered to be lower than nurses in most other cultures; nurses from Japan and Korea assessed pain the highest (Davitz and Davitz, 1985). Possible reasons to account for these differences could be related to the way different cultures deal with pain, as discussed earlier in the chapter. The British nurses may deal with pain in a more stoical way and expect the same from their patients.

Routine drug round

Some nurses tend to give out analgesia only on the routine drug round. This can lead to patients clockwatching for the next drug round and receiving pain relief only when the drug trolley appears (Walsh and Ford, 1989). Patients may not realise that they can have analgesia outside of the times of the routine drug round, as this is not always explained by the nurse. This is an example of patients in pain being expected to gear their pain relief requirements to hospital routines rather than to their individual needs. Good pain assessment should ensure that this does not happen.

Patients' characteristics

The patient's characteristics, such as gender, can influence the nurse's assessment of pain. The evidence base for the effects of patients' gender on pain assessment has produced mixed results. Cohen (1980) found that nurses tended to give less analgesia to female patients. She hypothesised that female patients may be viewed by female nurses as being better able to cope with pain. Some people suggest that due to the biological makeup of females (childbearing, menstruation), they are seen as having a greater ability to deal with pain.

Pain threshold and pain tolerance

When assessing a patient's pain, it is important to be aware of the concepts of pain threshold and pain tolerance, and the subtle differences between the two. The International Association for the Study of Pain (IASP) defines the pain threshold as 'The least experience of pain which a subject can recognise'. For example, if a large number of volunteers are tested to see how hard a clamp must be applied to a finger, or how hot a probe applied to the forearm needs to be, before the subject says that it is painful, this is the pain threshold, and it is found to be fairly constant from one person to another. The temperature pain threshold is usually about 44 °C.

Pain tolerance is defined as the greatest level of pain that the subject is prepared to tolerate. The pain tolerance level, which differs widely between people, is a far more important concept than pain threshold in medicine and nursing, as it is usually when pain has gone beyond a certain tolerance level that a person seeks professional help.

This section on pain perception and the many factors that can influence highlights how difficult it can be to assess a patient's pain accurately. However, if nurses are aware of the effects of these factors, they can at least develop a more shared perception of patients' pain (Figure 7.5).

Recap Questions

1. What factors can influence the patient's perception of pain?
2. What factors can influence the nurse when assessing a patient's pain?
3. Why is it important that the nurse is aware of these factors when assessing a patient's pain?

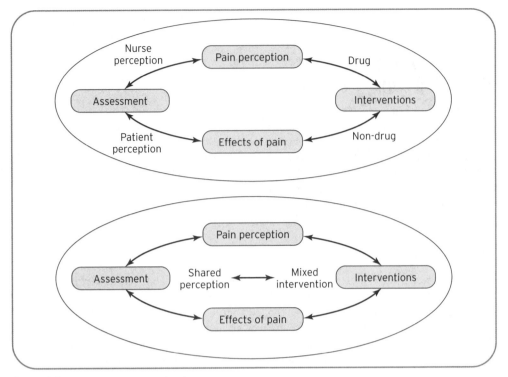

Figure 7.5 Shared perception of pain

Pain management

The nurse plays a major role in managing pain, mainly in terms of determining how best to deal with a patient's pain on an individual basis. This includes deciding, in liaison with the doctor, on the most appropriate analgesia for the patient. McCaffery highlighted six main aspects of the nurse's role in the administration of medication for pain relief (Exhibit 7.1).

+ The nurse determines whether and when analgesia should be given
+ The nurse chooses the appropriate analgesic when more than one is prescribed
+ The nurse evaluates the effectiveness of the analgesia at regular or frequent intervals following administration
+ The nurse should be aware of, and alert to, the possibility of certain side effects from the analgesia
+ The nurse reports promptly and accurately to the doctor when a change of analgesia is needed
+ The nurse may need to advise patients about the use of analgesics, both prescription and non-prescription

Exhibit 7.1 The nurse's role in pain relief
Adapted from McCaffery (1983)

Pain management decisions are inextricably linked with accurate assessment of patients' pain. Inappropriate analgesia decisions may have a detrimental effect on a patient's recovery and progress. It is vital that the nurse gives the correct type of analgesia to relieve pain and ensures that the drug given is effective; this can be monitored by frequently assessing the patient's pain.

There are many types of analgesia that can be given to control varying degrees of pain, ranging from mild to very severe pain. We consider these, along with the pharmacokinetics (drug circulation) and pharmacodynamics (drug action) of the drugs, in the following sections.

To think about

What types of analgesia have you seen given in clinical practice? Make a note of the names of the drugs, how they work and their possible side effects. Try to distinguish between weak and strong analgesics. Identify why certain drugs were chosen.

Non-opioid analgesics

These analgesics are generally used to control mild to moderate pain. They contain no opioids (which we consider later in this section).

Paracetamol

This analgesic is commonly used to relieve mild pain. It does not have to be prescribed and patients often self-medicate with this drug. Paracetamol is thought to work both centrally (in the brain and spinal cord) and peripherally (at the point of pain) by inhibiting the production of prostaglandins (pain-producing chemicals; Exhibit 7.2). Paracetamol has only a weak anti-inflammatory effect, but it is useful as an antipyretic (to lower the patient's temperature).

Prostaglandins are hormone-like substances that induce inflammation, pain and fever, support platelet function and protect the stomach lining. They are produced by the enzyme cyclo-oxygenase (COX). There are two types of COX: COX-1 and COX-2. Both types promote inflammation, pain and fever, but only COX-1 produces prostaglandins that protect the stomach lining and support platelet function.

Non-steroidal anti-inflammatory drugs (NSAIDs) inhibit COX-1 and COX-2. By blocking the action of COX-1, NSAIDs may damage the stomach lining, leading to gastrointestinal bleeding and ulcers, and altered platelet function.

A new class of NSAIDs – COX-2 inhibitors – suppress only COX-2. These agents reduce the risk of gastrointestinal problems and altered platelet function because they spare COX-1.

Exhibit 7.2 Prostaglandins

Paracetamol can be used to relieve headache, muscle aches and general pain and to reduce fever. It can also be given in combination with an opioid to help control **breakthrough pain.**

Paracetamol can have a toxic effect on the liver if taken in overdose. A person needs to take only nine tablets at any one time to cause some toxicity in the liver. There is a risk of accidentally overdosing if common cold remedies (which contain paracetamol) are mixed with paracetamol tablets.

Aspirin

This analgesic is a popular choice for mild to moderate pain. It can be bought over the counter. It is used mainly to relieve pain and inflammation and to reduce fever. Aspirin is not effective in the relief of visceral pain (pain arising from body organs or smooth internal muscles) or severe pain associated with trauma. Aspirin is a salicylate – this means it contains salicylic acid, which is manufactured from a substance called salicin derived from poplar trees.

Aspirin acts by inhibiting prostaglandin production in a similar way to paracetamol (see Exhibit 7.2).

Gastrointestinal bleeding is an important side effect of aspirin. Aspirin has a reduced therapeutic effect when given with non-steroidal anti-inflammatory drugs (NSAIDs).

Non-steroidal anti-inflammatory drugs

This group of analgesics includes a wide range of drugs, many of which can be bought over the counter. NSAIDs are often prescribed for osteoarthritis and rheumatoid arthritis and can be used to manage some aspects of cancer pain, particularly for pain related to bone cancer. Some examples of NSAIDs are:

+ Diclofenac
+ Ibuprofen
+ Ketoprofen
+ Naproxen
+ Piroxicam

Most NSAIDs are absorbed quickly and act peripherally (i.e. at the point of pain). They also work by interfering with prostaglandin production (see Exhibit 7.2). They are very effective in the treatment of inflammation, menstrual cramps, and mild to moderate pain after certain types of surgery.

Side effects of NSAIDs include gastrointestinal bleeding, liver toxicity, drowsiness, headache, dizziness, confusion, tinnitus, vertigo, depression and kidney problems. The risk of these adverse reactions is greatly decreased with short-term, low-dose and single-dose use.

Breakthrough pain is pain that occurs when the effects of opioid analgesia have started to wear off.

Opioid analgesics

Opioids include derivatives of the opium (poppy) plant and synthetic drugs that 'mimic' the action of natural opioids. All opioids act on the CNS (brain and spinal cord). They reduce the perception of pain by actively binding to opiate receptor sites in the CNS. Here, they mimic the effects of endorphins (naturally occurring opiates that are part of the body's own pain relief system). Opioids are classified as weak or strong in action.

Weak opioids

Codeine is classified as a weak opioid. It has a moderate potency and is effective for relieving moderate to severe pain. Codeine can be given alone or in combination with an NSAID or paracetamol.

The main side effect of codeine is constipation. Light-headedness, nausea and drowsiness are also reported.

Strong opioids

Most opioids fall into this group due to their high potency. By affecting the perception of pain, strong opioids are able to change the patient's emotional response to pain. Opioids can be administered alone or with an NSAID and/or paracetamol. Some examples of strong opioids are:

+ Morphine
+ Diamorphine
+ Buprenorphine
+ Tramadol
+ Fentanyl

Due to their high potency, these drugs have several side effects. By binding to receptor site, the drugs cause analgesia but also cough suppression, respiratory depression, drowsiness, euphoria, nausea, vomiting, hypotension and constipation.

Tolerance, dependency and addiction

In addition to relieving pain, opioids, particularly strong opioids, help to reduce anxiety and produce a pleasant somnolence. Unfortunately, this has led to their abuse and the development of drug addiction. Addiction occurs only if the drug is being used for its hallucinogenic effects rather than for pain relief; if a drug is used initially to relieve pain but the patient continues to use it after the pain has gone, this can be classed as addiction.

A patient receiving opioid treatment for a long period of time can develop a tolerance to the drug. This means that a higher dose is required in order to achieve the same therapeutic effect. Patients can also develop a psychological and physical dependency. Abrupt cessation of opioids may lead to a withdrawal syndrome characterised by fever, chills, nausea, vomiting and insomnia. Tolerance and dependency are not the same as addiction.

Some nurses have a fear of causing opioid addiction in their patients. This may be attributed to inadequate education being given on the pharmacology of opioid analgesia and the actions of opioid drugs. As a result, misconceptions about the side effects of opioid analgesia abound (Exhibit 7.3).

+ Narcotics given to relieve pain will lead to addiction in a large percentage of patients
+ Physical dependence on narcotics can be life-threatening
+ Tolerance to narcotics develops uniformly in all patients; for example, if narcotics are started too soon or escalated too fast, doses will become fatal or a ceiling on analgesia will be reached
+ Large or frequent doses will lead to respiratory depression
+ Low doses are safe and going beyond a certain dose in any patient is unsafe

Exhibit 7.3 Misconceptions about the side effects of narcotic analgesia
Adapted from McCaffery and Beebe (1989)

Administration of analgesia

This section considers the various methods by which analgesia can be given (Figure 7.6), including the advantages and disadvantages of each method.

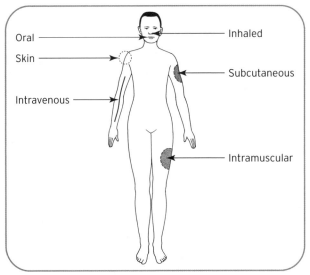

Figure 7.6 Different routes of analgesia administration

Oral administration

This is the simplest and most convenient way to give analgesia. Oral analgesics are available in tablet, capsule and liquid forms. After ingestion, they are absorbed by the gastrointestinal tract. The rate at which the drug is absorbed is dependent on factors such as whether the drug is formulated for immediate or controlled release. Liquid preparations tend to be absorbed faster than solid preparations.

The main advantage of this method is it is quick and easy. However, an important disadvantage is that it takes time for the drug to be effective in relieving pain.

Intramuscular administration

This involves the injection of the drug into the muscle, usually into the upper leg (quadriceps muscle) or the upper outer quadrant of the buttock (gluteus maximus muscle); note, however, that the ventrogluteal route is now recommended instead of the buttock. The intramuscular route tends to be used less often nowadays. It has several disadvantages, including patients' dislike of needles, local trauma to the injected muscle, and variation in pharmacokinetics in different patients. The advantages of intramuscular administration are that the drug acts more quickly than when given by the oral route, and it can be used in patients who are unable to take oral medication.

Intravenous administration

This involves the drug being given directly into a vein. Intravenous analgesia can be given as a bolus and/or an infusion.

An intravenous bolus is a large undiluted dose of analgesia (usually an opioid). It is given by a doctor or qualified nurse. This delivery method is used mainly in the operating theatre by the anaesthetist and in the recovery room by the anaesthetist and recovery nursing staff. A small bolus of diluted opioid, prescribed by the anaesthetist, is usually given to control pain during the surgical procedure. During the administration, the patient's response to the opioid is monitored closely by the qualified nurse. The patient's consciousness level, vital signs and pain relief are recorded. The advantage of this method is that it provides the patient with quick and effective pain relief, but a qualified nurse must be present at all times during administration because of the potency of the dose.

Intravenous infusion involves the continuous delivery of an opioid drug in a dilute solution into the patient's circulation through an intravenous cannula. This method is commonly used in intensive care and high dependency units. Its main advantage is that it delivers a constant supply of analgesia to the patient. The main disadvantage is that it takes several hours for the plasma concentration of the drug to be stable and reach a steady state, which can lead to ineffective pain relief. However, this can be overcome by giving an initial intravenous bolus dose (as described above) before commencing the intravenous infusion; as before, this must be monitored closely by a qualified nurse. Plasma concentrations can continue to rise, leading to side effects such as **respiratory depression** and **hypoxia**; this can apply to any intravenous infusion but is more of a problem when the drug is given as a bolus dose.

Patient-controlled analgesia

Patient-controlled analgesia (PCA) has become popular in the UK only recently. PCA systems deliver opioids at a rate controlled by the patient. The major problem with the traditional intermittent opioid regime of intramuscular injections prescribed every 4-6 hours, or 'PRN' (as necessary), is nurses interpreting this to mean 'as little as possible'. This can lead to a lack of effective pain relief. The basis of PCA is that the patient, rather than the nurse or doctor, regulates the amount of opioid given to achieve good analgesia with minimal side effects.

PCA devices consist of a pump and a timing device. When the patient feels pain, they press a button connected to the pump, which delivers a prescribed dose of opioid analgesia, usually intravenously but sometimes **subcutaneously** or via an arterial or epidural infusion. The risk of overdose is reduced by a lockout device, which ensures that no further doses are delivered for a preset interval, which is usually 5-10 minutes, depending on the drug and dosage.

Respiratory depression is a reduced respiratory rate.

Hypoxia is a low level of oxygen in the patient's bloodstream.

Subcutaneous means just below the skin layers.

The major advantage of PCA is patient satisfaction due to control over pain relief. Patients report feeling less anxious and have less discomfort as the analgesia is readily available and there is no delay in receiving it. The patient cannot overdose, opioids as the amount is preset by the anaesthetist or nurse. Several studies have reported improved efficacy, reduced dosage of opioid and earlier discharge compared with routine intramuscular therapy (Curry *et al.*, 1994; Thomas *et al.*, 1990, 1995).

Some patients are unable to use PCA devices due to physical disability or cognitively impairment. Other patients do not like being in control of the device and prefer a nurse to administer pain relief using more conventional methods.

Spinal opioids

Opioid receptors are present in the spinal cord. When administered, opioids may produce analgesia by acting on these sites. Opioids can be injected into the subarachnoid space containing cerebral spinal fluid, which surrounds and protects the spinal canal; this is called intrathecal administration. Alternatively, the opioid can be given into the epidural (extradural) space, between the dura mater and the bone of the spine; this is termed epidural administration. A catheter can be inserted into the epidural space to provide continuous infusions of opioids. These structures are illustrated in Figure 7.7.

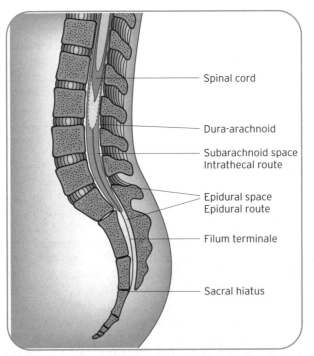

Spinal cord

Dura-arachnoid

Subarachnoid space
Intrathecal route

Epidural space
Epidural route

Filum terminale

Sacral hiatus

Figure 7.7 Lower end of the spinal cord, showing intrathecal and epidural routes of administration of spinal opioids
Source: Bruce (1992)

The main advantage of spinal analgesia is that good pain relief can be obtained with small doses. In the UK, this method is popular during and after Caesarian section for childbirth and postoperatively following thoracic and upper abdominal surgery.

Disadvantages of spinal analgesia include instances of incomplete analgesia and large inter-patient variability in response. The technique is time-consuming, there may be technical difficulties, and infection of the epidural space is a possibility. There is also a high incidence of nausea and vomiting, pruritus and urinary retention. Finally, potentially fatal respiratory depression can occur several hours after injection, and so close monitoring of the patient is required for some time after the procedure.

Transdermal opioids

With the transdermal route, the drug is absorbed through the skin. The drug, which is lipid-soluble, is usually supplied in the form of a transdermal patch. Certain creams and ointments can also be absorbed via the skin. One of the most well-known transdermal systems is the fentanyl patch (Durogesic®), which is 75 times more potent than morphine. The main advantage of using patches is they provide a steady concentration of opioid without the need for venous access or syringe pumps.

An important disadvantage of transdermal delivery is that doses cannot be titrated or altered to patients' individual needs, as the dose is preset within the patch. It also takes several hours to achieve effective plasma concentrations, which then fall slowly after the patch is removed. This could be a problem if overdose occurs. Furthermore, there is the potential for development of rashes and allergic reactions in some people.

Sublingual administration

Sublingual administration involves the giving of analgesia under the tongue. The route provides rapid and convenient pain relief. Buprenorphine and morphine can be given via this route. Some studies have found sublingual buprenorphine to be satisfactory; however, it is not as effective as morphine. Nausea, vomiting and sedation can be troublesome if the sublingual route is used to give opioids.

Rectal administration

Analgesia can be given via the rectum in the form of suppositories. The drug is absorbed quite quickly into the anal canal and then into the bloodstream. The main advantage of this method is that analgesia can be given if the patient is unable to take anything by mouth or they are needle-phobic. However, giving drugs via the rectal route can be uncomfortable or painful.

Local analgesia

Local analgesia (anaesthetic) works by blocking the conduction of impulses along nerves/pain fibres. The most common local analgesics in the UK are lidocaine (lignocaine), prilocaine and bupivacaine. Most local analgesia last about 2-3 hours. The main advantages of local analgesia are that the pain relief is profound and the drugs have no opioid-like side effects.

Side effects of local analgesia include numbness of the mouth and tongue, light-headedness, tinnitus, visual disturbances, slurring of speech, muscular twitching, irrational conversation, unconsciousness, grand mal convulsions, coma and respiratory arrest. These effects tend to occur when the drugs are given in high doses. Because of this toxicity, the volume of drug that can be given is limited. Unfortunately, the volume of solution required to block nerves supplying painful areas may be greater than the safe dose. The short duration of action of local analgesia is also a drawback.

Inhaled analgesia

Analgesia may be given in the form of nitrous oxide administered via a facemask in oxygen 50% (Entonox®). This is used routinely in childbirth and by first-aid workers. It is a quick and efficient method of pain relief and has minimal side effects if given in short, sharp bursts and titrated properly. It can also be useful for short periods of severe postoperative pain, during physiotherapy, and during painful procedures such as removal of drains and dressings.

The main disadvantages of inhaled nitrous oxide are the side effects of prolonged sedation and depression of bone marrow. There is also concern regarding the toxic effects on staff and the long-term influences on the environment.

Efficacy (effectiveness) of analgesia

The efficacy, or effectiveness, of analgesia is dependent on the delivery of the correct amount of analgesia to the correct site of action. This is greatly influenced by the type of drug given and the route of administration. In order to achieve maximum pain relief, the preparation must achieve the correct level of drug in the blood. Each drug has a minimum and maximum therapeutic effect (Figure 7.8). If the dosage given does not reach the minimum therapeutic effect, then the patient will be under-medicated. Conversely, if the dosage of the drug exceeds the maximum therapeutic effect, then the patient will experience toxic symptoms arising from overdosage.

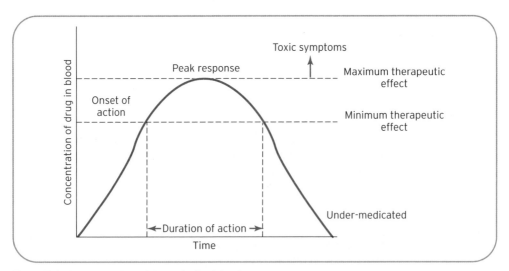

Figure 7.8 Concentration of drugs in the blood

The route of administration affects the action of the drug given. For example, if the drug is given intravenously, it will have a quicker effect than if it is given intramuscularly; the effect will be even slower if the oral route is used. Figure 7.9 illustrates the effect of the route of administration of a drug on the plasma concentration after a single dose.

Different types of analgesia operate at different levels within the CNS and peripheral nervous system. Figure 7.10 shows where the different forms of analgesia can influence pain.

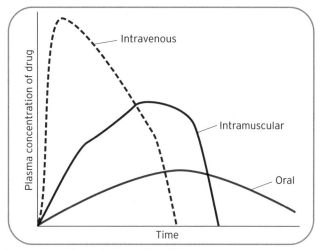

Figure 7.9 Effect of route of administration of a drug on the plasma concentration after a single dose

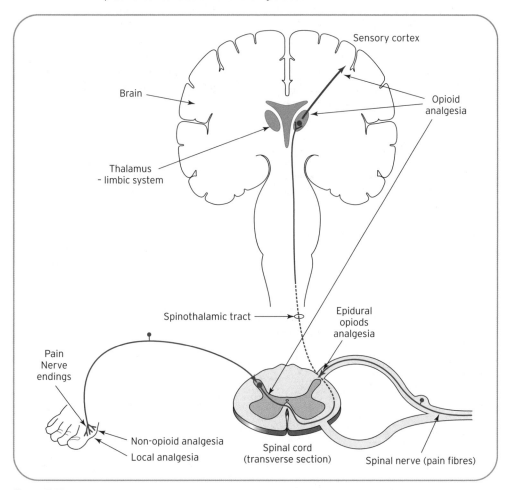

Figure 7.10 Neural pain pathways and action site of different types of analgesia

Now you have become more familiar with the different types of analgesia, consider Case study 7.3.

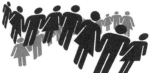

Case Study 7.3

Mrs Hopkin is a 67-year-old woman with terminal cancer. Currently her pain is controlled by modified-release morphine (30 mg every 12 hours). Mrs Hopkin's pain has been under control with this regime for 2 weeks. You are helping Mrs Hopkin to wash one morning, and she complains of severe pain.

What can you do to help the patient with her pain management?
What co-analgesics could be prescribed?

Discuss these issues with a colleague or a qualified nurse in your clinical placement. Jot down some notes as a result of your discussion.

Mrs Hopkin's pain will need to be re-assessed regularly to decide what changes need to be made to her medication. It is possible that the morphine dose the patient is receiving is inadequate for the severity of her pain. Would she be better with a continuous dose of morphine via an intravenous pump? Would it help to give co-analgesics such as paracetamol or an NSAID in conjunction with the opioid drug to relieve breakthrough pain? Ideally, breakthrough pain should not occur; if the appropriate analgesia is given regularly, then a constant therapeutic level of analgesia should be maintained, thereby ensuring optimum pain relief.

Analgesic ladder

How does the nurse decide which analgesia the patient requires when there are so many available? The World Health Organization (WHO) has devised an analgesic ladder to help nurses in their decision-making (Figure 7.11).

Recommended analgesia for adult patients

		Pain score 3 (severe pain)
	Pain score 2 (moderate pain)	Paracetamol 1g 4-6 hourly (maximum 8 tablets daily) + codeine 30-60mg 4-6 hourly ± ibruprofen 400mg 6-8 hourly
Pain score 1 (mild pain)	Paracetamol 1g 4-6 hourly (maximum 8 tablets daily) + codeine 30-60mg 4-6 hourly ± ibruprofen 400mg 6-8 hourly	or Morphine 10mg hourly ± NSAIDs
Paracetamol 1g 4-6 hourly (maximum 8 tablets daily)		

Figure 7.11 Analgesia ladder

This section has considered the various types of analgesia available and the different routes in which they can be given. Both the nurse and the doctor have to decide which analgesia, route and frequency are best to manage an individual patient's pain, taking into account the side effects of the drug. The WHO analgesic ladder can help with some of the decision-making. Regularly assessing and monitoring pain relief is important. It is also useful for the nurse to know the potency and side effects of the analgesia given, so that potentially fatal side effects such as respiratory depression can be detected early.

Recap Questions

1. What are the main types of analgesia?
2. What factors may influence the doctor when deciding what analgesia to give?
3. What are the most common methods used to administer analgesia?
4. When should the analgesic ladder be used?

Other methods of pain relief

Research suggests that many nurses rely on a single method approach to pain management (Field and Adams, 2001). However, other methods are available to relieve or mediate pain, and we consider these below.

To think about

Have you seen any methods of pain relief, other than analgesia, in your clinical placement? Ask your colleagues or a qualified nurse whether anyone has used alternative/complementary therapies to relieve pain.

Relaxation

Relaxation techniques, such as meditation, guided imagery and passive relaxation, can help to relieve muscular and mental tension, which exacerbate pain. The main goal of relaxation is to clear the mind and release pent-up muscular tension. Relaxation techniques aim to break the pain–anxiety–pain cycle (Figure 7.12).

Hypnosis

Modern hypnotic techniques originate from the nineteenth century, when there was great interest in the use of hypnosis to produce analgesia for major surgery. A lot of research has indicated the effects of hypnosis on experimentally induced pain, but there is little evidence from controlled clinical trials to show that hypnosis is effective for chronic pain. Hypnosis does not work for everyone: certain personality types, accounting for about a third of the population, are more susceptible than others to being hypnotised.

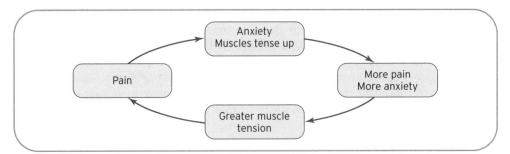

Figure 7.12 Pain-anxiety-pain cycle

Distraction

Diverting the patient's attention away from the pain is a useful technique. The adoption of methods such as deep breathing exercises and the use of pleasant imagery can help to distract the patient. The aim is to shield the sensation of pain by increasing sensation input via another sensory route such as the ear (auditory) or eye (visual) or through touch (tactile).

Transcutaneous electrical nerve stimulation

TENS applies a controlled level of low-voltage electricity to the body in order to relieve pain. This technique has long been used in physiotherapy, mainly for patients with chronic pain. TENS is thought to work by stimulating the large rapidly conducting A beta nerve fibres, thereby 'closing the gate' in the dorsal horn of the spinal cord. TENS is also thought to stimulate production of endorphins. It can be effective in painful situations such as childbirth. Figure 7.13 shows a TENS machine.

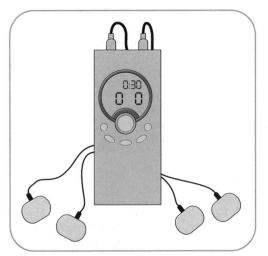

Figure 7.13 Transcutaneous electrical nerve stimulation (TENS) machine

Massage

Massage is an ancient form of non-invasive pain relief. It relies on the easing of muscle tension to relieve pain. Massage is usually carried out using cream or oil; sometimes aromatherapy oils are used (see below). The cream or oil is massaged into the body using a range of techniques, including stroking, percussion, kneading and pummelling (O'Hara, 1996). There is no single explanation as to how massage may relieve pain, but it is thought to activate some of the gate-control mechanisms and release endorphins. Massage also helps to distract the patient from pain and improves the nurse–patient relationship as the nurse spends more quality time with the patient (Vale, 1998).

Aromatherapy

Aromatherapy uses aromatic oils derived from a variety of plants known for their medicinal properties. Specific oils have either relaxing or stimulating effects. Oils that are thought to reduce pain include basil, eucalyptus, geranium, lavender, rosemary and tea tree. When these oils are absorbed, it is believed they interact with hormones and enzymes to produce changes in blood pressure, pulse rate and other physiological functions. It has been suggested that aromatherapy can affect the limbic system - the part of the brain associated with emotion and memory.

Acupuncture

Acupuncture involves the insertion of thin metal needles, just under the skin at specific points. The WHO has identified over 100 conditions that have been helped by acupuncture, including:

+ Arthritis
+ Back pain
+ Dental pain
+ Headaches
+ **Peripheral neuropathy**
+ **Trigeminal neuralgia**

A similar technique that does not require the use of needles can be used in people who are needle-phobic. Pressure is applied to acupuncture points on the skin, bringing about effects that are similar to those produced by the insertion of needles.

Peripheral neuropathy occurs when there is damage to peripheral nerves. It causes neuropathic pain characterised by unusual pain sensations such as shooting, burning and electrical pains.

Trigeminal neuralgia occurs when there is inflammation to the trigeminal nerve that supplies part of the face. The pain associated with trigeminal neuralgia is often described as excruciating.

Reflexology

Reflexology consists of applying small pressure movements to the surfaces of the foot and around the ankle. The movements follow a 'map' that relates parts of the body to corresponding reflex points on each foot. This has a relaxing effect and can be beneficial in giving pain relief.

Case study 7.4 encourages you to consider non-pharmacological strategies to help relieve pain.

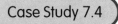

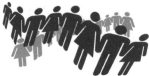

Case Study 7.4

You accompany the community nurse, who is visiting 57-year-old Miss Marr at home. Miss Marr has severe rheumatoid arthritis. Although she is taking a weak opioid, she has some pain occasionally. She insists she is happy with the treatment she is receiving and requires no change in her pharmacological management.

What other strategies could she use to reduce pain?
When should non-pharmacological strategies be used?
What strategies are available?

Discuss this with a colleague or qualified nurse in your clinical placement. Jot down some points for discussion.

Find out whether Miss Marr is aware of any non-pharmacological strategies that she could use. If not, tell her about them and how she might be able to access them via an alternative/complementary clinic. By giving her this information, she can make an informed choice as to whether she wants to try other methods to help relieve her pain.

Legal aspects of complementary/alternative therapies

When the multidisciplinary team is deciding on treatment for a patient, the team should consider the use of complementary therapies. Very often this does not happen in practice, and medication seems to be the main choice. Patients, nurses, doctors and pharmacists should be aware of the contribution that complementary therapies can make to care, particularly in relation to pain control.

When a nurse administers any kind of treatment or care to a patient, the nurse is governed by the Nursing and Midwifery Council (NMC) Code of Professional Conduct. This code sets the standards for conduct, performance and ethics and also applies when a nurse gives any of the complementary/alternative therapies outlined above.

Nurses wishing to administer any complementary/alternative treatments must have undertaken approved courses and be deemed competent to offer such treatments. Although the NMC regulates the practice of nurses, it does not have responsibility for the standards of other bodies that offer education and training in professional or complementary therapies. Therefore, nurses are advised to seek guidance from one of the various professional bodies representing complementary practices when choosing to undertake a specific course in this area. It is the nurse's responsibility to judge whether the qualification awarded has given them a level of competence to use that skill in patient care. Self-evaluation of competence and accountability are extremely important, particularly when the nurse is working independently. It is important for the nurse to ensure that any treatments given are not contraindicated with any medications that the patient is taking.

Local policies to provide a framework for the use of complementary therapies by nurses and other health professionals should be provided by hospital and community trusts. Any nurse using any of the complementary therapies outlined above must be aware of the extent of insurance cover their membership organisation provides in relation to the use of complementary therapies. Finally, nurses remain accountable when practising complementary or alternative therapies. The NMC Code states:

You must ensure that the use of complementary or alternative therapies is safe and in the interests of patients and clients. This must be discussed with the team as part of the therapeutic process and the patient or client must consent to their use.

Recap Questions

1. What is meant by 'other methods of pain relief'?
2. How are relaxation and distraction methods thought to help relieve pain?
3. How do massage and aromatherapy help to alleviate pain?
4. What legal aspects does the nurse need to be aware of when giving complementary/alternative therapies?

Summary

This chapter has considered the essential aspects of good pain management, from defining pain to discussing various ways to successfully relieve pain. The journey has been a little complex, particularly when looking at the processes that occur when pain is felt. Trying to define pain is not straightforward, as it involves sensory, emotional and cognitive dimensions. Melzack and Wall's gate control theory has helped greatly with our understanding of the process of pain perception and the variable relationship between injury/nociceptive (pain) stimuli and the degree of pain felt.

As the concept of pain is so complex, this can make the assessment of pain more difficult. We cannot feel another person's pain. We also know that pain reports are subjective and that the patient's perception of pain can be influenced by a plethora of factors, including gender, culture and past experiences of pain. Similarly, the nurse brings their own biases to the process of assessing pain, and ultimately this can give rise to differences in pain assessment between nurses and patients.

Pain is viewed from two perspectives – that of the patient and that of the nurse. Inevitably, this can lead to a variance in the assessment of pain. The aim when assessing pain is for the nurse and the patient to have a shared perception of pain. When assessing pain, the differentiation between pain threshold and pain tolerance must also be considered; if this is ignored, your patient may suffer pain needlessly.

Inaccurate assessment of pain can lead to the patient receiving inadequate or inappropriate analgesia. For example, a patient with pain from terminal cancer requires a strong analgesic, such as an opioid; to offer a mild analgesic such as paracetamol or aspirin would be inappropriate and lead to ineffective pain relief. Pain is an individual experience and patients may require different amounts of analgesia in similar situations (see Case study 7.2). Reference should be made to the analgesic ladder when deciding which analgesia to give. Knowledge of the pharmacodynamics and pharmacokinetics also helps in the decision-making process.

The route of administration has important implications in the management of pain. For example, a patient with severe abdominal pain needs to be given analgesia by the quickest route, probably intravenously, to give fast pain relief. Nurses have considerable power and responsibility in relation to the giving of analgesia, and they should ensure that their analgesia decisions are not influenced by unrealistic fears of opioid addiction. Therefore, it is important that the distinction between tolerance, dependency and addiction is understood so that adequate analgesia is always given.

Finally, there is a place in healthcare for alternative methods of pain relief. The use of massage, aromatherapy, reflexology and TENS can all complement the effects of analgesia and help to promote relaxation and a feeling of wellbeing in the patient. These complementary/alternative methods are often underused, possibly because of the legal aspects relating to the administration of these treatments in relation to accountability and competence to practice.

Key Points

1. It is difficult to define pain and to reach a consensus. This is due to the complex nature of the pain experience.

2. Assessment of pain is complex, because the patient experiencing the pain and the nurse assessing the pain will have different perceptions. Many factors, such as age, gender and culture, influence this assessment. The aim is to have a shared perception of pain and for this to lead to a more accurate assessment of pain.

3. Many types of analgesia are given to relieve pain. The nurse and the doctor must be aware of the action and side effects of analgesics in order to ensure that they make the best analgesia decisions. The WHO analgesic ladder provides guidance on this.

4. Nurses must be aware of the methods of administration of analgesia when deciding the best way to relieve different types of pain.

5. Complementary/alternative methods of pain relief, such as relaxation, massage and TENS, can be used in conjunction with pharmacological intervention to ensure optimum pain control.

Points for debate

Now that you have come to the end of this chapter here are a few points that you may wish to think about when you are in practice. You may wish to discuss these with your work colleagues or fellow students.

'Pain is what the patient says it is'
(McCaffery, 1968).

When assessing a patient's pain, many nurses are influenced by their own beliefs and values about pain.

Many nurses fear they will cause addiction in patients who are prescribed opioids for pain relief. Therefore, they are reluctant to give maximum doses, even though the patient is still in pain.

Links to Other Chapters

Chapter 2 Dignity and privacy
Chapter 3 Basic observations
Chapter 10 Record-keeping

Further reading

Arntz, A and Schmidt, J (1989) Perceived control and the experience of pain. In: Steptoe, A and Appels, A (eds) *Stress, Personal Control and Health*. Chichester: John Wiley & Sons.

Cowan, T (1997) Patient-controlled analgesia devises. *Professional Nurse* **13**, 119-124.

Epps, C (2001) Recognizing pain in the institutionalised elder with dementia. *Geriatric Nursing* **22**, 71-79.

Facett, J, Gordon, N and Levine, J (1994) Differences in postoperative pain severity among four ethnic groups. *Journal of Pain and Symptom Management* **9**, 383-389.

Field, L (1995) The role of the nurse in the assessment and relief of postoperative pain. Unpublished master's thesis. Warwick: University of Warwick.

Fordham, M and Dunn, V (1994) *Alongside the Person in Pain: Holistic Care and Nursing Practice*. London: Baillière Tindall.

Helme, R and Gibson, S (1996) Pain in the elderly. Plenary address at the Eighth World Congress on Pain. Vancouver, 17-22 August 1996.

Herr, K and Mobily, P (1991) Complexities of pain assessment in the elderly: clinical considerations. *Journal of Gerontological Nursing* **17**, 12-19.

Hirsh, M and Liebert, R (1998) The physical and psychological experience of pain: the effects of labeling and cold pressure temperature on three pain measures in college women. *Pain* **77**, 41-48.

Johnston, M (1976) Communication of patients' feelings in hospital. In: Bennett, AE (ed) *Communications between Doctors and Patients*. Oxford: Oxford University Press.

Lander, J, Fowler-Kerry, S and Hill, A (1990) Comparison of pain perceptions among males and females. *Canadian Journal of Nursing Research* **2**, 39-49.

Mackintosh, C (1994) Do nurses provide adequate pain relief? *British Journal of Nursing* **3**, 342-347.

McCaffery, M and Pesaro, C (1999) *Pain Clinical Manual*, 2nd edn. St Louis, MO: Mosby.

McCaffery, M and Pasero, C (eds) (1999) *Pain: Clinical Manual*, 2nd edn. St Louis, MO: Mosby.

Melzack, R and Wall, P (1988) *The Challenge of Pain*, 2nd edn. London: Penguin.

Owen, H, McMillan, V and Rogowski, D (1989) Postoperative pain therapy: a survey of patients' expectations and their experiences. *Pain* **41**, 303-307.

Salmon, P and Manyande, A (1996) Good patients cope with their pain: postoperative analgesia and nurses' perceptions of their patients' pain. *Pain* **68**, 63-68.

Schilling, J and Moreau, D (2003) *Pain Management made Incredibly Easy*. London: Lippincott Williams & Wilkins.

Scott, I (1994) Effectiveness of documented assessment of postoperative pain. *British Journal of Nursing* **3** 494-501.

Skevington, S (1995) *Psychology of Pain*. Chichester: John Wiley & Sons.

Sofoar, B (1983) Pain relief: the core of nursing practice. *Nursing Times* **79**, 34-40.

Sofoar, B (1998) *Pain: Principles, Practices and Patients*, 3rd edn. Cheltenham: Stanley Thornes.

References

Adams, N and Field, L (2001) Pain management 1: psychological and social aspects of pain. *British Journal of Nursing* **10**, 903-911.

Balfour, S (1989) Will I be in pain? Patients' and nurses' attitudes to pain after abdominal surgery. *Professional Nurse* **5**, 28-33.

Briggs, E (2003) The nursing management of pain in older people. *Nursing Standard* **17**, 47-53.

Carr, E (1990) Postoperative pain: patients' expectations and experiences. *Journal of Advanced Nursing* **15**, 89-100.

Closs, S (1990) An exploratory analysis of postoperative analgesic drugs. *Journal of Advanced Nursing* **15**, 42-49.

Cohen, F (1980) Post surgical pain relief: patients' status and nurses' medication choices. *Pain* **9**, 265-274.

Cottle, S (1997) Nurses' undermedication of analgesia in cardiac surgical patients: a personal exploration. *Nursing Critical Care* **2**, 146-149.

Curry, P, Pacsoo, C and Heap, D (1994) Patient controlled epidural analgesia in obstetric anaesthetic practice. *Pain* **57**, 125-128.

Dalton, J (1989) Nurses, perceptions of their pain assessment skills, pain management: practices and attitudes towards pain. *Oncology Nursing Forum* **16**, 225-231.

Davies, E, Male, M, Turner, M and Wylie, K (2004) Pain assessment and cognitive impairment: part 1. *Nursing Standard* **19**, 39-41.

Davitz, L and Davitz, J (1985) Culture and nurses' inferences of suffering. In: Copp, L (ed) *Recent Advances in Nursing (Perspectives on Pain)*. Edinburgh: Churchill Livingstone.

Department of Health (2003) *Essence of Care: Patient-Focused Benchmarks for Clinical Governance*. London: The Stationery Office.

Department of Health (2005) *Integrated Services to Treat People with Long-Term Conditions*. London: The Stationery Office.

Erickson, C (1992) Assessment and management of pain. In: Friedman, S, Fisher, M and Schonberg, S (eds) *Comprehensive Adolescent Health Care*. St Louis, MO: Quality Medical Publishing.

Ferell, B (1991) Pain management in elderly people. *Journal of the American Geriatric Society* **38**, 64-73.

Field, L (1996a) Are nurses still underestimating patients' pain postoperatively? *British Journal of Nursing* **5**, 778-784.

Field, L (1996b) Factors influencing nurses' analgesia decisions. *British Journal of Nursing* **5**, 838-844.

Field, L and Adams, N (2001) Pain management 2: psychological and social aspects of pain. *British Journal of Nursing* **10**, 903-911.

Fowler-Kerry, S and Lander, J (1991) Assessment in sex differences in children's and adolescents' self-reported pain from venepuncture. *Journal of Paediatric Psychology* **16**, 783-793.

Harkin, S (1988) Pain in the elderly. In: Dubner, R, Gebhart, G and Bond, M (eds) *Pain Research and Clinical Management*, Vol. 3. Amsterdam: Elsevier.

Hayward, J (1975) *Information: A Prescription Against Pain*. London: Royal College of Nursing.

International Association for the Study of Pain (1986) Classification of chronic pain: descriptions of chronic pain syndromes and definitions of pain terms. *Pain* **3** (suppl), 1-226.

Levine, F and De Simone, L (1991) The effects of experimenter gender on pain report in male and female subjects. *Pain* **44**, 69-72.

McCaffery, M (1968) *Nursing the Patient in Pain*. Cambridge: Lippincott and Harper and Row.

McCaffery, M (1983) *Nursing the Patient in Pain*, 2nd edn. Cambridge: Lippincott and Harper and Row.

McCaffery, M and Beebe, A (1989) *Pain: Clinical Manual for Nursing Practice*, 2nd edn. Toronto: Mosby.

Melzack, R and Wall, P (1965) Pain mechanisms: a new theory. *Science* **150**, 971-979.

Melzack, R and Wall, P (1982) *The Challenge of Pain*. London: Penguin.

Melzack, R and Wall, P (1988) *The Challenge of Pain*, 2nd edn. London: Penguin.

Melzack, R and Wall, P (1996) *The Challenge of Pain*, 3rd edn. London: Penguin.

O'Hara, P (1996) *Pain Management for Health Professionals*. London: Chapman & Hall.

Pasero, C *et al.* (1999) Pain in the elderly. In McCaffery, M and Pasero, C (eds) *Pain: Clinical Manual*, 2nd edn. St Louis, MO: Mosby.

Schofield, PA (2006a) Talking to older people in care homes: what are their perceptions of pain and their preferred management strategies? A pilot study. *British Journal of Nursing*, 509-514.

Schofield, PA (2006b) *International Journal of Disability and Human Development* **5**, 53-59.

Seers, K (1987) Pain, anxiety and recovery in patients undergoing surgery. Unpublished PhD thesis. London: University of London.

Thomas, V, Heath, M and Rose, F (1990) Effect of psychological variables and pain relief system on postoperative pain experience. *British Journal of Anaesthesia* **64**, 388-389.

Thomas, V, Heath, M, Rose, F and Flory, P (1995) Psychological characteristics and the effectiveness of patient controlled analgesia. *British Journal of Anaesthesia* **74**, 271-276.

Vale, A (1998) Fibromyalgia and pain. In: Carter, B (ed) *Perspectives on Pain: Mapping the Territory*. London: Arnold.

Walsh, M and Ford, P (1989) It can't hurt that much! *Nursing Times* **85**, 35-38.

Weis, O, Sriwatanakal, K, Alloza, J, Weintraub, M and Lasagna, L (1983) Attitudes of patients, housestaff and nurses towards postoperative analgesia care. *Anaesthetic Analgesia* **62**, 70-74.

Whipple, B (1990) Neurophysiology of pain. *Orthopaedic Nursing* **9**, 21-32.

Chapter 8
Pressure ulcers

Case Study

Mr Patel was a 70-year-old man with learning difficulties. He had lived until recently with his brother, who had helped care for him since their mother had died 10 years earlier. Mr Patel's brother had been taken ill and subsequently died. Mr Patel continued living in the home that he had shared with his brother. His GP visited every few months and was becoming concerned about Mr Patel's health. The GP contacted the district nursing service and asked them to visit. The district nurse found Mr Patel to be malnourished and fairly immobile. Mr Patel chose to sit in a chair all day, every day. The district nurses visited daily, as Mr Patel was incontinent and at risk of developing pressure ulcers. Mr Patel refused any help with washing and dressing, but he accepted help with meals from other members of his family.

Mr Patel became poorly and was taken into hospital. On admission, he was found to have septicaemia, which had developed as a consequence of pressure ulcers. Mr Patel did not respond to treatment and died.

Introduction

Consider the case study above. Why do you think this happened? The nurses and care workers failed Mr Patel. At the coroner's inquest held following Mr Patel's death, it was reported that Mr Patel had died through neglect and that the nurses had failed to protect Mr Patel from himself. He should have been treated earlier; if necessary, the nurses and other health professionals should have ensured this, even if it meant Mr Patel was detained temporally under the Mental Health Act. This case study demonstrates the importance of the prevention and treatment of pressure ulcers and the role of the nurse in this. In this chapter, we consider the care and prevention of pressure ulcers.

LEARNING OBJECTIVES

By the end of this chapter you will be able to:

1. Demonstrate an awareness of pressure ulcers
2. Identify the risk factors associated with the development of pressure ulcers
3. Understand the need for risk assessment and the use of scoring tools, and develop ways of integrating these into practice
4. Develop strategies to prevent pressure ulcers
5. Understand the different types of pressure-relieving equipment

Revision

Before reading this chapter, you need to revise the anatomy and physiology of the skin. Figure 8.1 shows the different layers of the skin.

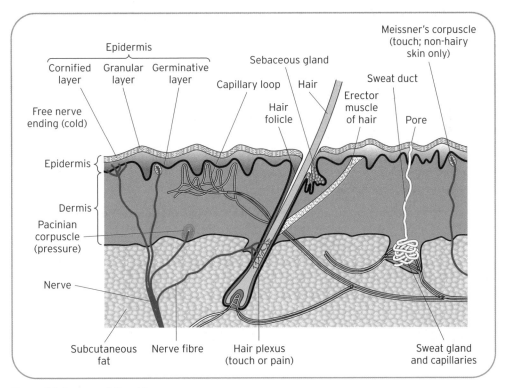

Figure 8.1 Layers of the skin
Source: Machean and Janes (1990)

Why study pressure ulcers?

Pressure ulcers can be prevented; if they do occur, they can be treated successfully. Britain has one of the highest prevalences of pressure ulcers in Europe (Hoban, 2004); it has been suggested that in certain care settings, in Britain nearly a third of residents have developed some type of skin damage due to the mismanagement of pressure area care (Bonomini, 2003). Therefore, it is very important that all health and social care workers know what a pressure ulcer is, how ulcers develop, how they can be prevented and how they can be treated. Nurses need to be able to determine patients who may be at high risk of developing ulcers and be able to understand why this is so.

There is a wide variation in practice with regard to pressure ulcer prevention, assessment and care, despite national guidelines being produced for the prevention and treatment of pressure ulcers (National Institute for Clinical Excellence, 2001). The *Essence of Care Toolkit for Clinical Practice Benchmarking* included a section on pressure ulcer prevention and care (Department of Health, 2003). It has been suggested that because pressure ulcer care has been placed within basic care rather than specialist care, it has lost its importance as a speciality (Hoban, 2004). However, as with all aspects of fundamental care, this is the care that underpins all nursing duties.

Pressure ulcers cause pain and discomfort, delay rehabilitation, and can lead to disability and even death (Grandis *et al.*, 2003). Nurses have a responsibility to know when to inspect the skin, what they are looking for, why they are doing this, what preventive measures can be taken, what equipment is available and what treatment can be given. The first step in prevention of pressure ulcers is to identify patients who may be at risk. The second is to implement measures that will reduce the likelihood of the person developing a pressure ulcer (Timby, 2005).

What is a pressure ulcer?

A pressure ulcer is an area of skin that has been damaged due to pressure. The *Essence of Care Toolkit* defines a pressure ulcer as follows:

> ... *identified damage to an individual's skin due to the effects of pressure together with, or independently from a number of other factors, for example; shearing, friction and moisture.*
> **(Department of Health, 2003)**

Pressure ulcers are usually caused by the patient sitting or lying down in one position for too long without moving. A pressure sore can develop in only a few hours. The ulcer appears initially as colour changes to the skin; the skin may be redder or darker than usual. If appropriate action is not taken at this stage, the area can develop into an open blister and then, if not treated, a deep hole in the flesh. Pressure ulcers are often grouped into four different stages, each stage indicating the amount of damage to the tissue. Early-stage pressure ulcers can and do develop into more serious ulcers if appropriate intervention is not made (Timby, 2005). The Stirling scale shown in Exhibit 8.1 identifies the four stages in pressure ulcer development.

Pressure ulcers are also known as bed sores, pressure sores and decubitus ulcers.

Stage 1: reddened area of skin

Stage 2: the area is red and blistered; a skin tear may be present, caused by shearing the skin against another surface such as a sheet

Stage 3: shallow skin crater, extending to subcutaneous tissue, which may be accompanied by leaking fluid (serous drainage)

Stage 4: deeply ulcerated area, extending to the muscle and sometimes exposing bone; this is potentially life-threatening due to the risk of the patient developing sepsis because of the presence of dead and infected tissue

Exhibit 8.1 Stirling scale: stages of pressure ulcer development

Cost of pressure ulcers

The costs associated with pressure ulcers can be divided into the cost to the patient and the cost to the treating organisation.

Cost to the patient

The pain, discomfort and loss of dignity caused by pressure ulcers are immeasurable. In Case study 4.6 in Chapter 4, Mr Brown was a fit and independent man before he developed pressure ulcers on his heels. These pressure ulcers affected his mobility (he was unable to drive until they were healed) and prevented him from following an activity that he enjoyed (dancing). His mental state was already fragile due to his recent bereavement, but his loss of independence and not being able to follow his hobby added to this. The combination of these factors hampered his recovery from surgery. For Mr Brown, the development of pressure ulcers had a detrimental effect on his health that could and should have been avoided. The cost of developing pressure sores for Mr Brown was extremely high.

Organisational cost

A study in 2004 found that the estimated cost in the UK of pressure ulcers was £1.4–2.1 billion, or 4% of the total NHS expenditure (Bennett *et al.*, 2004). It has been estimated that a third of hospital patients in the UK are at risk of developing pressure sores, and one in five patients already have a pressure ulcer (National Institute for Clinical Excellence, 2001). Once a pressure ulcer develops, it is expensive to treat: a stage 4 pressure ulcer (see Exhibit 8.1) can cost about £40 000 to heal.

To think about

Why do you think pressure sores occur?

Usually pressure sores occur because a person has a health requirement that needs to be taken into consideration or addressed.

> ## Recap Questions
>
> 1. Describe a pressure ulcer.
> 2. What are the four stages of pressure ulcer development?
> 3. What are the costs of pressure ulcers for the patient?

How and why pressure ulcers develop

> ## To think about
>
> Where are pressure ulcers likely to develop?

Pressure ulcers are most likely to develop on the parts of the body that take the weight of a person and where the bone is close to the surface. The areas most at risk are the following (Figure 8.2):

+ Back of the head
+ Ears
+ Shoulders
+ Elbows
+ Base of the spine
+ Bottom
+ Hips
+ Knees
+ Ankles
+ Heels

Consider Case study 8.1.

> ## Case Study 8.1
>
>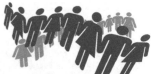
>
> Mr Red was 35 years old. He was admitted to a six-bedded unit on a general medical ward with an acute urinary tract infection, for which he was treated with antibiotics. He also was clinically depressed. Mr Red refused to leave his bed and lay on his side, facing the wall. Mr Red refused most treatment and drank and ate only minimal amounts. After a few days, Mr Red was found to have developed a pressure ulcer on the top of his left ear. This was extremely painful and added to Mr Red's general despondency.
>
> Why do you think this pressure ulcer occurred?
> What could have been done to prevent the ulcer from occurring?

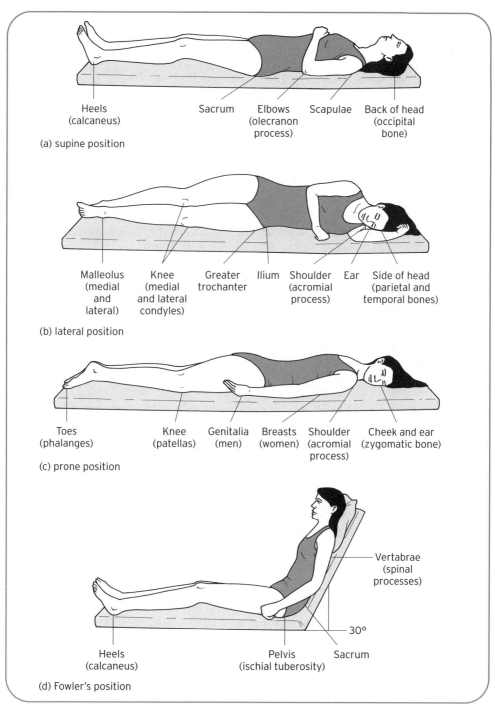

Figure 8.2 Areas of the body that are at risk of developing pressure sores

It was assumed wrongly by the staff on the ward that Mr Red, being a youngish man, would not be at risk of developing pressure sores. His depression and his placement on a six-bedded ward increased his risk of developing a pressure sore (he did not wish to communicate with other patients and therefore spent most of the time facing the wall), but these factors were not taken into account.

The development of pressure ulcers is dependent on many factors, which can be categorised as internal (intrinsic) and external (extrinsic). These factors influence why certain patients are more likely to develop pressure ulcers and how quickly ulcers may develop. Any patient plan needs to be centred on the correction or minimisation of intrinsic and extrinsic factors (Department of Health, 2003).

Intrinsic factors

Intrinsic factors are often related to immobility, age and illness. They include the following (Bonomini, 2003; Department of Health, 1994; Grandis *et al.*, 2003):

+ *Reduced mobility or immobility*: this is considered to be one of the most significant risk factors and, in the absence of other factors, is the primary cause of pressure ulcers

+ *Age*: people over the age of 65 years are at greater risk of developing pressure ulcers; this may be due to increased incidence of disease and changes in the elasticity of the skin in this age group. Young infants and children can also be at risk due to their skin still maturing and their head and body weight being disproportionate

+ *Illness*: for example:
  • Acute and chronic infections causing general debility and sometimes changes in levels of consciousness, thereby reducing the patient's awareness of the need to relieve pressure
  • Severe chronic illness, leading to multi-organ failure, poor **perfusion** and immobility
  • Vascular disease
  • Terminal illness

+ *Sensory impairment*: this results in reduced sensation and insensitivity to pain, therefore leading to a lack of stimulus to move or relieve pressure

+ *Neurological factors*: for example, paralysis

+ *Poor nutritional status*: malnutrition may increase the risk of developing ulcers and hampers the healing process

+ *Dehydration*: this causes a reduction in the skin's elasticity

+ *Body weight*: obese people may find it more difficult to move about, while very thin people have less fat over bony prominences and therefore the skin has less natural protection

+ *Anaesthesia*: this can cause **vasoconstriction**, shock and a lowering of blood pressure

Perfusion is the passage of fluid through an organ.
Vasoconstriction is constriction of the blood vessels.

Extrinsic factors

Extrinsic factors involved in the development of pressure ulcers include the following (Department of Health, 1994; Grandis, et al. 2003):

+ Pressure to areas of the body due to sitting or lying down
+ Friction due to the skin rubbing against another surface
+ Shearing (bones and tissues moving in opposite directions)
+ Inadequate support surfaces
+ Poor hygiene
+ Poor positioning
+ Poor moving and handling techniques
+ Prolonged sitting without adequate support
+ Medication, particularly steroids, anti-inflammatories and opiates
+ Moisture from sweating and incontinence

Who is most likely to get a pressure ulcer?

All patients are at risk of developing pressure ulcers, including children and young people. Therefore, all patients should be assessed for pressure ulcers. The NICE guidelines state that every patient, regardless of their age or condition, should use a pressure-relieving mattress (National Institute for Clinical Excellence, 2001). However, a person is more likely to get a pressure sore if any of the following apply:

+ Bed-bound
+ Wheelchair-bound
+ Spends long periods sitting in an armchair
+ Difficulty moving about
+ Elderly or weak
+ Serious illness
+ Problems with continence
+ Sensitivities due to other illnesses, such as diabetes, or following a stroke
+ Heart disorder and/or poor circulation
+ Not eating a balanced diet or drinking enough

Patients who cannot change position without help are at greatest risk of developing pressure ulcers. Patients who are less mentally aware, for example because of heavy sedation or due to a disorder such as Alzheimer's disease, are more prone to having problems with tissue viability. Consider Case study 8.2.

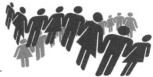

Case Study 8.2

Mrs Diane Forman was a 59-year-old woman with young-onset dementia. She had been diagnosed with dementia 6 months previously. Her progress through the disease had been very rapid, starting with short-term memory loss to her becoming aggressive. Mrs Forman was being cared for by her husband, but she had become reluctant to move. She spent the majority of her time in an armchair, despite being encouraged to walk. She was helped into bed each night, but after only a couple of hours in bed she would insist on getting up and return to the armchair.

Mr Forman was tired and distressed, and he was worried that Mrs Forman would develop pressure sores. Mr Forman contacted his GP, who asked the district nurses, community psychiatric nurse and social worker to visit. Together with Mr and Mrs Forman, the team was able to devise a package of care. Pressure-relieving equipment was delivered for Mrs Forman's chair and bed, and Mr Forman was given assistance to ensure that Mrs Forman was helped to reposition every few hours.

Fortunately, this problem was resolved, at least in the short term. The help and advice given to Mr and Mrs Forman, together with the pressure-relieving equipment, helped to avoid Mrs Forman developing pressure ulcers.

Recap Questions

1. Name five areas of the body where a person may develop pressure ulcers.
2. Who is likely to develop a pressure ulcer?
3. What factors influence the formation of a pressure ulcer?

Avoidance of pressure ulcers

Prevention is always better than cure. The best way to avoid a patient developing pressure ulcers is to ensure the person moves about, either alone or with help.

To think about

Consider some of the ways in which pressure ulcers can be avoided.

If the patient is unable to move alone, they should be helped to reposition. The benchmark of best practice for pressure ulcer prevention by repositioning is: 'the patient's need for repositioning has been assessed, documented, met and evaluated with evidence of ongoing assessment' (Department of Health, 2003). The need to assist a patient to reposition does not apply only to patients being cared for in bed; it also applies to patients in chairs, on emergency room trolleys, and in theatre undergoing or recovering from surgery. Appropriate equipment should always be used to avoid any damage to the patient or the carer as a result of repositioning (Department of Health, 2003). Moving and handling equipment needs to be available, and staff must be trained in how to use it. If hoists are used, the patient must be clear of the surface of the bed or chair, and the correct sling size must always be used (see Chapter 9). If a health professional is unsure how to use a certain piece of equipment, it is their responsibility to find out how to do so, either by working with a member of staff or carer who is familiar with the equipment or by contacting the manufacturer. All staff should attend regular moving and handling training.

People of all ages can develop pressure ulcers. Children are less likely than adults to develop pressure ulcers because they move about more and often recover quicker than adults following surgery; however, babies and children can and do develop pressure ulcers sometimes. Consider Case study 8.3.

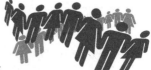

Case Study 8.3

Luke Grant was a 2-year-old boy with **acute lymphatic leukaemia**. The progression of the disease had been very quick and he was in the terminal stages. He was nursed in a children's ward. He was semi-conscious but appeared peaceful in his cot. Luke was not having any medication: whenever a nurse tried to give him any care, such as to tend to his hygiene needs, he screamed and became very distressed. Consequently, the nurses became reluctant to touch him.

How should the nurses care for Luke?

Luke needed nursing care. It was not appropriate for him to be left, however peaceful he appeared. If he was left uncared for, he could have developed pressure sores within a few hours. He was very poorly, reluctant to move, malnourished and incontinent. Luke should have been given regular pain relief.

Pressure ulcer care and prevention if the person is in bed

If the patient is in bed, repositioning them regularly is essential. All patients should use an appropriate pressure-relieving mattress, but it is important to note that the use of such a mattress does not remove the need to change the patient's position regularly. Manufacturers of pressure-relieving mattresses give recommendations for how long a patient can be left in the same position on a particular product. Consider Case study 8.4.

Acute lymphatic leukaemia is a malignant disease of the bone marrow.

> ## Case Study 8.4
>
> Nicola Mullin was 12 years old. She had recently had glandular fever and had appeared to make a good recovery. However, she then became increasingly lethargic, was eating very little and was spending more and more time in bed. She was diagnosed with chronic fatigue syndrome, or **ME**. She was nursed at home, and her family were given support from the children's district nursing team. Nicola was given an airflow mattress and an airflow cushion for her chair following assessment of her skin and calculation of her risk of developing pressure ulcers. Nicola was able to sit for short periods at first, and then for longer as her condition improved. She was encouraged to drink plenty of fluids. Following a full nutritional assessment, her diet was supplemented with high-protein and high-carbohydrate drinks. Despite being in this debilitated state for 5 months, she did not develop any pressure ulcers. This was due to her expert nursing care, the full assessment of her skin and the use of pressure-relieving equipment.

As demonstrated in Case study 8.4, the patient's position must be changed regularly, alternating between their back and sides. The 30-degree tilt should be used (Figure 8.3). Research has shown that if patients are nursed in bed at this angle, they can be moved less often – up to every 3 hours rather than every 2 hours – and they are less likely to develop skin damage than if they lie flat on bony prominences such as hips, sacrum or heels (Bonomini, 2003). Care should be taken not to drag the patient's skin along other surfaces such as bedsheets. Some people use pillows to position knees and ankles so that they are not touching. The use of a duvet rather than a heavy blanket can relieve pressure on the patient's legs, making it easier for the patient to move. A bed cradle or similar device is useful for keeping the weight of the bedclothes off the patient. Bedsheets made from synthetic materials should be avoided because they have a tendency to make the skin hot and sticky. Bedsheets should be changed regularly, especially if the patient sweats a lot. Special care should be taken to avoid creases in the bedclothes and crumbs in the bed.

The use of pressure-relieving equipment is essential. All patients confined to bed for longer than usual and patients who are unwell must have a skin risk assessment carried out and the appropriate pressure-relieving equipment used.

Pressure ulcer care and prevention if the person is in a wheelchair or armchair

Sitting in a chair for long periods can precipitate the development of pressure sores (Bonomini, 2003). The NICE guidelines do not specify which type of pressure-relieving equipment/cushion is recommended for patients sitting for long periods, as research has shown that no type of cushion outperforms another. Bonomini (2003) suggests that the type of chair rather than the type of cushion is of more significance. The chair should allow a 90-degree angle at the knees, be wide enough for the person, and be designed so that the spine,

ME, short for myalgic encephalomyelitis, is a disease that causes extreme tiredness and depression.

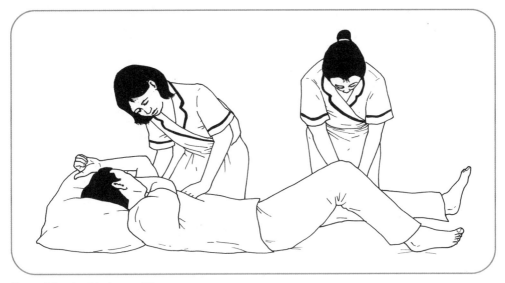

Figure 8.3 The 30-degree tilt

shoulders and head are supported. It is important that a qualified practitioner such as an occupational therapist or physiotherapist assesses the patient and their chairs (National Institute of Clinical Excellence, 2001).

If possible, the patient should be encouraged to relieve the pressure on their buttocks every 15 minutes or so by leaning forward and pushing up on the arms of the chair. Or they can roll from cheek to cheek for a short while. Assistance should be given to enable seated patients to stand when possible.

Recap Questions

1. What is meant by repositioning, and why is it important?
2. What is a 30-degree tilt?
3. Can people develop pressure ulcers sitting in a chair?

Screening and assessing the possibility of skin damage due to pressure

As we have already discussed, the cost of pressure ulcers to both the patient and the treating organisation is huge. Therefore, all patients must be assessed for their likelihood of developing pressure ulcers. Screening should be undertaken when the patient is first assessed, so that the nurse can develop a plan of care to prevent or treat any skin damage. The nurse initially screens the patient by identifying any risk factors that may be present; this screening process leads to a more detailed assessment, and the plan of care can then take into account and, where possible, minimise relevant factors. Screening involves identifying patients who may already have or are at risk of developing a pressure ulcer. The nurse who makes this initial screening must have sufficient knowledge of what a pressure ulcer is and why an ulcer may develop in order to make the necessary clinical judgement.

Scoring tools used in the risk assessment of pressure ulcers

Patients identified as high risk for pressure ulcers require a further, more comprehensive assessment. This is a formal and systematic process in which a range of specific methods and tools are used. The Norton scale (Table 8.1) is a scoring tool that assesses a patient's level of risk of developing a pressure ulcer. The Norton Scale was one of the first of its type; it was developed in the 1960s following research into problems that had arisen when nursing older people. The Norton Scale has been hugely influential in the development of later scoring tools that are still used today (Grandis *et al.*, 2003). The Waterlow score (Figure 8.4) was developed later and has been used extensively in hospital and community settings.

Table 8.1 Norton scale Score

Physical condition	Score	Mental condition	Score	Activity	Score	Mobility	Score	Incontinent	Score
Good	4	Alert	4	Ambulant	4	Full	4	Not	4
Fair	3	Apathetic	3	Walk/help limited	3	Slightly	3	Occasionally	3
Poor	2	Confused	2	Chairbound limited	2	Very urine	2	Usually/	2
Very bad	1	Stuporous	1	Bedfast	1	Immobile	1	Doubly	1

It is crucial that the nurse also uses clinical judgement when using any of the scoring tools. Research has shown that screening tools are effective only when they are used as part of a more comprehensive assessment; they are not adequate to be used alone.

> ## To think about
>
> What would you do if you thought a patient needed pressure-relieving equipment?

It is important that you act quickly. You could approach the team leader and ask for an assessment to be made. Consider Case study 8.5.

WATERLOW PRESSURE SORE PREVENTION/TREATMENT POLICY
RING SCORES IN TABLE, ADD TOTAL. SEVERAL SCORES PER CATEGORY CAN BE USED

BUILD/WEIGHT FOR HEIGHT	★	SKIN TYPE VISUAL RISK AREAS	★	SEX AGE	★	SPECIAL RISKS TISSUE MALNUTRITION	★
AVERAGE	0	HEALTHY	0	MALE	1	e.g. TERMINAL CACHEXIA	8
ABOVE AVERAGE	1	TISSUE PAPER	1	FEMALE	2	CARDIAC FAILURE	5
OBESE	2	DRY	1	14 - 49	1	PERIPHERAL VASCULAR DISEASE	5
BELOW AVERAGE	3	ODEMATOUS	1	50 - 64	2	ANAEMIA	2
		CLAMMY (TEMP)	1	65 - 74	3	SMOKING	1
		DISCOLOURED	2	75 - 80	4		
		BROKEN/SPOT	3	81+	5		

CONTINENCE	★	MOBILITY	★	APPETITE	★	NEUROLOGICAL DEFICIT	★
COMPLETE/CATHETERISED	0	FULLY	0	AVERAGE	0	e.g. DIABETES, M.S, CVA	4-6
OCCASION INCONT	1	RESTLESS/FIDGETY	1	POOR	1	MOTORSENSORY	4-6
CATH/INCONTINENT OF FAECES	2	APATHETIC	2	N.G. TUBE/FLUIDS ONLY	2	PARAPLEGIA	4-6
DOUBLY INCONT	3	RETRICTED	3	NBM/ANOREXIC	3		
		INERT/TRACTION	4			**MAJOR SURGERY/TRAUMA**	★
		CHAIRBOUND	5			ORTHOPAEDIC BELOW WAIST SPINAL	5
						ON TABLE > 2 HOURS	5

MEDICATION	★
CYTOTOXICS, HIGH DOSE STEROIDS, ANTI-INFLAMMATORY	4

SCORE	10+ AT RISK	13+ HIGH RISK	20+ VERY HIGH RISK

Figure 8.4 The Waterlow score (a)

247

REMEMBER TISSUE DAMAGE OFTEN STARTS PRIOR TO ADMISSION, IN CASUALTY, A SEATED PATIENT IS ALSO AT RISK

ASSESSMENT: (See Over)   IF THE PATIENT FALLS INTO ANY OF THE RISK CATEGORIES THEN PREVENTATIVE NURSING IS REQUIRED. A COMBINATION OF GOOD NURSING TECHNIQUES AND PREVENTATIVE AIDS WILL DEFINITELY BE NECESSARY.

WOUND CLASSIFICATION
Stirling Pressure Sore Severity Scale (SPSSS)
Stage 0 - No clinical evidence of a pressure sore.
S.1 - Healed with scarring.
S.2 - Tissue drainage not assessed as a pressure sore. (a) see below

Stage 1 - Discolouration of intact skin.
1.1 - Non blanchable erytherons with increased local heat.
1.2 - Blue/purple/black discolouration – The sore is at least Stage 1 (a or b).

Stage 2 – Partial-thickness skin loss or damage.
2.1 Blister   2.2 Abrasion
2.3 Shallow ulcer, no undermining or adjacent tissue.
2.4 Any of these with underlying blue/purple/black discolouration or induration.
The sore is at least Stage 2 (a, b or c+d for 2.3, e for 2.4)

Stage 3 – Full thickness skin loss involving damage/necrosis of sub-cutaneous tissue, not extending to underlying bone, tendons or joint capsule.
3.1 – Crater, without undermining of adjacent tissue.
3.2 – Crater, with undermining of adjacent tissue.
3.3 – Sinus, the full extent of which is uncertain
3.4 – Necrotic tissue marking full extent of damage.
The sore is at least Stage 3 (b, +/- e, f, g, +h for 3.4)

Stage 4 – Full thickness loss with extensive destruction and tissue necrosis extending to underlying bone, tendons or capsule.
4.1 Visible exposure of bone tendon or capsule.
4.2 Sinus assessed as extending to same (b+/-e, f, g, h, i).

Guide to types of Dressings/Treatment
a. Semi-permeable   f. Alginate rope/ribbon
b. Hydrocolloid   g. Foam cavity filler
c. Foam dressing   h. Enzymetric debridement
d. Alginate   i. Surgical debridement
e. Hydrogel

PREVENTION:
PREVENTATIVE AIDS:
Special Mattress/
Bed:
10+ Overlays or specialist foam matTresses
15+ Alternating pressure overlays, matresses and bed systems.
20+ Bed Systems: Fluidfeed, bead, low air loss and alternating pressure mattresses.
Note: Preventative aids cover a wide spectrum of specialist features. Efficacy should be judged, if possible, on the beds of independent evidence.

Cushions:
No patient should sit in a wheelchair without some form of cushioning. If nothing else is available – use the patient's own pillow.
10+ 4" Foam cushion.
15+ Specialist Gel and/or foam cushion
20+ Cushion capable of adjustment to suit individual patient.

Bed Clothing:
Avoid plastic draw sheets, isco pads and tightly tucked in sheets/sheet covers, especially when using specialist bed and mattress overlay systems.
Use Duvet - plus vapour permeable cover

NURSING CARE
General: Frequent changes of position, lying/sitting. Use of pillows.
Pain   Appropriate pain control.
Nutrition   High protein, vitamins, minerals
Patient Handling: Correct lifting techniques – Hoists – Monkey Pole – Transfer Devices

Patient Comfort Aids: Real sheepskins – Bed Cradle.
Operating Table: 4' cover plus adequate protection.
Theatre/A&E Trolley
Skin Care: General Hygiene, NO rubbing, cover with an appropriate dressing.

IF TREATMENT IS REQUIRED, FIRST REMOVE PRESSURE

Figure 8.4 The Waterlow score (b)

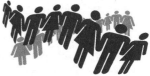

Case Study 8.5

Mrs Carter was a 72-year-old woman with acute myoblastic leukaemia; she was in the end stages of the disease. She had been nursed at home by her husband, with assistance from other family members and the district nursing service. The district nursing sister assessed Mrs Carter's vulnerability to pressure ulcers using the Waterlow scoring tool. The score indicated that Mrs Carter should have a foam mattress, designed for use in patients with minimal vulnerability to developing pressure ulcers. The nurse did not take into account the nature of Mrs Carter's disease; this type of leukaemia is rare and many health professionals do not fully understand its implications. As a result of the disease, Mrs Carter's white and red blood cell counts were very low. This meant that she was severely anaemic and prone to infection and had hardly any clotting ability. If Mrs Carter developed any broken skin areas, she could have developed an acute infection or bled to death.

The nurse failed her patient. She did not take into account the nature of Mrs Carter's disease when using the scoring tool to assess which pressure-relieving equipment should be used. Although this was a rare type of leukaemia, Mrs Carter was being treated by a specialist hospital team and GP, and the nurse could have found out more about the possible consequences of the disease. The nurse should have used the Waterlow scoring tool as only part of the assessment and then used her clinical knowledge to make decisions when treating and caring for her patient.

There is debate over the effectiveness of these tools in children. Research has concluded that it is more effective to use a tool that has been designed specifically for children, such as the Glamorgan paediatric pressure ulcer risk assessment scale (Wilcock, 2007); the researchers concluded that this tool was able to predict a child's risk of developing a pressure ulcer more accurately than a scale that had been designed specifically for use in adults.

Any assessment must take into account the patient's age, nutritional status, circulatory status, mobility, dependence level and mental awareness (Grandis *et al.*, 2003). An holistic individual assessment of the patient should be made, taking into account all the factors that may influence the patient's vulnerability to developing pressure ulcers. The scoring tools can play a vital part in pressure ulcer prevention by directing the healthcare worker in their choice of pressure-relieving equipment; for example, a high Waterlow score indicates that the patient requires an alternating-pressure mattress such as an airflow one.

Pressure ulcers are caused by a combination of intrinsic and extrinsic factors, and all of these influence a person's tissue tolerance (Bonomini, 2003). Any decisions made regarding pressure-relieving devices should always be made following an in-depth assessment that includes the patient's risk factors, comfort and general state of health. This assessment needs to be ongoing and carry the option to change the pressure-relieving device if the patient's condition alters (Bonomini, 2003). This was not done for Mrs Carter in Case study 8.5; the nurse did not use the risk assessment scale properly and failed to take into account all of the patient's risk factors.

The benchmark of best practice for the clinical benchmark for pressure ulcers in the *Essence of Care Toolkit* is: 'For all patients identified as "at risk" screening progresses to further assessment' (Department of Health, 2003). The Toolkit recommends that an assessment tool is used. It is important that the components of the screening assessment are adequate.

Scoring tools are constantly being developed and improved; the health professional should ensure that they are aware of these developments, that their knowledge is current and that they use evidence-based practice at all times. The Toolkit stresses that the screening assessment should be clearly recorded, and that the staff involved understand what they are assessing and why they are making the assessment.

The need for re-assessment is important. Again, the healthcare worker needs to know when this is required. Re-assessment should be carried out in response to changes in the individual's physical or mental condition (Bonomini, 2003) and not in a ritualistic manner.

The assessor should have the specific knowledge and expertise to enable them to undertake the assessment in an appropriate way. Therefore, ongoing education and training of the assessor is vital. Many organisations have access to specially trained tissue viability teams who give advice and training to practitioners and carers. The registered practitioner is ultimately accountable for assessing and screening the patient, although other health and social care workers can be trained to become competent to assess. The assessor must consider the impact of intrinsic and extrinsic factors, which influence the development of pressure ulcers, in those people they consider to be at risk and must know what choices to make in order to ensure that the individual receives the appropriate advice and treatment.

Plan of care

Each person assessed should have an individualised plan for the prevention and treatment of pressure ulcers. The benchmark for best practice is that there this individualised plan is documented and agreed by the multidisciplinary team working in partnership with the patient and/or carers with evidence of re-assessment. All treatments, interventions, goals and targets should be negotiated and agreed, and underpinned with best practice evidence. All plans need to be reviewed and evaluated at regular intervals (Department of Health, 2003).

Skin inspection

Skin should be checked for signs of damage. How often this is done depends on the patient's condition and influencing factors. Skin inspection may need to be undertaken several times a day (Grandis *et al.*, 2003).

To think about

What should you be looking for when inspecting a person's skin?

+ Look out for discoloured skin, especially red, purple or blue areas, and for skin that does not return to its normal colour after weight has been taken off it
+ Localised heat
+ Hardness of the area (induration)
+ Swelling
+ Persistent redness on light-coloured skin

Patients can be taught to inspect their own skin for signs of ulcers. For areas that are hard to see, a mirror can be used. The patient should be given information in a format that meets their particular needs about the causes, prevention and treatment of pressure ulcers. The patient should be discouraged from lying or sitting on skin that is redder or darker than usual and to wait until the skin has returned to its normal colour. All findings from skin inspections should be documented clearly – including if the skin is found to be intact (Hoban, 2004).

Skin care

The following points regarding skin care should be remembered:

+ Keep skin clean and dry
+ Limit the use of perfumed soap
+ Avoid the use of talcum powder, because this soaks up the skin's natural oils and dries it out
+ Avoid rubbing or massaging skin too hard, especially over the bony parts of the body
+ Pat skin dry with a soft towel
+ Moisturise dry areas with an aqueous cream
+ Small amounts of a barrier cream, such as zinc and castor oil, may be applied
+ If the patient is incontinent, the skin should be kept as clean and dry as possible
+ The patient should be encouraged to eat a healthy diet and drink plenty of fluids, and expert advice sought from a dietician or pharmacist

Pressure-relieving equipment

Two main types of equipment are used to help relieve pressure: static overlays and mattresses that alternate pressure, usually by way of air (Grandis *et al.*, 2003). The static devices that are available include high-specification foam mattresses and gel-filled mattresses. It is important for the carer and the patient to be familiar with the equipment being used and to be aware of what other equipment is available. Any equipment used needs to be installed correctly and checked regularly. The time and date such equipment is used for each patient should be documented (Hoban, 2004). To prevent cross-infection, pressure-relieving equipment must be cleaned effectively; equipment manufacturers give cleaning instructions, and advice can be sought from an infection control team.

If the patient requires an alternating-pressure mattress for their bed, they will also require an alternating-pressure cushion for their chair.

Pressure-relieving equipment is defined in the *Essence of Care Toolkit* as equipment that redistributes pressure and assists in spreading the patient's body weight in order to minimise the effects of pressure (Department of Health, 2003). The benchmark of best practice for this is: 'patients at risk of developing pressure ulcers are cared for on pressure redistributing support surfaces that meet individual needs, including comfort' (Department of Health, 2003). Meeting this benchmark can present something of a challenge, as patients do not always want to use pressure-relieving equipment, for various reasons. The noise generated by airflow mattresses can be very disturbing, while overlay mattresses add considerable height to a bed – unless the bed can then be lowered, the patient may find it difficult or even impossible to get in and out of bed unaided, leading to loss of independence and in some cases incontinence.

1. Why should patients be screened for pressure ulcer development?
2. What tools can be used to assess the risk of developing pressure ulcers?
3. Why is ongoing assessment important?

Pressure ulcer healing

A pressure ulcer is a wound – defined as an injury to the body that involves a break to the tissues or body structures (Norris *et al.*, 1998). Wounds are classified into four categories:

✛ Contusions (bruising)

✛ Abrasions (grazes)

✛ Lacerations (tears)

✛ Incisions (cuts)

Pressure ulcers are generally considered as abrasions and lacerations.

Some pressure ulcers take months to heal. NICE classes pressure ulcers as chronic wounds because they tend to heal slowly, unlike clean surgical wounds, which heal quickly. Wound healing can be divided into four stages (British National Formulary, 2006; Grandis *et al.*, 2003), as shown in Exhibit 8.2.

Stage 1: Inflammatory process where cells are released to help clot formation

Stage 2: Granulation

Stage 3: Epithelialisation

Stage 4: Remodelling/maturation – this stage can take anything from a few days to a few years, depending on the severity of the ulcer. Blood cell activity decreases, collagen fibres form and mature and the appearance of granulation tissue changes from red to white, this new tissue is scar tissue

Exhibit 8.2 Wound healing process
Source: Grandis *et al.* (2003)

If a pressure ulcer occurs, it should be treated as any other wound would be. The ulcer should be assessed, measured and recorded accurately. Some practitioners photograph the area, with the patient's permission. Pressure ulcers need to be examined carefully so that the extent and depth of tissue damage can be assessed. A transparent grid can be used to measure the ulcer accurately.

A number of dressings are available both to protect the skin from developing pressure ulcers and to aid healing of pressure ulcers. The purpose of the dressing is to keep the wound moist, free from infection, free from toxic chemicals, particles and fibres, and at an optimum temperature in order to promote healing.

The type of dressing used depends on the type of ulcer, the amount of damage and the stage within the healing process. The dressings are prescribed by a nurse or doctor, often following advice from a specialist tissue viability nurse. Manufacturers can supply healthcare workers with information and recent research papers on the effectiveness of their dressings.

Like any other wound, pressure ulcers should be dressed following an aseptic technique. Regular inspection and assessment are then continued throughout the healing process, and the wound is managed accordingly. If the ulcer shows signs of infection (red, painful, foul-smelling discharge), the nurse must report this to an advanced prescriber (doctor or nurse) so the patient can receive antibiotic treatment.

Recap Questions

1. What should the nurse do if they think the patient has developed a pressure ulcer?
2. What are the signs of infection in a pressure ulcer?
3. What are the stages of healing?

Summary

The cost of pressure ulcers is very high, and therefore it is essential that steps are taken to prevent pressure ulcers occurring. A pressure ulcer can develop into a chronic wound that is difficult and lengthy to heal. Preventing the development of pressure ulcers is essential and specialised work, and the patient depends on the nurse to be an expert in this field.

The nurse has an important role to play in educating the patient and their family and care-givers in all aspects of skin care (Grandis *et al.*, 2003). It is the nurse's responsibility to keep up to date, be knowledgeable and use evidence to support their practice. The nurse should understand what a pressure ulcer is, and how pressure ulcers can be assessed, prevented and treated. Interdisciplinary assessment gives a coordinated approach to pressure ulcer care and prevention.

It is important to note that pressure ulcers are unlikely to heal unless pressure is removed. It is essential to the healing process that as many of the predisposing problems that caused the ulcer are removed (Grandis *et al.*, 2003). Poor moving and handling of patients plays a major part in the development of pressure ulcers; therefore, adequate training in this and in positioning the patient is essential for all healthcare workers. Manual handling devices should be used appropriately.

Patients of any age can develop pressure ulcers. Timely and expert care should always be given, with special attention paid to identifying risk, so that pressure ulcers can be avoided. This is especially important with older people, because they tend to have a slower wound healing abil-ity. Regeneration of healthy skin can take twice as long in an 80-year-old than in a 30-year-old, due to diminished blood supply, collagen and skin elasticity. With age, the skin becomes thinner, and this can be heightened by drug therapy such as steroids and long-term exposure to ultravio-let rays; this puts the person at risk of shearing injuries. Older patients are also more likely to have a condition such as diabetes that impairs the circulation and nervous system, therefore reducing touch sensation so that the person is not aware of skin damage (Timby, 2005).

There are many tools available to help identify patients at risk of developing a pressure ulcer. The choice of tool depends on the age of the patient and local preferences. When using any scoring tool, it is important to remember that the tool is only part of the screening and assessment process. Such tools are useful as aide-memoirs and to alert the assessor to cer-tain issues, but it is argued that some of the tools are not evidence-based.

> ## Key Points
>
> 1. People of all ages can be at risk of developing pressure ulcers.
> 2. Appropriate assessment of the patient's skin and general health and the use of risk assessment tools or scales are essential components of pressure ulcer prevention and care.
> 3. Assessment tools are useful but have limitations, and they should form only part of a more comprehensive and holistic assessment.
> 4. The use of appropriate equipment is essential in the prevention and treatment of pressure ulcers.

Points for debate

Now that you have come to the end of this chapter here are a few points that you may wish to think about when you are in practice. You may wish to discuss these with your work colleagues or fellow students.

Children do not develop pressure ulcers.

People develop pressure ulcers because they do not or cannot move about.

> ## Links to Other Chapters
>
> Chapter 4 Hygiene
> Chapter 5 Nutrition
> Chapter 6 Fluid balance and continence care

Further reading

Royal College of Nursing (2001) *Pressure Ulcer Risk Assessment and Prevention Recommendations*. London: Royal College of Nursing.

Royal College of Nursing (2004) *The Use of Pressure-Relieving Devices (Beds, Mattresses and Overlays) for the Prevention of Pressure Ulcers in Primary and Secondary Care*. London: Royal College of Nursing.

Royal College of Nursing (2005) *Management of Pressure Ulcers in Primary and Secondary Care*. London: Royal College of Nursing.

References

Bennett, G, Dealey, C and Posnett, J (2004) The cost of pressure ulcers in the UK. *Age and Aging* **33**, 230–235.

Bonomini, J (2003) Effective interventions for pressure ulcer prevention. *Nursing Standard* **17**, 45–50.

British National Formulary (2006) *British National Formulary*. London: British Medical Association and Royal Pharmaceutical Society of Great Britain.

Department of Health (1994) *Your Guide to Pressure Sores*. London: The Stationery Office.

Department of Health (2003) *Essence of Care*. London: The Stationery Office.

Grandis, S, Long, G, Glasper, A and Jackson, P (2003) *Foundation Studies for Nursing*. Basingstoke: Palgrave Macmillan.

Hoban, V. (2004) Updating practice in pressure area care. *Nursing Times* **14**, 23-24.

National Institute for Clinical Excellence (2001) *Pressure Ulcer Risk Assessment and Prevention*. London: National Institute for Clinical Excellence.

Norris, C, Freshwater, D and Maslin-Prothero, S (eds) (1998) *Blackwell's Nursing Dictionary*. Oxford: Blackwell Science.

Timby, B (2005) *Fundamental Nursing Skills and Concepts*, 8th edn. Philadelphia, PA: Lippincott Williams & Wilkins.

Wilcock, J (2007) A risk assessment scale for pressure ulcers in children. *Nursing Times* **103**, 14.

Chapter 9
Rehabilitation and self-care

> ## Case Study
>
> Mr Cooper awoke with a severe pain in the left side of his head. At first he could not think where he was. He felt confused and frightened. The place seemed unfamiliar and his head hurt. He gradually became aware of a woman's voice and realised it was one he knew. He tried to move but found this difficult: only part of him would move, and his right arm and leg felt very heavy. He tried to talk but he could not say what he wanted: words came out of his mouth wrongly and in the wrong order. He was vaguely aware of his wife talking on the phone. Mr Cooper felt afraid.
>
> The next thing he remembered was waking up in hospital. A nurse came to see him and explained what had happened. She told him that over the next few days other clinicians would be coming to see him to find out what had happened and to assess the extent of any damage. The clinicians involved included doctors, nurses, occupational therapists, physiotherapists, speech and language therapists and dieticians. Later the clinicians met with Mr Cooper and his wife, and together they devised a plan of action that would help Mr Cooper to regain the use of the affected parts of his body. Mr Cooper was helped so he could follow the plan of action. Gradually he regained his independence and was ready to return home. Mr Cooper was relieved to find out that the rehabilitation programme was to be continued when he left hospital. This programme was likely to take several months.

Introduction

It is likely that Mr Cooper had suffered a **stroke**. He needed an extensive treatment programme because of the amount of damage caused by the stroke. It was important that his swallowing reflex was assessed as soon as possible to see whether he could swallow fluids without the risk of choking; this assessment is usually undertaken by a speech and language therapist or a nurse who has been specially trained in **dysphagia** awareness. His speech was affected, and so he needed treatment from the speech and language therapist. The physiotherapist assessed Mr Cooper's ability to walk and sit. The occupational therapist assessed his ability to undertake everyday activities, such as washing and dressing, and whether he needed specially adapted cutlery and crockery for eating and drinking or any other types of equipment. The dietician advised on appropriate meals and whether these were to be prepared in liquid form or semi-formed. The nurses were responsible for all care of Mr Cooper, including his physical, emotional, spiritual and cultural needs. They also assisted and encouraged him to achieve the goals set for him. The nurses were also responsible for continually assessing, monitoring and evaluating Mr Cooper's progress. This programme of rehabilitation was continued when Mr Cooper returned home, so he still had the support of many health and social care professionals, such as his GP, domiciliary physiotherapist and occupational therapist, district nursing service, social workers and rehabilitation support workers.

In this chapter we explore the underlying principles of rehabilitation, and what is meant by disability, independence and self-care. We look at a framework for rehabilitation nursing, teamworking and patient participation. We consider the services and equipment that are available and the impact of the patient's environment on their rehabilitation.

LEARNING OBJECTIVES

By the end of this chapter you will be able to:

1. Recognise the importance of promoting rehabilitation and self-care
2. Explore issues of rehabilitation in the context of practice
3. Identify the roles of the nurse and other health professionals and explore the value of interdisciplinary work
4. Discuss involving patients and carers in planning and evaluating care/treatment programmes
5. Explore physical, emotional and spiritual aspects of rehabilitation
6. Identify aids and equipment to be used in the rehabilitation setting

What is rehabilitation?

To think about

Before reading the next section, think about what rehabilitation means to you. Make some notes of what would be important to you if you lost the use of your dominant arm. What help would you need? Try to go about your normal business for an hour without using your dominant arm.

A **stroke**, also known as a cerebral vascular accident (CVA) or cerebral vascular event, results from a blood clot or bleeding into part of the brain.

Dysphagia is difficulty in swallowing.

How did this feel? What difficulties did you encounter? Think about the emotions you experienced: were you frustrated or angry? Did you have to ask for help from someone else? Rehabilitation is a way of helping a patient to manage a disability or impairment. Rehabilitation is about maximising the individual's potential for independence. It is an educational, problem-solving process aimed at reducing disability and handicap, so that the person can cope with all aspects of their daily life (Barnes and Ward, 2005). It is a process that aims to restore personal autonomy in those aspects of everyday living that are considered to be the most relevant by the individual patient or service user concerned. In addition to the patient's needs, those of the family and carer also require some consideration (Sinclair and Dickinson, 1998).

Purpose of rehabilitation

Rehabilitation can be seen as having three main purposes:

+ To enhance and maintain the patient's quality of life by reducing disability; this is an ongoing process that may take place over many years

+ To restore physical, psychological and social functioning to the patient through the promotion of independence to a level that is acceptable to that person, which in turn gives the person empowerment. The person is encouraged to take part in making decisions that concern their treatment programme

+ To prevent further disease and illness

The ultimate aim of rehabilitation is to maximise the person's wellbeing and enable the person to cope with changes in life circumstances. Rehabilitation ensures that problems are solved effectively and in a timely manner. Rehabilitation is always patient-centred, such that the individual is at the centre of their care/treatment programme and all decisions are made to suit the individual. These decisions take into account the person's spiritual, emotional, physical, mental and cultural wellbeing. Rehabilitation is often a long journey that involves the patient and health and social care personnel working together.

Key factors of rehabilitation

It is essential that all people who need rehabilitation are able to access it, regardless of their age or disability (Department of Health, 2001a). However, in reality, financial cost will always have a bearing on what services are available. The patient's needs must be taken into account when planning, implementing and evaluating the care/treatment programme; the nurse has an important role in making sure this happens. For some patients, rehabilitation involves major changes to their everyday life. Sometimes, rehabilitation involves learning completely new skills, or relearning basic skills such as tying shoelaces. Rehabilitation may involve adapting to a new way of life or a new environment; this may require the person to develop a different set of physical, practical and emotional skills. Emotional support for the patient is crucial to the success of the rehabilitation programme, but this is often overlooked or considered only from a superficial point of view. Peer support is also an invaluable component of emotional rehabilitation.

As we saw in the case study of Mr Cooper, one of the key factors of a successful rehabilitation programme is for clinicians to work together to plan the patient's treatment and care. This programme must always be planned in full consultation with the patient so that the rehabilitation team can find out what is important to the patient and then identify how the patient's goals can be met. The first step is to assess the patient's ability; this should be done throughout every stage of treatment or care. It is important that the person is able to make informed decisions. The aim of any rehabilitation programme is to help the patient regain some control of part of their life, although this may not always be at the level they once had. It is imperative that the patient is allowed to take risks; much work needs to centre on both enabling the patient to take informed risks and encouraging the patient's informal and formal carers to agree with the patient on an acceptable level of risk. Support for the patient is essential throughout this time. Regular meetings are required so that the programme can be evaluated.

To think about

What skills do you use everyday?

We use a variety of basic skills everyday to dress ourselves, keep ourselves clean, prepare and eat food, and go to the toilet when we need to. We often take these tasks for granted.

What is disability?

The Disability Discrimination Act 1995 defines disability as follows:

A person has a disability if he has a physical or mental impairment which has a substantial and long-term adverse effect on his ability to carry out normal day-to-day activities. **(Department of Health, 1995)**

The Act states that the term 'disabled person' means a person with impairment. However, below are some definitions that have been devised by people with disabilities:

Impairment is the loss or limitation of physical, mental or sensory function on a long-term and permanent basis.

Disablement is the loss or limitation of physical, mental or sensory function on a long-term and permanent basis.

To understand disability, we need to look much further than the label and the medical facts. Consider the following two models of disability:

+ *Medical model of disability*: this model considers disability as an illness (Figure 9.1). The disabled person is one who needs to be cured so that they can fit into 'normal' society. The emphasis is on the impairment or condition rather than the person. The medical model looks at what is wrong with the person and searches for ways to fix it. With this model, the professionals working in the field of disability are perceived as being the experts. This has led to such professionals having control over people with disabilities, which may result in disabled people feeling that they are disempowered and segregated from society.

+ *Social model of disability*: this model was created by people with disabilities (Figure 9.2). The social model looks at the person's life experiences rather than focusing on the person's impairments. The model sees solutions to the person's problems, such as barriers created by society, lack of access, lack of understanding, lack of awareness and oppressive behaviours. The social model stresses that support to enable people to take part in society should be given as a right and not as a favour. The social model focuses on the person rather than the condition or disability.

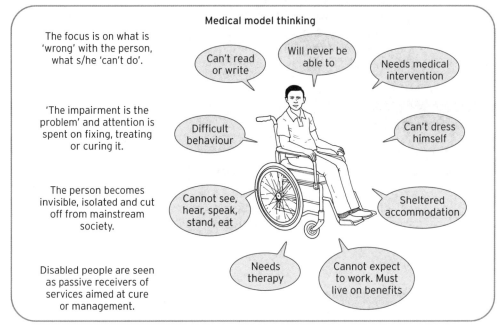

Figure 9.1 Medical model of disability
Source: Commission of Equality and Human Rights

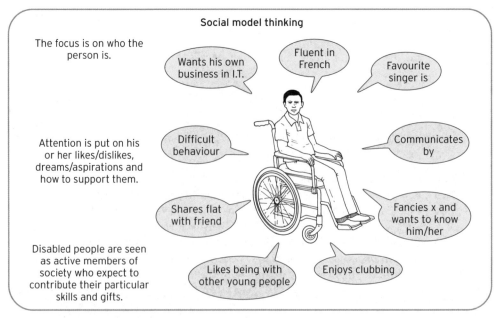

Figure 9.2 Social model of disability
Source: Commission of Equality and Human Rights

These two models have very different approaches. Traditionally, healthcare professionals have worked more towards the medical model approach, but they are now much more likely to use both models and therefore take a more holistic approach to rehabilitation.

History of rehabilitation

Rehabilitation emerged as a specialty during and following the First World War, when thousands of men returned from the war with impairments. Segregated institutions were set up to provide rehabilitation, care, housing and employment. During the Second World War, the 1944 Disabled Employment Act was passed, with an emphasis on employment provision for disabled people. Traditionally, rehabilitation has been led by therapists (predominant physiotherapists and occupational therapists), with nurses having a lesser role and providing care rather than promoting independence. However, more recently, the nurse's role in working with the patient and other therapists in the process of rehabilitation has been recognised as vitally important. Nursing models such as Activities of Daily Living (Roper *et al.*, 2000) and Self Care (Orem, 1991) have given structure to rehabilitation nursing. Nurses provide round-the-clock care, making them ideally placed to implement and evaluate the patient's treatment. Nurses are able to work in partnership with the patient to assess the effectiveness of the treatment programme.

Recap Questions

1. Why do we rehabilitate?
2. What are the differences between the medical and social models of disability?

Independence and self-care

Independence

Traditionally, care provided for patients lacked any reference to independence. It was often accepted that the health professional knew what was best for the patient, resulting in the patient having little choice in their own care. Fortunately, this is generally no longer the case.

To think about

What does independence mean to you?
What is important to you, and how can you achieve it?
What factors influence your independence?

Smith (1999) describes independence as 'an individual having choice of how to live his life within his capacity and means, which takes into account the individual's own values and preferences'. In order to help the patient regain independence, it is necessary for the rehabilitation team to work with the patient and for the individual patient to have choices regarding their treatment. In addition, for a patient to fully achieve their potential, they often need some degree of social and economic autonomy as well as physical and mental independence. Promoting independence, partnership working and patient participation are essential aspects of rehabilitation. These are the underlying principles to effective rehabilitation work. It is important that all members of the rehabilitation team work together and with the patient to follow these principles. Giving choices is one of the key aspects of person-centred care.

Self-care

Self-care is about having control of one's own care. For the purposes of health, it is about the person being able to decide how and what actions need to be taken, and by whom, in order to sustain their care/treatment. Self-care is about the choices a person makes and the actions they take to maintain their health and wellbeing (Department of Health, 2003). Self-care can be given in a number of ways, by the patient and their family, friends, formal and informal carers and related community groups. Self-care is about the individual being actively involved in finding effective ways to deal with their identified problems and to enable them to achieve their goals (Creek, 2003).

The DH includes the promotion of self-care in the *Essence of Care Patient-Focused Benchmarks for Clinical Governance* (Department of Health, 2003). The DH categorises self-care as follows:

+ *Self-management of health and lifestyle*: the person manages their own health by making informed health and lifestyle choices

+ *Self-management of health status information (monitoring and diagnosis)*: the person scrutinises their own health and wellbeing

+ *Self-management of choices and decisions*: the person makes decisions about their care and treatment

The benchmark for best practice is that patients are enabled to make choices about self-care and these choices are respected. The key word here is 'enabled'. The patient should be made an equal member of the team in their care delivery and management programme. The patient should be enabled to assess risk and evaluate the impact of risk identified on their care and treatment. Worst practice includes telling patients how care is to be delivered and practitioners deciding what is best for the patient.

To achieve best practice, patients need to be aware of all the self-care options available to them. These options need to be discussed with all agencies, including the patient and, if applicable, the patient's family, friends and carers. Decisions regarding care and treatment should be made at times and places that are acceptable to all parties. Information should be readily accessible so that an informed and educated programme of rehabilitation can be developed. The information should be evidence-based so that all members of the team are knowledgeable and consistent. Ongoing monitoring systems need to be in place to ensure that the patient participates fully in all aspects of their care and treatment.

Assessment must always take into account the patient's abilities and whether the patient wants to be involved in their treatment and care. The patient should contribute to this assessment. The assessment process should be ongoing and continuous. At best, the patient contributes to assessing their self-care abilities in an ongoing process that continually informs professionals and others in the patient's care management and treatment.

Best practice is achieved by considering how information is recorded and understood by all parties concerned with the patient's self-care abilities. This assessment informs and is reflected in the care and treatment programmes, so that care and treatment plans are based on informed decisions and used at all stages throughout the patient journey. Self-care assessment is integral to these individualised plans. Training should focus on the ability of patients and their informal and formal carers to enable patients to assess their self-care requirements and to inform the direct care and treatment provided. Education and training should lead to patients and carers gaining skills and sharing knowledge and expertise. Any education and training needs to be grounded in practice and underpinned by theoretical evidence.

Consider Case study 9.1a. Think about what may have influenced the decisions taken.

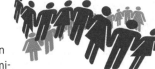

Case Study 9.1a

Mrs Main is a 62-year-old woman admitted to your rehabilitation ward following a CVA with a left-sided weakness. She is predominantly right-handed. Since her admission, she has been found to be diabetic. Her diabetes requires her to have insulin twice daily. Also since admission, Mrs Main has suffered a major bereavement – her husband has died. Mrs Main is reluctant to participate in any of her self-care needs. It has been decided by the ward team and Mrs Main's relatives that she will live in a purpose-built flat in her daughter's home and that her 18-year-old grandson, who is interested in training to be a paramedic, will give her insulin.

Can you see any possible problems with this scenario?
How might you have dealt with this differently?
Do you think the decisions taken were made in the best interests of the patient or of the service?

Mrs Main was a relatively young woman. She may well have been reluctant to accept her newly diagnosed conditions (diabetes and vascular disease), particularly as she was recently bereaved. Losing a life partner is a significant event in itself, but to then become incapacitated through illness must have had a massive influence on her recovery. Any decisions made at this time needed careful consideration with options for future discussion.

In the second part of the scenario in Case study 9.2b, see what happened to Mrs Main a few months later.

Exhibit 9.1 lists some aspects that you may wish to think about.

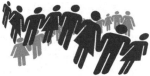

Case Study 9.1b

Mrs Main has been living at her daughter's house for the past 8 months. She has recently started to attend a day hospital as part of her treatment programme. During the short time that Mrs Main has been attending the hospital, Mrs Main has shown consistent improvement. However, the team has noticed that Mrs Main has become increasingly withdrawn and depressed. On questioning, it is apparent that Mrs Main's circumstances have changed. Her daughter has been promoted, and she now works long hours and increasingly stays away from home due to business commitments. Mrs Main's grandson has applied and been accepted for paramedic training.

What needs to be done?

How are you going to initiate and aid this change?

+ The multidisciplinary team, Mrs Main and Mrs Main's relatives need to work together to formulate a care/treatment plan
+ Mrs Main needs to decide what her goals are, and negotiate these with the team in order to formulate a plan of action
+ The plan needs to be evaluated regularly by all parties concerned so that Mrs Main can gain her independence at a level that is acceptable to her
+ Mrs Main's goals should be realistic and achievable

Exhibit 9.1 Points for consideration regarding Mrs Main's treatment (see Case studies 9.1a and 9.1b)

Case studies 9.1a and 9.1b show that when Mrs Main was first discharged from hospital, she was fully reliant on her family. However, her circumstances changed. Mrs Main was a relatively young woman who was expected to be dependent on others for a potentially long time. Eight months after her discharge from hospital, Mrs Main was eager to regain her independence; she had needed the support of her family but she was now physically and emotionally stronger. The case studies illustrate that rehabilitation can start at any time. For Mrs Main, it was inappropriate to commence rehabilitation and self-care in the earlier stages as she needed time to come to terms with her bereavement and illness; however, it was important for her to gain her independence at a later date.

Assessing possible risks when undertaking self-care

Most rehabilitation programmes carry some degree of risk to the patient. For example, when a patient is relearning a skill such as walking, there is a significant risk that the patient will fall. Together, health professionals and the patient need to be able to assess this risk and agree on what may be an acceptable level. Consider Case study 9.2.

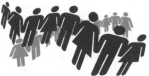

Case Study 9.2

Mrs Bless was admitted to the day hospital. One of her treatment goals was to be able to cook an evening meal. She had been unable to cook since her stroke, which had resulted in her not being able to use her right arm as well as she could before. Mrs Bless was helped in her everyday care by her husband. Following discussion, it became clear that Mr Bless was unwilling to let Mrs Bless cook, as he felt it was too dangerous.

How do you think this situation could be resolved?

The members of the day hospital rehabilitation team arranged to meet Mrs Bless and her husband. Mrs Bless's treatment goals were discussed. It was agreed that Mrs Bless should prepare and cook a meal at the day hospital, which she could then take home and share with her husband that evening. Mrs Bless was supervised and taught to use various kitchen aids by the nurses and occupational therapists. The physiotherapists helped Mrs Bless with her mobility and balance while she was cooking. Mrs Bless was soon able to cook independently at home, following a home assessment by the occupational therapist so that aids and adaptations could be made to Mr and Mrs Bless's kitchen. This was successful because the risk associated with cooking was assessed carefully by the rehabilitation team and by the patient and her husband, and this level of risk was found to be acceptable to all parties.

Risk assessment tools based on reliable research evidence can be used to assess levels of risk. Sometimes, however, as in the case of Mrs Bless, individualised risk assessment is used. Most important is that the patient understands the level of risk and has full knowledge to make an informed decision about their treatment. Health professionals need to remember that both the patient and the patient's circumstances can change; therefore, continual assessments are important. The frequency of when and how often safety is assessed must be tailored to the individual patient's needs.

The patient's understanding and collaboration must always be sought, and their acceptance of risk should be documented. Most practitioners, carers and patients will require some level of education and training in relation to risk and whether the level of risk is acceptable for both the patient and the organisation. Critical incidents and complaints may arise, and therefore robust systems must be in place such that events and complaints are recorded, monitored, analysed and acted upon.

Recap Questions

1. What does rehabilitation mean to you?
2. In what ways can you encourage a person to be independent?

Framework for rehabilitation nursing

This is a structured approach that provides the patient with a framework for their rehabilitation. The nurse is key to the coordination of the patient's treatment and to the services that the patient may require. The framework contains components that take account of essential everyday skills, such as keeping oneself clean. In addition to these skills, the framework takes into account the education of the patient and the information the patient needs and facilitates the patient to develop any additional knowledge. During the rehabilitation programme, the nurse acts as the patient's advocate, giving advice and counselling when required to do so. The patient is at the centre of this framework (Figure 9.3).

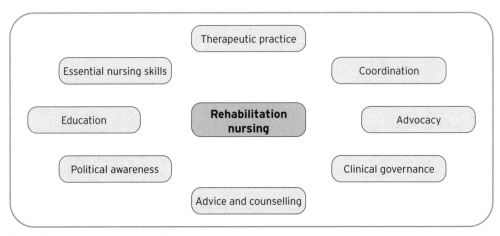

Figure 9.3 Framework of rehabilitation nursing

Successful rehabilitation uses a framework to make an integrated care pathway in which the patient, the interdisciplinary team members and the formal and informal carers can be involved. One of the most difficult challenges facing nurses is to ensure that the individual's needs dominate within the hospital or healthcare professional's programme (Smith, 1999), which can be very difficult to achieve due to financial constraints.

The rehabilitation process, like most healthcare in the UK, may be driven by political influences. The *National Service Framework for Older People* emphasises the importance of rehabilitation and the availability of rehabilitation services; this framework has had a huge effect on the provision of rehabilitation treatment to older people since 2002 (Department of Health, 2001a). Acute and primary care trusts are obliged to provide intermediate care services for people who need them. The aim of such services is to maximise the person's level of independence, thereby reducing hospital admissions and length of stay in hospital.

Rehabilitation can be a lifetime activity: very few cases of rehabilitation are time-limited. Rehabilitation service provision varies from region to region and at different times within a person's lifetime. The provision of holistic rehabilitation can be financially costly; but not providing emotional rehabilitation can be devastating for the patient.

The rehabilitation team

We now consider the different people who make up the rehabilitation team. Successful rehabilitation is about teamwork and often involves a large number of different professionals (Figure 9.4).

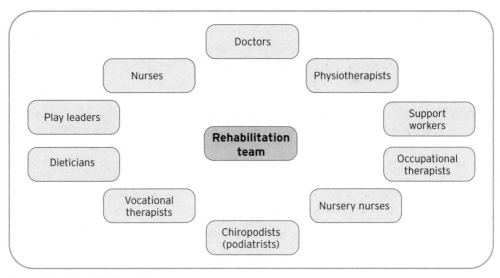

Figure 9.4 Rehabilitation team

Rehabilitation teams work in a variety of settings, including general and specialist hospitals and the community. Although the members of the team come from different disciplines, their primary aim must be to work together and with the patient to treat and rehabilitate. Agreement of goals and outcomes is integral to successful teamworking. Most patient-centred goals will require the involvement of more than one discipline at any one time. It is important that all team members work together to achieve patient-centred goals rather than trying to achieve only those goals that are specific to the discipline in which they work. For example, in Case studies 9.1a and 9.1b, Mrs Main needed help to be able to dress independently. A number of disciplines were involved in helping her to achieve this goal:

+ A physiotherapist ensured Mrs Main could sit up and was able to balance while dressing.

+ An occupational therapist taught Mrs Main to use certain equipment and adaptations to assist.

+ Ward nurses and rehabilitation support workers assisted with Mrs Main's personal hygiene, washing and dressing and continued the programmes set by the physiotherapist and occupational therapist.

Rehabilitation teams work in various ways:

+ *Multidisciplinary teamworking*: each discipline (e.g. physiotherapy) has specific goals to be achieved (e.g. for physiotherapy, to increase the patient's mobility; for occupational therapy, to maximise the patient's ability to be able to wash and dress independently). The health professionals work alongside each other and with the patient's doctors and nurses, but each health professional sets separate goals for the patient. There are clear boundaries between the disciplines involved. The outcomes of care and treatment are the sum of the efforts of each discipline. Effective communication between the team members is key to the success of this type of team. This is a more traditional approach to teamworking.

+ *Interdisciplinary teamworking*: the team members collaborate with each other to identify patient goals. The team works closely to solve problems by looking at how goals can be achieved by each professional; these professionals then work together to help the patient to achieve specific aims. Thus, more than one health professional assists the patient to achieve one goal. The health professionals work together on each goal rather than setting separate discipline-specific goals. The team members need to be flexible and prepared to work across boundaries. The team members share their respective goals with each other, the patient and the patient's family (Kumar, 2000).

+ *Trans-disciplinary teamworking*: the boundaries between the health professionals are blurred. There is cross-training and flexibility between the different disciplines, which minimises duplication. The health professionals work together and support one another to help the patient attain their goals through maximising functional ability. Specific boundaries between the different health professionals are not so apparent, and it may not be immediately apparent which discipline each team member is from (Kumar, 2000). Trans-disciplinary team working is still relatively uncommon, although some intermediate care teams are moving towards this ways of working.

Interdisciplinary and trans-disciplinary working demands a higher degree of group interaction and focused treatment effort.

To think about

Which professionals and informal carers may be involved with a patient's treatment and care?

A large number of people may be involved in a rehabilitation team, including health and social care professionals, voluntary agency staff, charitable agency staff, and support workers such as healthcare assistants and rehabilitation assistants.

The role of the support worker in a rehabilitation team, and in successfully implementing the rehabilitation programme, is an important one. Support workers are in a unique position to establish therapeutic relationships with their patients, as much of their time is spent in the delivery of care and treatment: the support worker may assist the patient with nursing, physiotherapy, occupational therapy, dietetics, podiatry and speech and language. The coordinator of the rehabilitation programme is often a nurse, and it is therefore essential that the nurse is familiar with the full extent of the support worker's role and ensures that the support worker has the necessary skills to complete these tasks. It is also important that the knowledge of the support worker is acknowledged and they are given full opportunity to contribute to setting goals and evaluating treatment.

Education should support the development of support workers. Such education reflects the context of the national agenda for the modernisation of health and social care – that is, promoting the independence of patients. All members of the rehabilitation team, including support workers, should have access to ongoing educational training to ensure that the workforce is competent to support all stages of the patient's journey. Government initiatives such as the *National Framework for Older People* (Department of Health, 2001a) promote the development of generic roles for all health and social care workers, with special emphasis on the support worker role.

Patient participation in treatment programmes and service development

Patient partnership is about the patient influencing every level of the services that they receive. This means that all care and treatment plans should be formulated in full partnership with the patient. This gives the patient equal power with all the other members of the rehabilitation team and those who plan, deliver and evaluate services. The DH actively promotes patient participation, as demonstrated in the National Service Frameworks and the NHS Plan (Department of Health, 2001b). The challenge for health practitioners is how to involve patients in the everyday management of services. The NHS Plan created a vision for a patient-centred NHS, shifting the balance of power to patients and frontline staff and away from service leaders and managers (Department of Health, 2001b). True patient partnership demonstrates mutual respect between the patient and health and social care professionals.

To think about

How can patients be involved in the development and evaluation of services?

By involving patients in the development and evaluation of services, this shows that they are being treated and respected as equal partners in decision-making. The patient's voice can be heard through:

+ Patient forums
+ Patient Advocacy and Liaison Service (PALS)
+ Patient surveys
+ Clinical practice benchmarking
+ Patient representatives on various strategic groups, such as a professional executive committee (PEC)

The key concepts of patient involvement, participation and partnership are central themes of any rehabilitation programme. The important point is that all members of the rehabilitation team understand the patient's perspective.

It is important to distinguish between the terms 'user involvement' and 'patient participation'. Patient participation is about patients being fully involved in decisions about their treatment and the services that are provided. User involvement tends to mean that patients are the users of services that have been provided for them by others.

The decision as to who has responsibility for all or parts of care and treatment should be a consensus between the patient and the practitioners working with the patient. This can be achieved only through inter-professional and inter-agency work and is best demonstrated through comprehensive assessment in a single assessment format – that is, patient-centred assessment, whereby the patient is a full member of the process and has direct input into any decisions made regarding their care and treatment. This partnership process needs continual monitoring in order to ensure maximum equality of responsibility.

Service provision

Best practice requires users to participate in the planning and evaluation of their services at every stage. The patient should be at the centre of the service. The patient's views should be actively sought and services then planned with these views in mind. All the agencies involved in care, treatment, service development and delivery should be seen to be working together and with the patient. Service development depends on patient satisfaction and on any complaints being addressed appropriately. Best practice requires patients and their carers and advocates to understand and to have access to the services provided. A key aspect of the patient's journey is that early discharge from hospital is not prevented by slow access to resources and services.

To think about

Consider the rehabilitation services that are available to people aged over 65 years compared with those available for young adults.

Healthcare practitioners interact with vulnerable people and often in sensitive situations. It is essential that they are able to treat clients and colleagues in an equal and appropriate way. Health professionals have considerably power over the lives of their patients. Consider Case study 9.3.

Case Study 9.3

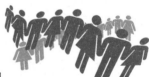

Mrs Brown was an 82-year-old widow. She lived in a bungalow and was self-caring until she had an accident that resulted in her left leg being amputated below the knee. Her recovery was fairly slow, and she was moved from an acute hospital to a rehabilitation hospital. She progressed with her rehabilitation programme to become wheelchair-independent; she was then able to transfer independently from bed to chair, chair to chair, and chair to toilet. She was looking forward to returning home. A home visit was arranged. Those taking part in the visit were Mrs Brown, an occupational therapist and a social worker. The professionals decided that the bungalow was unsuitable for wheelchair access, as the hallways were too narrow. They discussed the situation with Mrs Brown. Even though Mrs Brown desperately wanted to go home, it was decided that residential care would be a better option for her, as alterations to the bungalow would be too expensive and no grants were available to help her. Despite further rehabilitation to get Mrs Brown mobilising on crutches, this was not achieved; therefore, Mrs Brown reluctantly agreed to go into residential care.

Unfortunately, older people are often discriminated against with regard to housing issues. The health and social care professionals considered the option of making alterations to Mrs Brown's bungalow as not being cost-effective. Their main argument was that, because of her age, Mrs Brown was likely to have deteriorating health and would likely need full-time care in the near future. Mrs Brown did have other health issues, including unstable diabetes and coronary heart disease, but perhaps a different rehabilitation programme could have been initiated – or perhaps Mrs Brown may have been willing to release equity in her bungalow to finance the alterations needed.

Ideally, the patient's environment should help to promote their independence. Some situations do fail to support self-care, but practitioners should work together with the patient to promote self-care within such an environment. Service users should be encouraged and involved to ensure that the environment promotes self-care and takes into account any cultural or religious needs – essential components of many people's wellbeing.

Equipment

The availability and provision of equipment is an integral part of patients being able to achieve self-care. Having the right equipment can be crucial to independent living; for example, a walking stick or a wheelchair can enable the person to move about. Healthcare workers should know what type of equipment is available and be able to help the patient access it. In order for patients to access resources that meet their individual needs, sufficient resources must be available, but this depends on the organisation's finances. Patients should have an input into decisions concerning service and equipment provision. They also need to be familiar with any barriers to the availability of resources and understand why these are so.

Equipment can by obtained from various sources, including social services departments, the NHS, education services, Jobcentre Plus and voluntary organisations. Social services and the NHS usually supply equipment on loan, in some areas from a joint equipment loan store. Most of the equipment provided by the NHS and social services is supplied following an assessment by an occupational therapist, technical therapist or rehabilitation support worker. The type of equipment provided depends on the person's needs. Some simple items make it safer and easier for the person to deal with everyday tasks, such as preparing food or managing their own personal hygiene. Other equipment and adaptations are more complex, such as stair lifts, computer-aided lights and door-opening systems. Most UK regions have specialist equipment loan stores and specialist shops, and information about these can be found in local libraries, council offices and GP surgeries, and on the Internet.

Some people prefer to buy their own equipment rather than borrow it from the NHS. The patient should always contact an occupational therapist or physiotherapist before making a major purchase of equipment. Second-hand equipment is also available, but again consultation with a therapist is recommended before using. People with disabilities do not have to pay VAT on equipment for daily living.

Disabled living centres (DLCs), based around the UK, aim to increase people's opportunities to live independently. DLCs offer disabled people the chance to see and try out a wide range of products to find those that suit their needs. DLCs offer independent advice about the equipment and services that are available, including costs and where they can be obtained. These centres also provide training for disabled people, carers and professionals.

In the checklist below, we consider some of the more common pieces of equipment and explain how to keep the equipment safe for the patient. This checklist can be used for assessing each piece of equipment.

Wheelchairs

✢ Check the wheelchair is suitable for indoor and/or outdoor use

✢ Ensure footrests are attached when transporting the patient

✢ Ensure the brakes are on when the patient is moving from into or out of the chair

✢ Check the wheels for damage and signs of wear and tear

✢ Check there is adequate air in the tyres

✢ Check the condition of the brake pads and that brakes are working

✢ Check the general condition of chair

✢ Use pressure-relieving equipment when required

Walking sticks

Wooden and metal walking sticks are available (Figure 9.5). Some people buy walking sticks privately, but it is important that all patients using a walking stick on a regular basis have a health professional such as a physiotherapist or rehabilitation support worker check that they are using the stick appropriately and that the equipment is in a safe condition:

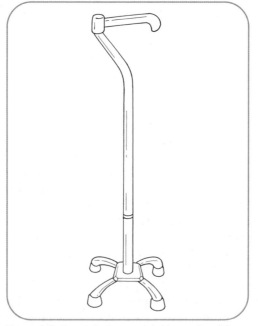

Figure 9.5 Quad device: a metal type of walking stick

✢ Check the stick is the correct height for the patient; this should be done by a suitably trained professional, such as a physiotherapist

✢ Inspect ferrules (rubber cap on the end of the stick) regularly for signs of wear and tear; replacement ferrules are available from physiotherapy departments, specialist equipment shops and large pharmacies

+ On metal walking sticks, check that spring catches are located in the hole correctly

+ Check the plastic grip handles for wear and tear

Walking frames

Most people who use a walking frame will have had this issued by a health professional. The walking frame may be a standard frame with four legs and ferrules, or a wheeled frame with two wheels at the front and two legs with ferrules at the back (Figure 9.6). The following checks should be made:

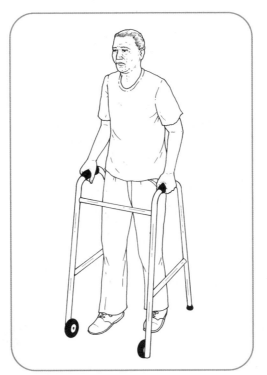

Figure 9.6 Two-wheeled walking frame

+ Check the height of the frame is correct for the patient; this should be done by a suitably trained professional, such as a physiotherapist

+ Inspect the ferrules for signs of wear; replacement ferrules are available from physiotherapy departments, specialist equipment shops and large pharmacies

+ Make sure the spring catches are located firmly in the holes

+ Check the plastic grip handles for signs of wear and tear

+ Ensure nuts and bolts are not loose

+ Explain to the patient that the frame should be used to carry only light items, such as spectacles, using the specially adapted basket; heavy items may cause the frame to tip

+ Check the wheels turn freely and are secure

+ Check the tread on the wheels for signs of wear

Crutches

+ Ensure crutches are the correct height; this should be done by a suitably trained professional, such as a physiotherapist

+ Check that the cuff is secured firmly and can pivot

To think about

What should be taken into consideration when a patient has an aid to mobility, such as a walking stick?

What makes a piece of equipment safe?

Mobilisation

Helping people to keep fit and healthy helps them to stay mobile and independent. Many conditions can be treated and sometimes even prevented by the patient becoming more active. The role of the healthcare practitioner is crucial in aiding mobilisation by ensuring that patients have encouragement, support and access to information. Age need not be a barrier to taking up new sports or activities. Extend classes are available for older people in many parts of the UK. This is a nationwide initiative that trains teachers to give movement to music classes for older or disabled people. Details of these classes can be obtained through Age Concern.

Changes to lifestyle such as diet and exercise programmes can improve suppleness and strength and are relevant for all ages. Encouraging people to eat healthily and if necessary to lose or gain weight can reduce restrictions to mobility; dietary advice is available through GPs and dieticians. Consider Case study 9.4.

Case Study 9.4

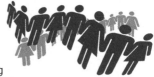

You visit Mrs Davis, an 83-year-old woman who has recently been having some mobility problems. You observe her using a walking frame incorrectly: she lifts it to get through small spaces and sometimes walks along with the frame off the ground. However, Mrs Davis still finds the frame beneficial. On discussion, you find she has borrowed the frame from a neighbour.

What is your plan of action?

Further discussion with Mrs Davis is needed regarding her mobility problem, when it started, and how it affects her ability to do the things she wants to do. With Mrs Davis' help, an action plan can be devised, including the following:

+ Discussion about the services and equipment that are available

+ Discussion about potential problems that may arise from using someone else's walking frame

+ Discussion regarding safety issues and why a referral would be advisable

+ Referral to a physiotherapist for full mobility assessment
+ Referral to her GP for investigations into her loss of mobility
+ Advice from the team leader
+ General check of the condition of the frame and its suitability for use in the short term

Recap Questions

1. Which health and social care practitioners may be involved with a person's rehabilitation?
2. Where can you and the patient obtain equipment for rehabilitation?
3. What is meant by a person-centred approach to rehabilitation?

Factors that impact on individual wellbeing

In this section we explore factors that may impact on a patient's rehabilitation programme. We consider the patient's wellbeing, spirituality, culture and ethical decision-making. A person undertaking a rehabilitation programme can find themselves having to adapt to a completely different way of life. They may find that they have to make considerable adjustments not only to their lifestyle but also to how they see themselves as a person. Different people cope differently with their illness or disability (Hoeman, 2002). It is important for the health professional to understand that the patient's goals may be different from their own and for the health professional to recognise any potential barriers to achieving these goals. The health professional needs to work with the patient to devise possible strategies to overcome these barriers. The patient's cognitive processes (how they think, whether they are able to solve a problem and how much they understand) is very important to the rehabilitation process, as is the patient's ability to communicate. The patient's knowledge about their illness or disability can also have an impact on their feeling of wellbeing. The level of impairment can mean different things to different people. As a nurse, you may see people with severe disabilities who appear to be able to cope far better than people with much less complex disabilities; however, the healthcare worker needs to be able to give the appropriate level of support to all patients. Family support is also crucial, as we saw with Mrs Bless in Case study 9.2: her husband stopped her from cooking because he was worried she would hurt herself – but although this was well meaning, it seriously curtailed her ability to rehabilitate fully. Now consider Case study 9.5.

Case Study 9.5

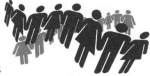

The health visitor for older people had been asked to visit Mrs Sheridan by her son. He had informed the health visitor that his mother was no longer capable of preparing and cooking her meals and needed meals on wheels. Mrs Sheridan was 85 years old and lived alone. During discussion, Mrs Sheridan told the health visitor that although she was getting frailer and sometimes dropped things and made mistakes, she enjoyed cooking for herself and wanted to continue to do so.

What would you have done if you were the health visitor?

Mrs Sheridan and the health visitor agreed jointly that Mrs Sheridan should continue preparing and cooking her own meals but that she would apply to have meals on wheels when she felt she was no longer able to do so. Mrs Sheridan was aware of the risk involved, but she wanted to take this risk. Mrs Sheridan was advised to discuss this with her son; the health visitor agreed she would meet with him if it was required. Sometimes family dynamics can have an effect on treatment.

Barnes and Ward (2005) based a study on behaviours associated with stress following illness or injury. These behaviours included anger, hostility and rebelliousness, with the patient refusing care and treatment. The patient may refuse to take part in self-care activities, learn new strategies or socialise by shunning family and friends. Some patients experience depersonalisation by avoiding or disowning altered body parts. This may be seen following a stroke that leaves the person paralysed in one side of the body; the person may ignore the affected side, and therefore much of the rehabilitation work needs to be centred on getting the patient to regain awareness of the affected side (see Case study 9.6).

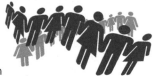

Case Study 9.6

Mr Blackburn had a paralysed right arm and leg following a stroke. It was apparent that he was ignoring his right side. The rehabilitation team, together with Mr Blackburn, devised a treatment plan that included ways of getting Mr Blackburn to become more aware of his right side. This included putting the bedside locker on the right-hand side of the bed, approaching Mr Blackburn from his right side and handing drinks from the right. This helped Mr Blackburn to become more aware of his right side and assisted in his rehabilitation by correcting his balance and body awareness.

Providing psychological support

The nurse can provide psychological support to the patient with injuries and significant disabilities by communicating in a person-centred way with the patient, using all of the communication skills such as active listening, looking for non-verbal cues and observing the patient closely, and allowing time for silence so that the person can reflect and perhaps open up deeper feelings. This person-centred approach to communication shows that you respect the patient's individuality and value that person (Tribal Education, 2006). Non-judgemental acceptance on the part of the healthcare practitioner encourages the patient and their relatives to acknowledge and build towards reconstruction of the patient's life. Active listening and empathy (rather than sympathy) for the patient are essential. Giving psychological support is time-consuming but time well spent. Healthcare professionals need to work collaboratively with patients in order to build up strong, supportive and empathic relationships.

Culture

The patient needs to be able to experience care and treatment in a manner that actively encompasses their culture – that is, their individual values, beliefs, personal relationships, rules of behaviour and lifestyle practices. The patient's culture defines how they think and influences how they behave. Culture is characterised by learning from birth, through language and socialisation. It is something that is shared by all members of the same cultural group. It is an adaptation to specific activities related to environmental and technical factors and to the availability of natural resources. It is a dynamic and ever-changing process (Andrews and Boyle, 2003).

Patients are also influenced by their own life experiences of health and illness. The nurse's own culture, with its beliefs, values and practices, can impinge on the care and treatment that they provide to others. A further influence on care is the culture of the setting in which the patient and caregiver meet, whether this is in hospital, the community or a family setting (Holland and Hogg, 2001).

Spirituality

Spirituality can be seen as a need to find meaning, purpose and fulfilment in life, suffering and death. It is the need for hope, the will to live, and belief in oneself, others and, for some people, God (Hoeman, 2002). All care and treatment is influenced to some degree by the patient's spirituality and system of beliefs. The nurse is in a unique position to assist in upholding the patient's system of beliefs. The nurse can ascertain what practices are meaningful to the patient and can help to facilitate these practices. Assessment of the patient's situation on their spiritual wellbeing is an important part of treatment, as the spiritual wellbeing will in turn have consequences on the patient's response to care and treatment. An assessment that helps the patient to maintain their spirituality takes into account the individual's life history and background; only then can the assessor gain the patient's trust and respect.

Ethical issues in rehabilitation

Rehabilitation can be defined as helping an individual to readjust to society after a period of illness or imprisonment. Rehabilitation includes the consideration of all aspects of the patient's life and wellbeing. Ethical decision-making influences assessment, goal-planning, and implementation and evaluation of care. The questions below help the nurse to make ethical decisions (Tschudin, 1992).

When assessing care and treatment, consider the following:

+ What does the patient want?
+ Who are the people directly involved (e.g. the patient, family, friends, health and social care workers)?
+ What facts are important or unimportant, and to whom?
+ Are there any aspects that enhance or go against the patient's conscience?
+ What expectations of the outcome does each person have? (Remember that the patient's expectations could be very difficult from those of health professionals.)
+ Is the problem actual or potential?
+ Are there any aspects that can or cannot be changed?
+ What other relevant considerations are there?

When planning care and treatment, think about the following:

+ What actions are possible?
+ What are the possible outcomes?

+ Who will be helped (e.g. the patient, family members)?

+ Will anyone be hurt by the outcome? If so, how?

+ Is there a time limit? If so, is it due to constraints on resources?

+ Is the action right?

+ Is there a question of professional responsibility? What principles are involved?

+ Is the workplace code of conduct involved? If so, does it change or influence the situation?

When implementing care and treatment, consider this question:

+ What is the action to be taken, who is going to take it, when and how?

When evaluating care and treatment, try to follow a reflective cycle and think about the following:

+ Did the decision taken solve the problem?

+ Were the expected outcomes realistic in practice? If not, why not?

+ If you had to take the decision again, would you make the same decision?

+ Have other people benefited?

+ Have further decisions become easier because of this one?

Use the checklists above to consider the following three scenarios:

Scenario 1: *Mr Young was admitted to hospital following an acute infection. He is very confused, especially at night. He is physically violent and verbally abusive to staff and other patients. Should he be restrained?*

Scenario 2: *A patient's husband is rude and verbally abusive to the care staff looking after his wife in their own home. How can this be addressed?*

Scenario 3: *Should a patient be sent home with a family member if it appears that the family member is not interested or supportive?*

Did the checklists help you to reach some decisions? Note that the scenarios above are to give you points for consideration and to stimulate discussion. You would never be expected to resolve these issues on your own; rather, these cases would involve all members of the rehabilitation team, the patients and their families.

Recap Questions

1. What are some of the behaviours associated with stress following illness and injury?
2. In what ways can the nurse provide psychological support to a person who has significant disabilities following an accident?
3. What is culture?

Summary

All disciplines play an important role in rehabilitating the patient. A team approach is important in order for the patient to gain maximum functional ability. Rehabilitation is about the patient and their family, the environment in which the patient lives, the patient's community, the patient's society and the patient's spiritual wellbeing. The rehabilitation process is about solving problems and setting and attaining goals; this can be achieved only by all professionals working together, with the patient being an equal stakeholder in their treatment. Nurses have a key role in rehabilitation; nurses are likely to have a 24-hour presence with the patient, and a nurse is often the coordinator of the treatment programme, liaising with other disciplines and either acting as a key worker or working very closely with the designated key worker. The nurse is able to work with the patient and their carers as the patient's advocate. The nursing role is a specialist one and a key component of this is to reinforce the input of others (Nolan *et al.*, 1997).

Rehabilitation is an increasing body of work for staff working within health and social services. Roles within nursing are evolving and developing in response to a number of influencing factors, including policy initiatives that reflect the demand for more patient-focused services. The work of this multi-professional team includes assessment, coordination and communication, implementing technical and physical care and treatment, therapy development, therapy integration, the continuation of therapy, and the provision of emotional support to the patient and their family. All of this should be done in conjunction with the patient and their family.

Support workers are crucial to patient care. They spend a large amount of time giving direct care to the patient and are therefore in a unique position to contribute to the assessment and evaluation processes of the patient's care and treatment.

Rehabilitation is delivered in a variety of settings within health, social services, voluntary and independent sectors. Roles within the rehabilitation team are similarly diverse, and responsibilities vary between settings, depending on the needs of the patient and the service. Different settings may have dissimilar team members; however, the constant member of the team is the patient.

The patient's needs and goals change over time, and the team needs to accommodate this. Rehabilitation is not time-limited but an ongoing process. It is essential that rehabilitation practice is underpinned with relevant theory and research. Finally, emotional and spiritual rehabilitation, and support for the development of practical skills, all form part of the patient's journey.

Key Points

1. The rehabilitation programme is person-centred and takes into account the individual's physical, mental, emotional, psychological, spiritual and cultural needs.

2. The nurse is a crucial member of the rehabilitation team. Nursing staff have a 24-hour presence with the patient and are the link between the patient and other members of the rehabilitation team.

3. Rehabilitation should be available to all people, regardless of their age and disability.

4. Assessment should be an holistic, ongoing and continuous process throughout the rehabilitation period. This may last from a few weeks to many years.

Points for debate

Now that you have come to the end of this chapter here are a few points that you may wish to think about when you are in practice. You may wish to discuss these with your work colleagues or fellow students.

Rehabilitation is costly and should be time-limited.

Nurses should concentrate on the caring and medical aspects of care.

Links to Other Chapters

Chapter 1 What is caring?
Chapter 2 Dignity and privacy
Chapter 5 Nutrition

Further reading

Department of Health (1995) *Disability Discrimination Act*. London: The Stationery Office.

Department of Health (2005) *Disability Discrimination Act*. London: The Stationery Office.

Department of Health (2005) *National Service Framework for Long-Term Conditions*. London: The Stationery Office.

Gilchrist, C (1999) *Turning Your Back on Us*. London: Age Concern.

References

Andrews, M and Boyle, J (2003) *Transcultural Concepts in Nursing Care*, 4th edn. London: Lippincott Williams & Wilkins.

Barnes, M and Ward, A (2005) *Oxford Handbook of Rehabilitation Medicine*, Oxford: Oxford University Press.

Creek, J (2003) *Occupational Therapy Defined as a Complex Intervention*. London: College of Occupational Therapists.

Department of Health (1995) *Disability Discrimination Act*. London: The Stationery Office.

Department of Health (2001a) *National Service Framework for Older People*. London: The Stationery Office.

Department of Health (2001b) *Involving Patients and the Public in Healthcare: Response to the Listening Exercise*. London: The Stationery Office.

Department of Health (2003) *Essence of Care Patient-Focused Benchmarks for Clinical Governance*. London: The Stationery Office.

Hoeman, S (2002) *Rehabilitation Nursing, Process Applications and Outcomes*. New York: Mosby.

Holland, K and Hogg, C (2001) *Cultural Awareness in Nursing and Healthcare: An Introductory Text*. London: Arnold.

Kumar, S (2000) *Multidisciplinary Approach to Rehabilitation*. Boston, MA: Butterworth-Heinemann.

Nolan, M, Booth, J and Nolan, J (1997) *New Directions in Rehabilitation: Exploring the Nursing Contribution*. Research report series no. 6. London: English National Board for Nursing, Midwifery and Health Visiting.

Orem, D (1991) *Nursing Concepts of Practice*, 4th edn. St Louis, MO: Mosby.

Roper, N, Logan, W and Tierney, A (2000) *The Roper Logan Tierney Model of Nursing*. Edinburgh: Churchill Livingstone.

Sinclair, A and Dickinson, E (1998) *Effective Practice in Rehabilitation: The Evidence of Systematic Reviews*. London: Kings Fund.

Smith, M (1999) *Rehabilitation in Adult Nursing Practice*. London: Churchill Livingston.

Tribal Education (2006) *Certificate in Palliative Care*. York: Network Publishing.

Tschudin, V (1992) *Ethics in Nursing: The Caring Relationship*. Oxford: Butterworth-Heinemann.

Acknowledgements

Pam Collett, Inspect-a-Gadget Specialist Equipment Shop, South Warwickshire Primary Care Trust

Jo Galloway, Consultant Nurse, Older People, Walsall

Physiotherapy Department, South Warwickshire Primary Care Trust

Hazel Ratcliffe, Ratcliffe Consultancy

Chapter 10
Record-keeping

Case Study

Simon Jennings, a 34-year-old electrician, is admitted to the emergency assessment unit (EAU). He is unconscious and believed to be in a diabetic coma: his blood results are showing very high blood glucose levels and he is wearing a Medic-Alert pendant indicating he has type 1 diabetes. On admission, Mr Jennings is unconscious, dehydrated and in a shocked state due to loss of fluid. The first priority is to assess his airway, breathing and circulation. He requires urgent fluid replacement and insulin intravenously to lower his blood glucose levels. His condition is critical and his relatives need to be informed.

The EAU is very busy and a record is not made of Mr Jennings' relatives' phone numbers, so they are not contacted about his condition. Furthermore, there is no record on his fluid balance chart of him receiving any intravenous fluids or insulin. His medication record does not indicate when or how much insulin Mr Jennings has been given.

Mr Jennings' vital signs (pulse, blood pressure, respirations and temperature) and ALERT score (conscious level) were recorded on admission, but there appears to be no record of any further readings. Furthermore, there are only two recordings of his blood glucose levels. Very high blood glucose levels could be fatal if they are not detected and treated. Mr Jennings is already unconscious and could lapse further into a coma and die.

After spending one and a half hours in the EAU, Mr Jennings is due to be transferred to the ward for close observation. The nurse receiving him on to the ward is extremely unhappy about his lack of documentation. She feels very strongly and intends to complain about the poor record-keeping and its consequences for the patient.

Introduction

Consider the above scenario and reflect on your reactions to it. It clearly demonstrates a case of poor record-keeping by the nurses caring for Mr Jennings in the EAU. Important information is omitted, such as how much and when insulin was given. There is no record of intravenous fluids being given, and there is only one recording of the patient's vital signs and consciousness level. It is imperative that such observations are recorded in a patient who is dehydrated and in a shocked state, as potentially the patient's condition could deteriorate rapidly and he could die.

Good record-keeping, whether written or computer-based, is essential for all nursing care given to any patient. Accurate records give direction to the care and treatment a patient receives and help to ensure that all members of the interdisciplinary team give coordinated and unfragmented care. Making and keeping records is an integral part of care and its provision. This chapter considers all the aspects of record-keeping, including the purpose of keeping records, the legal aspects, the types of nursing documentation available, and the use of information technology and electronic records.

LEARNING OBJECTIVES

By the end of this chapter you will be able to:

1. Show an awareness of the purpose of keeping records
2. Discuss the legal aspects of record-keeping in relation to the Nursing and Midwifery Council (NMC) and show an understanding of the importance of accountability and confidentiality when keeping records
3. Outline the various forms of nursing documentation
4. Consider the emergence of electronic records and the impact of information technology in healthcare
5. Show an understanding of the standards for record-keeping and the essential elements set out by the NMC
6. Explain what is meant by regulation and outline the Code of Professional Conduct

Overview of record-keeping

Good written or computer-based record-keeping is essential for all nursing care given to any patient. It encourages effective communication between healthcare professionals and provides a record of all the care given to a patient in a healthcare environment. Records are legal documents and are open to scrutiny by any legal organisation. Consequently, it is of paramount importance that all records are an accurate report of individual patient care. Since the introduction of the Patient's Charter (Department of Health, 1991), there has been a shift of attitudes within the nursing profession towards the importance of good record-keeping (Rodden and Bell, 2002). The Charter promotes the importance of patients' rights, including the right of patients and relatives to be involved in their care. More recently, this has been endorsed by Patient Focus and Public Involvement (Scottish Executive, 2001). This partnership approach has led to an increase in patients and relatives questioning the nursing and medical professions about their treatment and care. Consequently, comprehensive and robust complaints procedures have been developed by healthcare trusts.

All healthcare organisations have policies and protocols for the recording and reporting of patient data, and every nurse is accountable for practising within these established standards. At all times, the nurse is accountable for the care they give to the patient. If there are errors in this care, then an explanation is warranted; if the nurse has not recorded information correctly, then they may have to explain why the errors occurred to the NMC or a court of law. As Dr Ashton, medical director at BMI Healthcare stated: 'We live in a blame culture and there is an attitude of "Something bad happened to me – therefore it must be someone's fault".' Dr Ashton warned nurses that the only 'bullet-proof' way of defending themselves against legal wranglings is by faultless record-keeping (Gooding, 2004). For most nurses involved in legal proceedings, nursing records are the most crucial defence, with cases being won or lost based on the quality of the documentation. Case study 10.1 outlines how poor record-keeping led to a court case (Oxtoby, 2004).

Case Study 10.1

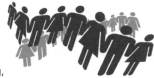

A nurse admitted a 45-year-old man for a **cholecystectomy**. The admission process was carried out correctly. The next morning, the same nurse was on duty and was responsible for the immediate preoperative preparation and providing the patient with a pair of anti-embolism stockings. The record does not show whether she measured the patient or the size of stocking she selected.

The patient had the operation. The following morning, the patient complained of a sore heel to the same nurse. Later, he alleged that the nurse did not remove the stockings or look at his heel. He described the ward as very busy. Two days later, the patient had a black heel (due to the stocking reducing the blood flow to the heel), which led to tissue loss and scarring.

The patient complained while in hospital but did not receive a satisfactory answer from the chief executive of the hospital. The patient then visited a solicitor, who investigated the case.

During the investigation, the nurse admitted that the team had been very busy. She said she had routinely measured the patient but had not recorded this. The nurse stressed that it was normal practice to remove the stockings each day and to wash and check patients' feet. She insisted that if she had not done this, she would have told the nurses at handover to do it. There was no record of this on the handover, however, and no evidence that it had been done.

What do you think was the outcome of this case?

The trust settled out of court for £35 000. It would appear, from the evidence presented, that no one had checked the patient's heel: the heel was black but no changes to the heel had been reported. This case study clearly demonstrates that without record-keeping, the nurse had no defence, even though she claimed that she had checked the patient's heel.

The nurse and all the trust's healthcare staff were sent on a retraining programme to ensure that all patients were measured correctly for their stockings and that this was recorded in the notes.

Cholecystectomy is removal of the gallbladder.

This case is an example of the health and financial costs of inadequate record-keeping, both to the patient and the trust. If the case had not been settled out of court, the costs incurred probably would have been even greater.

Inadequate record-keeping impacts upon the patient in many ways, including the following (Nursing and Midwifery Council, 2004a):

+ If medication or other treatment is not recorded, it may be duplicated or omitted.
+ Continuity of care between shifts and different nursing staff can be impaired if accurate records are not maintained.
+ There can be a breakdown in communication between staff if all care and treatment is not recorded, ultimately leading to patients receiving fragmented care.
+ Significant observations and conclusions can be missed if they are not recorded on the patient's observation chart, leading to a delay or omission in the giving of necessary treatment or care.
+ Failure to detect early signs of deterioration in a patient's condition can occur if vital signs are not recorded correctly. This can have serious outcomes for the patient, such as cardiac or respiratory arrest.

Communication flaws were cited as one of the major contributory factors in investigations into complaints and legal proceedings (Wilson, 2001). Poor communication was one of the main reasons for the record number of complaints reported by the Health Service Ombudsman in July 2006. This report criticised nurses' record-keeping and found that in some instances they had failed to detail adequate planning for the patient, record observations properly, or maintain accurate documentation (Oxtoby, 2004).

It has been suggested that many nurses consider the skill of record-keeping to be second to other clinical skills (Rodden and Bell, 2002). Very often, nurses have difficulty striking a balance between meeting the needs of clinical practice and management and administration (Currell et al., 2000). Nurses may feel that they do not have enough time to address both patient care and administration; the delivery of care to patients in clinical practice can be perceived to be a greater priority than recording the care given. However, recording of patient care should be viewed not as an administrative task but as an integral part of the holistic care package. Whatever the pressures of the job, maintaining accurate, up-to-date patient records is an essential part of nursing practice.

To think about

When you are next in practice, think about the priority you and your colleagues give to record-keeping. Is it seen as an integral part of nursing care or as a chore to be done at the end of a shift or before the nursing report is given?

Purpose of records

This section considers the main reasons why patient records are produced and kept.

Communication

Patient records serve as a basis by which all healthcare professionals who interact with patients can communicate with each other. This ensures that important information is passed on to all healthcare professionals caring for an individual patient. For example, any change in the patient's vital signs should be recorded and reported to the nurse in charge, who can then convey this information to the doctor. When planning a patient's discharge, the nurse needs information about the patient's home circumstances, so that continuing care can be planned accordingly.

Information, problem-solving and planning care

Records should provide accurate, current, comprehensive and concise information regarding the condition and care of the patient and their associated observations. These can then provide a baseline record against which any improvement or deterioration may be judged. For example, it is important to know the patient's vital signs at previous stages during care in order to notice any changes that could be significant to their health. Any problems that the patient encounters should be noted in the patient's records and appropriate action taken. The medical and nursing teams need to be aware of any changes in a patient's problems in order to decide what treatment and care the patient needs.

When deciding whether a patient is fit for discharge, it is imperative that any problems have been dealt with, otherwise this could result in a later re-admission. There should be a record of any physical, psychological and social factors that appear to affect the patient; such factors should not only be recorded in the patient's notes but also should be acted upon in order to ensure a satisfactory outcome for the patient while receiving care.

Healthcare professionals use data from the patient's records to plan the patient's care. This helps them to identify any problems that the patient has and what nursing interventions are needed to deal with those problems. For example, if a patient is experiencing some problems with breathing, nursing care will be planned around helping to relieve the breathing problems; the patient may be encouraged to sit upright as this assists with expansion of the chest and improves breathing. Medication may be prescribed to help assist the patient's breathing. The patient's respirations will be recorded at regular intervals to detect any changes in the breathing pattern. The colour of the patient will also be noted to indicate adequate gaseous exchange and to determine whether oxygen therapy is required. Once this care has been planned and administered, nurses can use baseline and ongoing data to evaluate the effectiveness of the nursing care plan – in other words, to determine whether the planned care has been effective in dealing with the patient's problem and if not then to review and change the care.

Education

Nursing and medical students and students from other health disciplines often use patients' records as an educational tool. The records can provide a comprehensive view of the patient, the illness, the treatment given and any factors affecting the outcome of the illness. However, it is important that confidentiality is maintained at all times, since patient records hold all information pertaining to the person's physical and psychological health. Students with access to patient information are bound by a strict ethical code to hold all information in confidence. This aspect of confidentiality and accountability is discussed in more detail later in this chapter.

Research

Information contained in records can be a valuable source of data for research studies. For example, the treatment plans for a number of patients with the same health problems can yield information helpful in treating other patients. Patients' records also provide the basis for research to support the care and treatment prescribed. The same aspects of confidentiality apply as for students (see above).

Evidence of care and chronology of events

Documentation provides the evidence of care required by the patient, along with the necessary intervention by healthcare professionals and the patient's responses to care given. On admission, the nurse should obtain essential information to provide this evidence of care. In other words, the records need to contain evidence of the ways in which a patient has been assessed and with what, if any, tools. For example, if a patient is admitted to the ward with abdominal pain, the nurse and doctor need to know the type and severity of the pain and whether the patient has taken anything to relieve it. The pain should be assessed using a pain assessment chart and a record made of any analgesia given and whether it was effective; this helps the nurse and doctor in deciding which analgesia is most appropriate to relieve the patient's pain.

Records are evidence of what has been done, when and why. They provide a chronology of events and the reasons for any decisions made in relation to the care given. This is important if the patient's records are ever revisited for legal reasons in relation to a complaint. All care given should be recorded accurately and any subsequent changes duly noted, along with the rationale for these changes. It is important to record any treatment or care given as soon as possible, as this helps to ensure documentation is up to date.

Recap Questions

1. Why do we keep records?
2. What should the nurse remember when recording any information?

Legal aspects of record-keeping

It is worth exploring why cases are taken to court in the first instance. Cases arise mainly following a complaint from either the patient or their relatives about some aspect of the care they received. The care may not have been adequate or mistakes may have been made that resulted in bad or even fatal consequences. If an investigation is instigated to explore all the issues related to the case, this could lead to the hospital or healthcare agency being sued for large amounts of money and resulting in bad publicity.

With this in mind, it is important for nurses to realise that any record documenting patient care may be used as evidence by a court or as part of an investigation or complaints procedure, at a local level, at an NMC hearing or for criminal proceedings, depending on the severity of the case (Rodden and Bell, 2002). Generally, nursing staff provide the majority of patient care and therefore have more entries on the patient's record. Nursing documentation should give an accurate and comprehensive account of patient care and therefore has the potential to inform the process of any enquiry. Generally in a court of law, most lawyers think that poor records mean a poor defence, while no records mean no defence. In other words, for legal purposes, it is assumed that if it is not recorded, then it did not happen.

Cases can take many years to come to court and therefore good and accurate record-keeping is essential for the recollection of events surrounding the case, i.e. the chronology of events (see above). If nurses are discredited by poor record-keeping, they may be discredited as professionals and the nursing profession may be viewed in a negative way (Rodden and Bell, 2002).

In order to avoid such situations, the NMC points out that all qualified nurses have both a professional and a legal duty of care when recording any aspect of patient care. Consequently, nurses' record-keeping should demonstrate the following (Nursing and Midwifery Council, 2006a):

✢ A full account of the assessment and care that has been planned and given

✢ Relevant information about the condition of the patient at any given time

✢ Measures taken by the nurse to respond to the patient's needs

✢ Evidence that the nurse has understood and honoured their duty of care – that is, that all reasonable steps have been taken to care for the patient and that any actions or omissions on the part of the nurse have not compromised the patient's safety in any way

✢ A record of any arrangements that have been made for the continuing care of the patient

To think about

Have a look at some patient records when you are next in practice. Are they written in a way that they are accurate and could be used successfully in a court of law/NMC hearing? If not, then think about why not. Discuss your findings with a colleague and identify ways the records could be improved. Also look for some examples of good record-keeping and determine what makes them good. Again, share your ideas with a colleague.

Case study 10.2 outlines a case presented to the Professional Conduct Committee (PCC) of the NMC in 2006.

Case Study 10.2

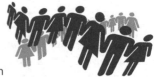

A registered mental health nurse (RMN) was working at a residential home for elderly mentally ill patients. He worked full time on night duty. Being the only trained member of staff on night duty, he was in charge of the night shift and the drug keys. Drug audits were carried out on a weekly basis and revealed a number of discrepancies in relation to the 2200 hours drug round at night and the 0800 hours drug round in the morning. The RMN could not explain why the records showed that some of the residents had not received their important medication for diabetes and severe pain.

What do you think happened next?

The RMN was found guilty of misconduct. He had admitted the charges and was found to be in direct contradiction of the NMC's Code of Professional Conduct. He had failed to give pre-scribed medication and therefore had not complied with this aspect of the Code. Second, and more relevant to this chapter, the RMN had failed to record that medication had not been given and thus he had failed to comply with the NMC's standards for records and record-keeping.

The RMN had previously been given verbal and written warnings for three disciplinary matters. On one of the occasions he was verbally cautioned for not disposing of medication appropriately, and on two separate occasions he had been given verbal and written warnings for drinking alcohol on duty.

The chair of the PCC announced that the PCC had decided to remove the RMN's name from the Register, with immediate effect. The RMN was found guilty of two charges:

+ Failure to administer prescribed medication
+ Failure to record that medication had not been given

To think about

What do your think of the PCC's decision? Do you think the PCC made the right decision? What sort of things did the PCC need to consider in this case? You may wish to discuss this case with your nursing colleagues and find out what they think.

The PCC and Fitness to Practice Panel consider many such cases. Extra funds have been made available to deal with a backlog of cases. In 2005-06 there were 370 cases waiting for hearing, with cases continuing to increase by an average of 22 each month (Nursing and Midwifery Council, 2006b). It is concerning that cases of misconduct are on the increase; however, it could be that healthcare professionals and patients feel increasingly that it is important to deal with examples of poor or dangerous practices appropriately, and conse-quently complaints about care have increased.

Accountability

Accountability applies directly to the process of record-keeping. The term 'accountable' means to be responsible for one's own actions and the subsequent outcomes of such actions. The term 'answerable' is also used to capture the essence of accountability. Nurses are answerable for the consequences of what they do in relation to patient care. The implications of such actions could lead to a trained nurse being removed from the Register if the actions result in death or damage to any patient they have nursed, as outlined in Case study 10.2. Nurses need to be clear about the reasons for any nursing actions taken and be able to explain any decisions made. The explanations should be based on sound knowledge and understanding of the ration-ale for actions taken rather than anecdotal 'This is how we have always done it' comments.

To think about

To whom do you think the nurse is accountable? Do you think accountability is important? You may like to discuss these issues with your work colleagues.

To whom is the nurse accountable?

Accountability in nursing is an essential part of professional practice, as the registered nurse frequently has to make decisions in a wide range of circumstances. The nurse is professionally accountable to four parties: the public, the patient, the employer and the profession. Each of these parties is protected by different parts of the law; for example, the public and the patient are protected by both criminal and civil law. (To simplify the issue of the patient and the public, they can be viewed as one party, since the patient is technically a member of the public.)

How does accountability relate to the law?

The nurse is accountable to criminal and civil law, just like any other citizen. Therefore, the nurse will answer to criminal law when there is an allegation that a crime has been committed. If there is evidence of negligence involving the care of a patient, such that the nurse is seen to have fallen below the legal standard of care and the patient wishes to take action, then this would be in a civil court rather than a criminal court. For negligence to exist, three factors must be present: a duty of care, a breach of that duty of care, and a direct foreseeable harm to the patient. Negligence refers to not only physical harm but also psychological harm.

Accountability to the employer

The nurse is accountable to the employer because when the nurse accepts the offer of a post, a contract comes into existence and the nurse is bound by its terms. The employer expects the nurse to be accountable for their own actions at all times. Any breaches in the contract of employment may be considered by an industrial tribunal (Semple and Cable, 2003).

Accountability to the nursing profession

The NMC regulates the nursing profession in order to protect the public and all registered professionals. It protects the public by setting standards for the education, training and professional conduct of all registered practitioners. Each individual qualified nurse is expected to work within a set of standards required by the whole profession. These standards are set out in the Code of Professional Conduct (Nursing and Midwifery Council, 2004b) and are discussed in more detail later in this chapter.

Consider Case study 10.3 and reflect on your reactions to it. Discuss it with your colleagues and find out their views.

Case Study 10.3

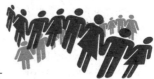

Miss Gloria Brown is a 38-year-old Afro-Caribbean woman admitted with **sickle cell anaemia**. She requires a blood transfusion. Regular monitoring of Miss Brown's vital signs every quarter of an hour is required in order to ensure that the blood is transfused safely.

Following the handover report, Student Nurse Parkes is asked to look after Miss Brown for the afternoon shift. She looks at the observation chart and discovers that Miss Brown's vital signs have not been recorded for the past one and a half hours and that the first and current second units of blood have not been recorded on the fluid balance chart. She reports these findings to the nurse in charge.

What do you think should be done?
What could be the consequences of these omissions?

> **Sickle cell anaemia** is a type of anaemia that occurs mainly in Afro-Caribbean people. The red blood cells form a sickle shape, which causes the blood to become more viscous. This can lead to clot formation in the blood.

Clearly this situation is not acceptable. Student Nurse Parkes did the right thing by reporting the omissions to the nurse in charge, who is ultimately accountable for all care given while on duty. It will be necessary to investigate the incident to identify who was responsible, and therefore accountable, for Miss Brown's care in the earlier shift. A full explanation will be required to establish why the vital signs were not recorded and why the units of blood were not written on the fluid balance chart. Miss Brown could have had a reaction to the blood transfusion and this would not have been detected. This is very unsafe practice and the nurses responsible for the omissions would have to provide statements indicating why Miss Brown's vital signs were not recorded and why the units of blood were not on the fluid balance chart. In this instance, all the nurses caring for Miss Brown would be accountable for their actions to the patient, their employer and their profession. Such an incident could be reported to the NMC, and the professionals involved could find themselves in front of the PCC or Fitness to Practice Panel.

Confidentiality

When discussing accountability, the issue of confidentiality needs to be addressed. Nurses have access to all personal information on the patients they come into contact with. A breach of confidentiality occurs if anyone employed by a trust or other agency with access to patient information divulges either deliberately or accidentally any information concerning a patient without the patient's or guardian's consent. It is vital that nurses never discuss any patient details with anyone not directly involved in the care and treatment of the patients.

Recap Questions

1. Why does the nurse need to be aware of the legal aspects of record-keeping?
2. What is meant by the term 'accountability'?
3. To whom is the nurse accountable?

Nursing documentation

The patient's records should reflect the patient's ongoing care and treatment and include the full range of the nursing process, including assessment, nursing diagnosis, and planning, implementing and evaluating care. Information is documented on a variety of forms, some of which are outlined in Exhibit 10.1. You may see additional assessment tools in use that are not mentioned here. The different forms are:

+ Admission assessment forms
+ Nursing care plans
+ Flow charts
+ Progress/evaluation forms
+ Nursing discharge/referral forms

+ Admission assessment form (Figure 10.1)

Name _____	GP _____
Address _____	Next of kin _____
Postal code _____	Allergies _____
	Past medical history _____

Observations   T.   P.   R.   BP. _____

Identification of problems - Roper model

	Problem		Problem
Breathing		Washing and Dressing	
Eating and Drinking		Spiritual/Religious	
Mobilising		Circulation	
Eliminating		Expressing Sexuality	
Sleeping		Working and Playing	
Communication		Pain	

Figure 10.1 Admission assessment form

+ Nursing care plan (Figure 10.2)

Patient problem	Aim of care	Nursing intervention/care prescribed	Outcome

Figure 10.2 Nursing care plan

+ Flow charts – recording vital signs, fluid balance, nutrition, pressure area care, medication sheets, etc. (Figure 10.3)

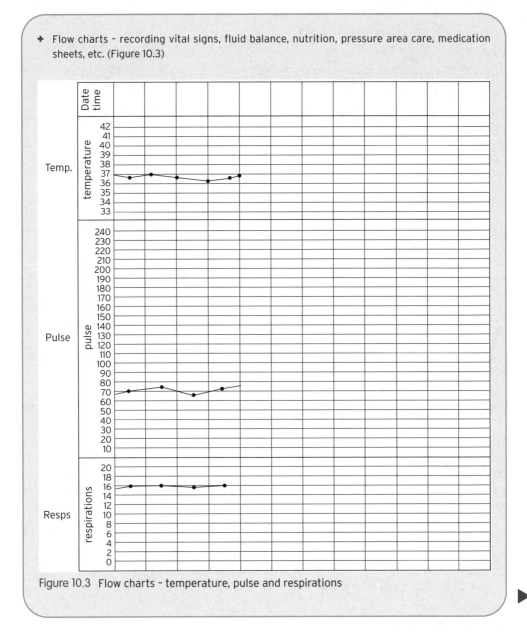

Figure 10.3 Flow charts – temperature, pulse and respirations

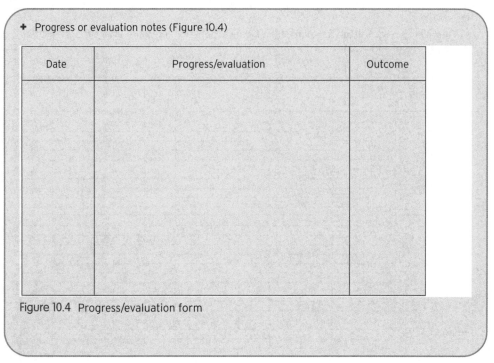

Figure 10.4 Progress/evaluation form

Exhibit 10.1 Nursing documentation

Admission nursing assessment

The nurse needs to carry out an initial comprehensive admission assessment when the patient has settled in after arriving on the ward. This assessment includes a full nursing history and a complete nursing assessment. The admission form can be organised according to body systems, functional abilities, health problems and risks, nursing model and type of healthcare setting (e.g. labour ward, paediatrics, mental health). Some nursing assessment forms use a nursing model such as that of Roper and colleagues (1990) as a framework on which the nurse can base their questions. It is useful to identify any problems that the patient has, such as difficulty with walking, problems with eating due to poorly fitting dentures, or problems with sleeping. Once a detailed nursing assessment has been carried out, the appropriate care can be planned.

Nursing care plans

The patient should have a care plan following the initial assessment. This usually incorporates nursing diagnoses and/or patient needs, nursing interventions, patient outcomes and evaluation. This process is formally known as the 'nursing process' and involves identifying the patient's problems and deciding what care is needed to address these problems. It is important to set outcomes by which the care prescribed can be evaluated and the care changed if necessary. All the essential information is set out in a nursing care plan, which is usually kept separate from the patient's charts and may be filed with the patient's progress notes or incorporated into a multidisciplinary plan of care or **patient pathway**. The main reason for keeping this information separate is related to maintaining patient confidentiality: if the patient's care plan containing all personal information is placed at the end of the bed, then anyone on the ward can access it. Having said that, some clinical areas display the plan of care in order to remind the nurses what care the patient needs, and then file away any confidential information.

Generally, there are two types of care plan: traditional and standardised. The traditional care plan is written for each individual patient. A record is made of the patient's problems and the appropriate nursing care prescribed. In order to save time in writing out a full individual care plan, the standardised care plan was developed. This includes a set of specific problems that are generally associated with a particular condition or surgical intervention. For example, for a patient undergoing surgery, the potential problems that may occur include **asphyxia**, haemorrhage and pain; by using a standardised care plan, the nurse does not need to write out these problems for each patient, consequently saving the nurse time on a busy surgical ward. However, the plan of care must still be individualised to ensure the individual's needs are addressed by adding them on to the standard care plan.

Flow charts/sheets

A flow chart allows the nurse to record nursing data quickly and concisely and provides an easy-to-read record of the patient's condition over time. Various charts are available, including the following:

+ *Graphic record*: this records body temperature, pulse, respiratory rate, blood pressure, weight and other significant data related to the patient's condition, such as bowel movements and appetite.

+ *Fluid balance record*: all routes of fluid intake and output are measured and recorded on this chart.

+ *Medication administration record*: all details of any medication given are recorded here, including the name and dose of the medication, the frequency of administration, the route and the nurse's signature.

+ *Pressure area/nutrition assessment record*: these provide information about the patient's nutritional status and skin integrity, such as whether the skin is broken or the patient is developing a pressure sore. Any ongoing treatment is also recorded.

+ *Progress/evaluation records*: the nurse makes progress notes relating to the patient care plan and whether the care prescribed is successful. In other words, using these records, the care can be evaluated and changed if necessary, and any further problems identified and added to the nursing care plan.

The **patient pathway** includes all the care the patient receives, from the point of admission to discharge, from all members of the multidisciplinary team.

Asphyxia is blockage of the airway, so that no air can enter the lungs. If not dealt with immediately, the patient dies from lack of oxygen.

Nursing discharge/referral records

These records are completed when the patient is discharged or transferred to another ward or institution. It is important that these documents are completed correctly, with the appropriate information written in understandable terms for the patient and their family if the patient is going home. When possible, records should be written with the patient and their carers present so they are involved in the care process from the start. For example, if the patient has been prescribed a certain treatment or medication, they need to be aware of when and how to take it. Patients often require ongoing care from a district nurse, practice nurse or GP, and therefore discharge information must be accurate and informative.

It is important to ensure that all nursing documentation shows continuity of care - that is, there should be clear links between the nursing care plan, flow charts and discharge/referral records. This is important not only for legal aspects but also to ensure that the patient's care is presented and carried out in a logical, systematic way.

To think about

When you are next in practice, have a look at the different nursing documentation. Is it being used correctly? Is it being referred to when discussing patient care at report time? Discuss your findings with a colleague. Look for good examples of completed nursing documentation and compare them with poorer examples.

Electronic patient records

Many nurses are now using information technology (IT) to record the planning, assessment and delivery of care. The same standards that apply to manual records also apply to computer-held records.

The NHS has tended to lag behind other public and private organisations in the adoption of IT, particularly in clinical areas. The DH has supported a National Project for Information Technology (NPFIT), resulting in a complete technical infrastructure being developed with data dictionaries (providing a source of terminology and common health language for medicines and devices used in healthcare) in the UK. Interestingly, computer training was one of the top ten priorities in the *Nursing Times'* 'nurses plan' (Munro, 2002). However, a more recent survey of more than 4000 nurses from across the UK found that 69% of nurses had not received any IT training at work (Royal College of Nursing, 2006), and so it would appear that more training is needed.

The government's ambitious plan to provide IT in healthcare is also lagging behind (Davidson, 2003). The government's target of each patient having an electronic health record by March 2005 has not been achieved. This is due partly to funding but also to the great need to train staff and to solve compatibility problems between hospital and primary care systems (Cooper, 2003).

A survey of RCN members (Royal College of Nursing, 2007) indicates that the health service needs to communicate more with frontline nurses if it wants them to be ready for the new electronic patient records (EPRs). Only half of the nurses surveyed believed that EPRs will improve patient safety, while a third felt that the security of the system would not be any better than that offered by the current paper records. Two-thirds of the nurses indicated that they had not been consulted about the introduction of EPR. Peter Carter, the RCN General Secretary, said it is vital to engage all nursing staff 'on the important issues of consultation' to help ensure EPR is successful in the field of professional practice.

Advantages of information technology in healthcare

Clinical information and patient records are still maintained on paper throughout most of the NHS. Once all records are held electronically, the NMC believes there will be no requirement to keep manual duplicates. Paper records can be lost easily, and therefore one of the main benefits of electronic records is the storage of information in a way that renders it difficult to lose. Furthermore, if all information is recorded and stored in one place, this enables all healthcare professionals, in different locations, to share and have direct access to the patient's information. Appointments for patients can also be made electronically; consequently, patients should be seen, diagnosed and treated more quickly and efficiently (Department of Health, 2000).

If necessary, patients can be given access to their electronic medical records. Information can be accessed easily for the purposes of clinical governance and risk management purposes, and practitioners could be updated on clinical developments quickly.

Potential disadvantages of information technology in healthcare

As with most new systems, there may be potential problems with using IT in healthcare. The systems used must be compatible between different clinical areas, in particular between primary and secondary care, so that information can be transferred easily between hospitals and GP practices. When developing an NHS-wide IT system, there are certain potential problems that need to be addressed:

+ The system must ensure that patient confidentiality cannot be breached
+ The system should be easy to use but sophisticated enough to meet the requirements of a range of healthcare professionals
+ There should be contingency plans to ensure that services can still function if system failure occurs

It is worth noting that the principles of confidentiality of information are equally important for computer-held records as for other records. Nurses are professionally accountable for ensuring that the system is fully secure. Clear local protocols will be available to specify which staff should have access to computer-held records.

Recap Questions

1. What are the different types of nursing documentation?
2. Why is it important to maintain continuity regarding all nursing documentation?
3. What are the advantages of using electronic patient records?

Standards for record-keeping

The NMC has set out important standards for nurses to follow when producing patient records. This section considers these standards in detail.

Principles of good record-keeping

The NMC believes that a number of key principles underpin good record-keeping, some of which relate to legal issues as discussed earlier and others of which relate to the content and style of the record. Consider Case study 10.4.

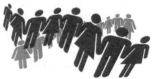

Case Study 10.4

You are new to the ward and have been asked to look after four patients. You decide to look at these patients' records to familiarise yourself with their care. After reading through the care plans, you decide to introduce yourself to your patients, but you are surprised to find that one of them has gone home for the weekend. You glean this information from another patient. There is no mention of weekend leave in the patient's care plan or case notes.

What would you do next?

Important information has been omitted from the 'missing' patient's records, and you need to discuss this with the nurse in charge. Omission of information is related to the content of the records, which should give an accurate account of patient care and other aspects related to the patient. Care study 10.4 shows an example of poor record-keeping, as important information has not been recorded.

Some of the key features of good record-keeping are as follows:

+ Records should be made as soon as possible after the events to which they relate. This ensures accuracy and prevents loss or distortion of facts due to problems with memory and recall. It also provides current information on the care and condition of the patient.

+ Records should identify any factors that may jeopardise standards or place the patient at risk. For example, if the patient has or is at risk of developing a pressure sore, then a record must be made so that the nursing staff are aware and can employ measures to reduce the risk of the problem or prescribe the appropriate care. Similarly, if a nutritional assessment reveals that the patient is malnourished or at risk of falling, then this should be recorded and acted upon.

+ Records should provide evidence for the need, in certain circumstances, for input from specialist practitioners.

+ Records should be factual, consistent and accurate. There is no need to record personal opinions about the patient, as these provide only unnecessary subjective data.

+ Records should assist the patient's involvement in their own care. The NMC stipulates that the patient should be an equal partner, whenever possible, in their own care. This means the patient should have access to records such as their care plan and be encouraged to discuss their care with the nurse on a regular basis.

+ Records should be written, wherever possible, with the involvement of the patient or their carer. This helps to ensure that the patient and the carer are aware of the care needed, which can improve cooperation and outcome of care.

+ Records should be written, where possible, in terms that the patient can understand.

Consider Case study 10.5 and reflect on your reactions to it. Discuss with your fellow students or work colleagues what you think the outcome should be. What decision would you make if you were a member of the PCC committee considering this case?

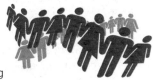

Case Study 10.5

Mrs Gregg is a 72-year-old woman with acute myeloblastic leukaemia. She is terminally ill, has a problem with blood clotting and is at risk of infection. She is in a debilitated state and is taking a limited diet and fluids. She is developing swollen ankles due to poor circulation, but her skin is intact. She is to be assessed for risk of pressure sores.

As Mrs Gregg is in her own home, the district nurse visits to carry out the assessment. The district nurse completes Mrs Gregg's pressure area assessment score. The district nurse knows that a certain mattress is available and consequently adapts the patient's pressure area assessment score to fit this particular mattress's requirements. Because Mrs Gregg was not given the type of mattress she really needed, she developed several pressure sores.

What do you think was the outcome of this case?

Mrs Gregg's relatives submitted a formal complaint to the NMC. The nurse in question was given a written warning (recorded in the nurse's record of employment) for falsifying a patient's records and was asked to attend several education sessions on pressure area care, with particular reference to assessment. Do you consider this to be the 'right' decision? The nurse had previously had an exemplary record. She said she was under a lot of stress and felt quite pressurised to give Mrs Gregg the mattress in question, as she knew it was available. She expressed that she was sorry for any pain and discomfort Mrs Gregg had suffered as a consequence of developing pressure sores. Mrs Gregg's relatives accepted the PCC's decision.

We have considered the standards of record-keeping that must be adhered to in order to avoid such incidents as the one outlined in Case study 10.5. We now look at what should be included in a patient's records.

What to include in records

The patient's record is a legal document and therefore may be used to provide evidence in a court of law or NMC inquiry. Consequently, the record needs to be legible, clear and understandable and meet the legal standards in the process of recording. The NMC lists a number of points to consider when completing any documentation. The NMC describes the following as the essential elements of good record-keeping:

> ### To think about
>
> What do your think the essential elements of good record-keeping are? You may like to discuss this with your work colleagues.

+ Records should always be completed correctly, with the correct date and time of the event, procedure or care given. Any additions to existing entries must be individually dated, timed and signed. The signature must be legible.

+ Records should identify problems that have arisen and the actions taken to rectify them. There should be clear evidence of the care planned, the decisions made, the care delivered and the information shared.

+ All handwritten entries must be legible and easy to read. Anything written in error must be scored out with a single black line, initialled, dated and timed correctly. Correcting fluid must not be used.

+ Any information that the nurse has forgotten to include on the record must state the correct date and time followed by a statement such as 'Omitted from yesterday' and signed appropriately.

+ Any additions or existing entries must be individually dated, timed and signed.

+ All entries on records must be made in black ink to ensure permanence and to aid photo-copying.

+ Abbreviations such as 'UTT' ('up to toilet') and meaningless phrases such as 'bath taken' should not be used unless they are followed by more detailed information. Offensive subjective statements not related to the patient's care should not be included in the records; for example, a patient who continually presses their call bell should not be labelled as a 'bell pusher', while a patient who does not participate in their own care should not be described as 'lazy' – the latter may in fact be depressed.

The use of initials for major entries is not acceptable; instead, the nurse must give their signature in full. Some local protocols do allow initials to be used in some cases, but this should be checked before signing.

> ### To think about
>
> When you are next in practice, have a look at some patient records and see whether all the standards we have discussed in this section have been included. If not, why not? Discuss your findings with a colleague.

Exhibit 10.2 summarises the important things to remember when producing patient records. It is worth using this as a checklist when you are next admitting a patient, devising a care plan or recording a patient's observations on a chart.

+ DO record information as you go along. This helps to prevent the build-up of a backlog of paperwork, ensures accuracy and ensures nothing is omitted.
+ DO make sure records are written with the patient where possible, as this helps with accurate perception of events and enhance partnership in care.
+ DO keep records legible. Make sure writing is clear, with any corrections signed and dated and the time noted.
+ DO audit your records regularly and update your training, as it is easy to pick up bad habits.
+ DON'T use abbreviations and jargon. Instead, ensure that everyone involved in care, including patients, can understand what is written.
+ DON'T be subjective or judgemental. Just stick to the facts.
+ DON'T just write. Act! Good record-keeping is more than writing – it is also about acting on what you have written.

Exhibit 10.2 Dos and don'ts of record-keeping
Adapted from Oxtoby (2004)

Code of Professional Conduct

We have referred to the Code of Professional Conduct in several parts of this chapter, and we focus on it here. The Code acts as a means of self-regulating the nursing profession. It has been devised by the NMC in order to protect the public. Each registered nurse is required to work within a set of standards that govern the whole nursing profession. These standards are set out in the Code of Professional Conduct (Nursing and Midwifery Council, 2004b) and are outlined in Exhibit 10.3.

As a registered nurse or midwife, you are personally accountable for your practice. In caring for patients, you must:

+ Respect the patient as an individual
+ Obtain consent before you give any treatment or care
+ Protect confidential information
+ Cooperate with others in the team
+ Maintain your professional knowledge and competence
+ Be trustworthy
+ Act to identify and minimise risk to patients

Exhibit 10.3 Code of Professional Conduct
Adapted from Nursing and Midwifery Council (2004b)

Nurses must adhere to this code when carrying out all forms of record-keeping, as outlined throughout this chapter.

The name of the Code has since been extended to the NMC Code of Professional Conduct: Standards for Conduct, Performance and Ethics. A review of the Code took place in 2006 in order for the Code to keep pace with changing medical and nursing procedures (Nursing and Midwifery Council, 2006c). It is important that nurses realise that the Code is not a constant but is subject to change over time.

In July 2006, the Foster Review set out the DH's radical plans to overhaul the regulation of nurses (Department of Health, 2006). This review could see the profession lose its right to self-regulate, a right that nurses fought to attain over a century ago. A former president of the NMC, Sir Jonathan Asbridge, believes that this would not be a good move for the nursing profession and suggests that fighting the Foster Review should be top of the NMC's agenda.

Recap Questions

1. What are the main standards for record-keeping set by the NMC, and why are they important?
2. What needs to be included in order to ensure good record-keeping?
3. What is the content of the Code of Professional Conduct, and why is it important for nurses to know about the Code when carrying out record-keeping?

Summary

This chapter has considered several aspects of good record-keeping, including the purpose of keeping records and nursing documentation and the standards set by the NMC to help ensure all records are legible, accurate and chronological, with any omissions and amendments addressed.

The important legal aspects of record-keeping have been discussed, with reference to courts of law and the role of the PCC of the NMC in dealing with complaints concerning inaccurate record-keeping. Some cases have been included to illustrate the dire consequences of poor record-keeping. Accountability and confidentiality are related directly to the process of record-keeping. The importance of regulation and adhering to the Code of Professional Conduct when keeping patient records has been discussed.

We have discussed the importance of record-keeping in the day-to-day duties of nurses and whether record-keeping is seen as a priority and an integral part of nursing care or as a secondary task to be completed as an 'add-on' to clinical care.

The adoption of electronic records has been noted, along with the advantages and disadvantages of using IT in healthcare and the effect of electronic records on nursing practice.

The emphasis throughout this chapter has been to highlight the consequences of poor record-keeping, which leads to poor practice. If this chapter has seemed rather negative at times, this is not intentional; rather, we hope to make readers aware of why good record-keeping is essential.

We hope that we are moving away from a blame culture. The NHS is actively trying to replace this approach with the need to learn from mistakes made. Mistakes should be dealt with in a constructive rather than a punitive way; this will encourage the reporting of near-misses, so that nurses and other healthcare professionals can learn from their errors rather than the mistakes remaining hidden and developing into major problems.

The nurse should remember that records must always be an accurate account of the patient's journey while receiving care, whether in a hospital setting or in the community. In the event of a complaint, records provide important evidence that ultimately could affect the nurse's professional future as indicated in the court cases discussed. Do not forget: if it is not recorded, then it didn't happen!

Key Points

1. There are several purposes for keeping patient records, including the provision of information and evidence of care, problem-solving, planning care, education and research.

2. Any patient record documenting patient care could be used to provide evidence in a court of law/NMC inquiry; therefore, the legal aspects of record-keeping are of vital importance.

3. Records should demonstrate a full account of the patient's planned care, relevant information about the patient's condition at any given time, and evidence that the nurse has honoured their duty of care through maintaining accountability and confidentiality.

4. There are several forms of nursing documentation, and it is important that continuity is maintained throughout all this documentation. Patient records are now beginning to be held electronically. This means that clinical information can be stored more efficiently.

5. The NMC has set out important standards for record-keeping, which the nurse must follow. These standards relate mainly to legal issues, the essential elements of good record-keeping, and the content and style of records.

6. The NMC has produced a Code of Professional Conduct, which governs the entire nursing profession. The nurse must adhere to this Code when carrying out all forms of record-keeping.

Points for debate

Now that you have come to the end of this chapter here are a few points that you may wish to think about when you are in practice. You may wish to discuss these with your work colleagues or fellow students.

Many nurses are not always fully aware of the legal and professional implications of poor record-keeping.

Litigation is becoming an occupational hazard in nursing and can result in nurses becoming somewhat complacent about any complaints they receive.

Nurses may have well-written patient records, but do they always act on them.

Links to Other Chapters

Chapter 2 Dignity and privacy
Chapter 3 Basic observations
Chapter 4 Hygiene
Chapter 5 Nutrition
Chapter 6 Fluid balance and continence care
Chapter 9 Rehabilitation and self-care

Further reading

Department of Health website: www.dh.gov.uk

Nursing and Midwifery Council website: www.nmc-uk.org

References

Cooper, K (2003) Electronic records target unlikely. *Nursing Standard* **17**, 7.

Currell, R, Wainwright, P and Urquhart, C (2000) Nursing record systems: effects on nursing practice and health care outcomes. *Cochrane Database Systematic Review* **2**, CD002099.

Davidson, L (2003) Making IT work for you. *Nursing Times Supplement* 6.

Department of Health (1991) *Patient's Charter*. London: The Stationery Office.

Department of Health (2000) *The NHS Plan: A Plan for Investment, a Plan for Reform*. London: The Stationery Office.

Department of Health (2006) *Foster Review: Regulation of Nurses*. London: The Stationery Office.

Gooding, L (2004) A nurse's best defence. *Nursing Standard* **19**, 12.

Munro, R (2002) What we need from Gordon Brown's millions. *Nursing Times* **98**, 10-13.

Nursing and Midwifery Council (2004a) *Guidelines for Records and Record Keeping*. London: Nursing and Midwifery Council.

Nursing and Midwifery Council (2004b) *Code of Professional Conduct*. London: Nursing and Midwifery Council.

Nursing and Midwifery Council (2006a) *A-Z Advice Sheet: Record Keeping*. London: Nursing and Midwifery Council.

Nursing and Midwifery Council (2006b) Backlog of fitness to practice cases. *NMC News* **17**, 15.

Nursing and Midwifery Council (2006c) The NMC code under review: let us know what you think. *NMC News* **14**, 5.

Oxtoby, K (2004) Is your record-keeping up to scratch? *Nursing Times* **100**, 18-20.

Rodden, C and Bell, M (2002) Record keeping: developing good practice. *Nursing Standard* **17**, 40-42.

Roper, N, Logan, W and Tierney, A (1990) *The Elements of Nursing: A Model for Nursing Based on a Model of Living*, 3rd edn. London: Churchill Livingstone.

Royal College of Nursing (2006) Nurses want more from NHS IT plans. *RCN Bulletin* **159**, 1.

Royal College of Nursing (2007) Nurses still unsure over benefits of EPR. *RCN Bulletin* **182**, 1.

Scottish Executive (2001) *Patient Focus and Public Involvement*. Edinburgh: Scottish Executive.

Semple, M and Cable, S (2003) The new Code of Professional Conduct. *Nursing Standard* **17**, 40-48.

Wilson, J (2001) Risk management in documentation and communication. *Health Care Risk* **September**, 17-19.

Index

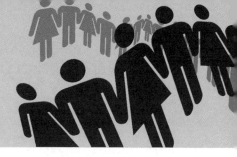

abuse
  assessment process, 21
  dignity and privacy, 40–51
    confidentiality, 50
    discrimination, 47
    financial abuse, 44–5
    indicators of abuse, 47–9
    institutional abuse, 47
    managing disclosure, 51
    neglect, 46–7
    overview, 40–1
    physical abuse, 42–3
    preventing abuse, 42, 49–50
    psychological abuse, 43–4
    sexual abuse, 45–6
    summary, 52
    what is abuse?, 41–2
accountability, 95, 228, 229, 284, 286,
      297, 302
acetate, 125
Action on Elder Abuse, 42, 43, 48, 50
activities of daily living, 93, 261
acupuncture, 198, 227
acute incontinence, 168, 171
acute lymphatic leukaemia, 243
acute pain, 205
addiction to opioids, 212, 217–18, 230
ADH see antidiuretic hormone
adrenal cortex, 152
afferent neurons, 197–8, 199
Age Concern, 4, 7, 9, 35, 93, 274
alcohol, 81, 107, 119, 125
aldosterone, 152
Allitt, Beverley, 32
alternative therapies, 225–9, 230
alveoli, 68, 69
amino acids, 119
analgesia
  administration of analgesia, 218–22
  analgesic ladder, 224–5, 230

efficacy of analgesia, 222–4
  non-opioid analgesics, 215–16
  opioid analgesics, 217–18
  overview, 193, 214, 215
  pain assessment, 200
  pain perception, 208, 209, 210, 211, 212
  record-keeping, 287
  summary, 229–30
angiotensin II, 152
anorexia nervosa, 125, 126
antibiotics, 112
anticholinergic medication, 160, 174
antidiuretic hormone (ADH), 152, 163
antiemetics, 159
anuria, 164
aphasia, 37
apical pulse, 60, 62, 63, 64
apnoea, 72
Aristotle, 194
aromatherapy, 227
arrhythmia, 65
Asbridge, Sir Jonathan, 302
asphyxia, 295
aspiration, 138, 139, 142
aspirin, 216
assessment process, 18–24, 42, 94–5
asthma, 73, 74
atonic bladder, 170
atonic colon, 186
atrial fibrillation, 65
Attendance Allowance, 45
audit, 9, 11
Audit Commission, 127
autism, 41
autonomic nervous system, 81, 202, 206
axilla temperature, 83, 84–5

Balance of Good Health Plate model, 123–4,
      136, 143
balanced diet, 122

basal metabolic rate (BMR), 79, 80, 124
basic observations, 56-90
   importance of, 57-9
   introduction, 56-7
   pulse, 59-68
   respirations, 68-77
   summary, 87-8
   temperature, 77-87
bed-bathing, 102-4
benchmarking
   dignity and privacy, 30-1, 32, 34, 38, 52
   hygiene, 94, 96
   quality of care, 10, 11, 12-15
   rehabilitation nursing, 269
benign prostatic hyperplasia, 170
betel quid, 107
Better Hospital Food project, 130, 131, 132
bile acids, 121
bladder, 161, 162, 163, 171, 174
blood gas analysis, 74, 75
blood glucose, 86
BMR see basal metabolic rate
body mass index (BMI), 127-8, 135, 136, 143
body weight, 124-5, 127-30, 136, 149, 240
bolus, 219
brachial pulse, 62, 63
bradycardia, 64, 65, 68
bradypnoea, 72, 73
breakthrough pain, 216, 224
Bristol stool chart, 181, 182
bronchoconstriction, 74
buprenorphine, 217, 221

calorific value, 124
cancer, 107, 128, 181, 201, 206-7, 216, 224, 229
cannulation, 159
carbohydrates, 118-19, 123, 124
cardiac arrest, 59
cardiac output, 60
cardiotonics, 61
care plans, 24, 96, 250, 292, 294-5, 299
care programme approach, 20, 21
caring, 1-26
   assessment process, 18-24
   dignity and privacy, 32-3
   introduction, 1
   quality of care, 9-18
   summary, 24

what do we mean by 'caring'?, 2-8
Caring Model™, 8, 28
carotid pulse, 62, 63
carpal tunnel syndrome, 33
Carter, Peter, 297
catalysis, 121
catheters, 172, 174, 176, 177-81
central nervous system (CNS), 196, 217
central venous pressure (CVP), 156
cerebral vascular accident (CVA) see stroke
CHAI see Commission for Health Audit
   Improvement
Cheyne-Stokes respiration, 72, 73
children, 24, 41, 70, 80, 153, 163, 249
Children's Act (1989), 24
cholecystectomy, 284
chronic incontinence, 169-70
chronic obstructive pulmonary disease, 74, 75
chronic pain, 205, 206-7
Climbie, Victoria, 21
clinical governance, 9, 10, 11-12, 297
clinical practice benchmarking see
   benchmarking
clinical supervision, 17-18
CNS see central nervous system
Code of Professional Conduct (NMC), 40,
   228, 229, 289, 290, 301-2
codeine, 217, 224
Commission for Health Audit Improvement
   (CHAI), 9
Commission for Patient and Public
   Involvement in Health, 132
common assessment framework, 20, 21
communication, 19, 36-40, 52
comorbidities, 141
compassion, 32-3, 34, 52
complaints, 10-11, 36, 265, 283-5, 287, 289,
   299, 302
complementary therapies, 225-9, 230
complete proteins, 119
compression stockings, 104-5, 284
conduction, 79, 80
conduction system, 65
confidentiality, 50, 51, 286-7, 291, 295, 297,
   301, 302
constipation, 183-6, 187, 188
continence care, 160-89 see also fluid balance
   catheter care, 177-81

dignity and privacy, 31-2
incontinence, 165-72
overview, 147-8
problems with elimination of faeces, 181-8
promoting continence, 173-7
summary, 188-9
urinary continence, 160-5
Control of Substances Hazardous to Health (COSHH), 112
convection, 79, 80
core temperature, 78, 81
court cases, 284, 287, 288, 302
COX see cyclo-oxygenase
Crede manoeuvre, 171-2
critical care outreach teams, 58
crutches, 274
culture, 35-6, 125, 126, 195, 209-10, 212, 213, 276-7
CVA (cerebral vascular accident) see stroke
CVP see central venous pressure
cyanosis, 66, 76
cyclo-oxygenase (COX), 215

Death by Indifference (Mencap), 6
decontaminating equipment, 111-12
deep vein thrombosis, 104
dehydration, 142, 147, 153, 158, 159, 240
dementia, 39, 104, 168, 242
dentures, 106, 107, 128
Department of Health (DH), 5, 12, 22, 28, 175, 200, 262, 269, 296, 301
depression, 125, 126, 209, 210, 238, 240
Descartes, René, 194, 195, 196
detrusor muscle, 162, 163, 171
DH see Department of Health
diabetes, 86, 128, 164, 253, 263, 282
diaphragm, 70
diarrhoea, 186-8
dignity and privacy, 27-55
communication, 36-40
continence care, 189
culturally sensitive healthcare, 35-6
dignity in care, 28-34
hygiene, 98
introduction, 27
pressure ulcers, 237
protecting individuals from abuse, 40-51
summary, 51-2

'Dignity on the Ward' campaign, 6
Dignity Security Opportunity, 35
Dingman, Sharon, 8, 28
disability, 41, 99, 258, 259-61, 271, 275
discrimination, 35, 47, 53
disinfection, 111-12
distraction, 198, 226
diuresis, 158
diuretics, 158, 163
DLCs (disabled living centres), 271
Dobson, Frank, 6
Donaldson, Sir Liam, 11
dorsalis pedis pulse, 62, 63
dyslexia, 41
dysphagia, 125, 128, 136-43, 144, 256, 257
dyspnoea, 72
dysrhythmia, 65
dysuria, 164

electrolytes, 148, 151-2, 153, 158
emergency assessment unit (EAU), 193, 282
empathy, 19, 29, 276
endorphins, 198, 217, 226
enemas, 186
enteral nutrition (EN), 134, 138
enuresis, 163, 164
epidural administration, 220
Essence of Care Toolkit, 12, 14, 36, 93-4, 175, 200, 236, 249-51, 262
essential amino acids, 119
essential care, 3-4, 94
evaluation of care, 9-10
evaporation, 79, 80
exercise, 60, 68, 70, 80, 274
expiration, 69
extended-spectrum beta-lactamases (ESBLs), 112
external respiration, 68
extracellular fluid, 150

faecal impaction, 185
faecal incontinence, 165, 188
faeces, elimination of, 151, 181-8
fat-soluble vitamins, 121, 122
fats, 119, 120, 123, 124
femoral pulse, 62, 63
fentanyl, 217, 221
fibre, 118

fight or flight syndrome, 70, 206
financial abuse, 44-5
A First Class Service: Quality in the New NHS, 5, 10
Fitness to Practice Panel, 289, 291
flow charts, 293, 295
fluid balance, 147-59 *see also* continence care
   anatomy and physiology, 149-50
   electrolytes, 151-2
   factors affecting fluid and electrolyte balance, 153
   fluid imbalances, 153-5
   fluid intake, 150
   fluid output, 150-1
   hormonal influences, 152
   kidneys, 152
   overview, 147-9
   recording fluid balance, 155-9, 295
   regulation of body fluids, 150
   summary, 188-9
food supplements, 129, 130, 132 *see also* nutrition
Foster Review, 301, 302
Fowler's position, 142
Framework for the Assessment of Children in Need and their Families, 24, 42
functional incontinence, 170, 172
Fundamentals of Care, 200

gag reflex, 140
gastrostomy, 134
gate control theory of pain, 196-7, 198, 210, 227, 229
gender, 60, 123, 153, 208, 213
General Medical Council (GMC), 9
Gibbs Reflective Cycle, 16, 17
governance *see* clinical governance
Grossman, Lloyd, 130, 131

haemoglobin, 74
handwashing, 108-9, 113, 180
Health Advisory Service (HAS), 6, 29, 94
Health Service Ombudsman, 36, 285
healthcare-associated infections (HCAIs), 112, 130, 180
Healthcare Commission, 132
hearing impairment, 37, 136

heart beat, 60
heat loss/production, 79-80
hepatitis, 110
HIV *see* human immunodeficiency virus
hoists, 243
homeostasis, 148, 149
hormones, 81, 152
hospital-acquired infections, 112, 130, 180
human immunodeficiency virus (HIV), 41, 110
hydrogenated fats, 120
hygiene, 91-115
   infection control, 107-12
   introduction, 91
   oral hygiene, 106-7
   personal hygiene, 92-106
      aids and adaptations, 99-100
      assisting with personal hygiene, 96-7
      bed-bathing, 102-4
      care-planning, 96
      compression stockings, 104-5
      environment, 97-8
      evaluation and re-assessment, 99
      information and education to support patients, 99
      person-centred approach, 94-5
      provision of toiletries, 98
      teamworking, 95
      washing and dressing, 101-2
      what is personal hygiene?, 92-4
   summary, 112-13
hyperventilation, 72
hypervolaemia, 153, 154
hypnosis, 225
hypothalamus, 80, 150, 152
hypothermia, 80, 82, 86
hypotonic bladder, 170
hypoventilation, 72
hypovolaemia, 61, 65, 153, 154-5
hypoxia, 219

iatrogenic incontinence, 170
ibuprofen, 216, 224
incomplete proteins, 119
incontinence, 31-2, 165-72, 183, 188
independence, 261-2, 264
infection control, 107-12
information technology (IT), 296
inhaled analgesia, 222

insensible fluid losses, 150, 151, 156
inspiration, 69
institutional abuse, 47
insulin, 86
interdisciplinary working, 267-8
internal respiration, 68
International Association for the Study of
    Pain (IASP), 195, 213
interpreters, 39, 40
intracellular fluid, 150
intracranial pressure, 70
intramuscular administration, 218-19, 222,
    223
intrathecal administration, 220
intravenous administration, 219, 222, 223
ions, 122, 151
IT see information technology

jejunostomy, 134

kidneys, 152, 153, 161

laboured breathing, 73
laxatives, 185-6
learning disabilities, 5, 6, 24, 41, 234
leukaemia, 243, 249, 299
limbic system, 198, 199, 227
lipids, 119-21
The Living Archive, 35
local analgesic/anaesthetic, 221
locus of control (LOC), 210
London Hospital pain observation chart,
    205, 207

McCaffery, Margo, 195, 201, 208, 212, 214
McGill-Melzack Pain Questionnaire, 203, 206
macrominerals, 122
Making a Difference (DH), 5
malnutrition, 117, 126-9, 131, 132, 135, 136, 142
massage, 227
ME (myalgic encephalomyelitis), 244
Medical Devices Agency, 112
medical model of disability, 259, 260, 261
meditation, 225
Melzack, R, 195, 196, 198, 207, 229
Mencap, 6
Mental Health Act, 234
metabolism, 78, 79, 80, 81, 124

methicillin-resistant Staphylococcus aureus
    (MRSA), 107, 112
methicillin-sensitive Staphylococcus aureus
    (MSSA), 107
microminerals, 122
micturition, 162-3
minerals, 118, 122
mobility, 10-11, 19, 20, 172, 237, 240, 271-5
monounsaturated fats, 119, 120, 121
morphine, 81, 193, 198, 217, 221, 224
mouth cancer, 107
mouth care, 106
MRSA see methicillin-resistant
    Staphylococcus aureus
MSSA see methicillin-sensitive
    Staphylococcus aureus
multi-agency assessment, 19-20, 21
multidisciplinary working, 19, 267
myalgic encephalomyelitis (ME), 244

nasogastric feeding, 134, 156
National Audit Office, 112
National Health Service see NHS
National Institute for Health and Clinical
    Excellence (NICE), 9, 132, 143, 241,
    244, 252
National Patient Safety Agency (NPSA), 132
National Project for Information Technology
    (NPFIT), 296
National Service Framework (NSF) for Older
    People, 5-8, 35, 94, 141, 172, 174,
    266, 268
National Service Frameworks, 5, 7-8, 22,
    200, 269
near-misses, 9, 10, 11
neglect, 46-7, 234
neurogenic bladder, 164
neurogenic shock, 202
NHS (National Health Service), 5, 175, 184,
    237, 271, 296, 297, 302
NHS Plan, 5, 12, 22, 130, 143, 269
NHS Quality Improvement Scotland, 200
NICE see National Institute for Health and
    Clinical Excellence
nitrous oxide, 222
NMC see Nursing and Midwifery Council
nocturia, 164
nocturnal enuresis, 163

nocturnal frequency, 163
non-ambulant patients, 177
non-English-speaking patients, 39–40
non-opioid analgesics, 215–16
non-steroidal anti-inflammatory drugs
      (NSAIDs), 215, 216, 224
non-verbal communication, 19, 37–8, 39
Norton Scale, 246
Not Because They Are Old (HAS), 6, 7, 29, 30
NPFIT *see* National Project for Information
      Technology
NPSA *see* National Patient Safety Agency
NSAIDs *see* non-steroidal anti-inflammatory
      drugs
NSF Older People *see* National Service
      Framework for Older People
Nursing and Midwifery Council (NMC), 9, 40,
      228, 229, 284, 287–91, 297–9, 301–2
Nursing and Midwifery Practice
      Development Unit, 200
nutrition, 116–46
    dysphagia awareness, 136–43
    essential nutrients, 118–22
    factors affecting nutritional choice, 124–6
    feeding patients, 133–6
    hospital nutrition, 130–3
    importance of good nutrition, 117–18
    nutritional assessment, 126–30
    nutritional requirements, 122–4
    overview, 116–17
    pressure ulcers, 240
    quality of care, 14, 15
    rehabilitation and self-care, 274
    summary, 143–4

obesity, 124, 128, 136, 240
Observer, 6, 94
occupational therapists, 95, 256, 261, 265,
      267, 271
oedema, 104
older people
    caring, 5, 6, 7, 8, 24
    dignity and privacy, 35, 38, 42, 44, 51, 53
    fluid balance and continence care, 153,
      160, 163, 174
    hygiene, 94
    nutrition, 123
    pain management, 209

pressure ulcers, 253
    rehabilitation and self-care, 266, 270
oliguria, 164
opioid analgesics, 217–18, 219, 220, 221, 230
oral administration, 218, 222, 223
oral hygiene, 106–7
oral temperature, 81, 82, 83–4
Orem model, 93
orthopnoea, 72
overflow incontinence, 170, 171–2, 183, 188
oxidation, 150
oxygen saturation, 74, 75, 76, 77

pain assessment tools (PATs), 202–5, 206,
      207
pain fibres, 197–8, 199
pain management, 193–233
    administration of analgesia, 218–22
    analgesic ladder, 224–5
    efficacy of analgesia, 222–4
    government policy developments, 200
    how is pain felt?, 196–9
    non-opioid analgesics, 215–16
    opioid analgesics, 217–18
    other methods of pain relief, 225–9
    overview, 193–4, 214–15
    pain assessment, 200–7, 229, 287
    pain perception, 207–14
    summary, 229–30
    what is pain?, 194–6
pain threshold, 213, 229
pain tolerance, 208, 213, 229
paracetamol, 193, 215–16, 224
parenteral nutrition (PN), 135
Partnership Hospital Sites Club, 131
Patient Advocacy and Liaison Services
      (PALS), 269
patient-centred approach, 4–5, 29, 172, 269,
      276
patient-controlled analgesia (PCA), 219–20
Patient Focus and Public Involvement, 283
patient participation, 269
patient pathway, 295
Patient's Charter, 283
PATs *see* pain assessment tools
pattern theory of pain, 196
PCA *see* patient-controlled analgesia
PCC *see* Professional Conduct Committee

penicillin, 112
penile sheaths, 174, 176, 177
percutaneous endoscopic gastrostomy
        (PEG), 134, 135
percutaneous endoscopic jejunostomy
        (PEJ), 134
perfusion, 240
peripheral neuropathy, 227
peripheral pulses, 60, 63
peripheral vasoconstriction, 80
peripheral vasodilation, 61, 80
peristalsis, 187
person-centred approach, 4–5, 29, 172, 269,
        276
personal hygiene see hygiene
personal protective equipment, 109
personhood, 29–30
physical abuse, 42–3
physiotherapists, 95, 256, 261, 265, 267, 271
pituitary gland, 152
PN see parenteral nutrition
pneumonia, 56, 57, 74
pneumothorax, 72, 73
polyunsaturated fats, 119, 120, 121
polyuria, 164
popliteal pulse, 62, 63
posterior tibial pulse, 62, 63
A Practical Guide for Disabled People or
        Carers, 99
pressure-relieving equipment, 243, 244, 246,
        249, 251–2
pressure ulcers, 234–55
    anatomy and physiology, 235
    avoidance of pressure ulcers, 242–5
    healing, 252–3
    how and why pressure ulcers develop,
        238–42
    nutrition, 129
    overview, 234
    record-keeping, 299
    screening and assessing skin damage,
        245–52
    summary, 253
    why study pressure ulcers?, 236–8
privacy see dignity and privacy
Professional Conduct Committee (PCC), 288,
        289, 291, 299
prognosis, 101

prostaglandins, 215, 216
proteins, 119, 123, 124
psychological abuse, 43–4
pulmonary oedema, 74
pulse, 59–68
    anatomy and physiology, 60
    assessment, 64–6
    factors affecting the pulse, 60–2
    frequency of recordings, 66–8
    overview, 59–60
    pain assessment, 201, 202
    recording the pulse, 62–4
pulse oximetry, 63, 71, 74
pyrexia, 82, 85, 86

qualitative research, 6
quality of care, 9–18
    benchmarking, 12–15
    clinical governance, 11–12
    clinical supervision, 17–18
    complaints procedures, 10–11
    overview, 9–10, 24
    reflective practice, 15–17
    what do we mean by 'caring'?, 4, 5–7

radial pulse, 62, 63, 64, 66
radiation, 79, 80
RCN see Royal College of Nursing
record-keeping, 282–304
    introduction, 282–3
    legal aspects, 287–91
    nursing documentation, 291–7
    overview, 283–5
    purpose of records, 285–7
    standards, 298–302
    summary, 302
rectal administration, 221
rectal temperature, 81, 83, 85
'red tray' systems, 132, 143
reflective practice, 9, 15–17
reflexology, 228
rehabilitation and self-care, 256–81
    factors that impact on individual
        wellbeing, 275–8
    framework for rehabilitation nursing,
        265–75
        equipment, 271–4
        mobility, 274–5

overview, 265-6
    patient participation, 269
    rehabilitation team, 266-8
    service provision, 270-1
  independence and self-care, 261-5
  introduction, 256-7
  summary, 279
  what is rehabilitation?, 257-61
relaxation techniques, 225
religion, 125, 126, 142, 143, 277
renal dialysis, 164
repositioning patients, 242-4
respirations, 68-77
  anatomy and physiology, 68-9
  assessment, 71-4
  factors affecting respiration, 70
  frequency of recordings, 75-7
  procedure, 75
  recording respirations, 71
respiratory depression, 219, 221, 225
retention catheter, 178, 179
Roper model of nursing, 93, 294
Royal College of Nursing (RCN), 108, 296
Royal College of Physicians, 131, 140, 141
Royal Marsden Hospital pain assessment
    chart, 204, 207

saturated fats, 119, 120, 121
Scally, Gabriel, 11
Scottish Intercollegiate Guidelines Network,
    140, 141
self-care, 93, 261, 262-5, 271
self-efficacy, 210
senile dementia, 39, 168
septicaemia, 57, 234
sexual abuse, 45-6
sharps, 109-11
Shifting the Balance of Power (DH), 32, 38
shower seats, 99
sickle cell anaemia, 290, 291
single assessment process, 21, 42
skin care, 235, 250-1 see also pressure ulcers
social model of disability, 259, 259-60
space blanket, 86
specificity theory of pain, 196
spinal analgesia, 220-1
spinal cord, 196, 197, 199, 206
spirituality, 277

spurious (false) diarrhoea, 185
SSDs (sterile service departments), 112
stair lifts, 99
Staphylococcus aureus, 107
sterilisation, 111, 112
Stirling scale, 236, 237
stoma, 67, 134, 156
stress, 61, 70, 81, 202
stress incontinence, 169, 171, 172
stridor, 74
stroke, 3, 23, 138, 141, 143, 170, 256, 257, 263,
    276
strong opioids, 217
subcutaneous (definition), 219
sublingual administration, 221
substantia gelatinosa, 196
supervision, 17-18
support workers, 268
suppositories, 186, 221
suprapubic area, 171
surface temperature, 78
surgical stockings, 104-5, 284
swallowing, 6, 137-8, 141 see also dysphagia
sympathetic nervous system, 81, 202, 206
sympathy, 29

tachycardia, 64, 67
tachypnoea, 72, 73
teamworking, 95, 266-8
temperature, 77-87
  anatomy and physiology, 78
  assessment, 81-2
  continence care, 188
  factors affecting body temperature, 80-1
  frequency of recordings, 85-7
  heat loss, 79-80
  heat production, 79
  overview, 77
  procedure, 83-5
  recording temperature, 81
  sites used for temperature recording,
    82-3
TENS see transcutaneous electrical nerve
    stimulation
thalamus, 198, 199
thermoreceptors, 82
thermoregulation, 80
thirst mechanism, 150

thyroxine, 79, 80
tidal volume (TV), 72
tobacco, 107
toiletries, 98
total parenteral nutrition (TPN), 135
TPR (temperature, pulse and respiration), 57
    see also pulse; respirations; temper-
    ature
trans-disciplinary working, 268
trans-fats, 120, 121
transcutaneous electrical nerve stimulation
    (TENS), 197-8, 226
transdermal opioids, 221
trigeminal neuralgia, 227
triglycerides, 119, 120
tympanic temperature, 83, 84

ulnar pulse, 62, 63
unsaturated fats, 119, 120
ureters, 161
urethra, 161, 162
urge incontinence, 170, 171
urgency, 164
urinalysis, 168
urinary continence, 160-5
urinary tract infections, 163, 180

urine output, 150, 151, 159
user involvement, 269

vasoconstriction, 72, 73, 240
vasoconstrictors, 152
venepuncture, 208
venous ulcers, 104
ventilation, 69
visual impairment, 37
vital signs, 56, 59, 87, 282, 286, 290, 291 *see
    also* basic observations
vitamins, 118, 121-2
vulnerable individuals, 40, 41, 51

walking frames, 273, 274
walking sticks, 271, 272-3
Wall, P, 195, 196, 198, 207, 229
waste management, 109-11, 113
water-soluble vitamins, 121
Waterlow score, 246, 247, 248, 249
weak opioids, 217
weight *see* body weight
wheelchairs, 244-5, 270, 271, 272
World Health Organization (WHO), 224, 225,
    227
wound healing, 252-3